Hand-Rearing Wild and Domestic Mammals

Hand-Rearing Wild and Domestic Mammals

Laurie J. Gage, DVM

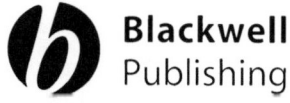
Blackwell Publishing

Laurie J. Gage, D.V.M., served as the Director of Veterinary Services concurrently at both Marine World Africa USA and The Marine Mammal Center from 1980 to 1994. She continued to hold that title at Marine World Africa USA until 1998, when the park became Six Flags Marine World. She also was the consultant veterinarian for Safari World in Bangkok, Thailand from 1992 to 1994, and has done consultant veterinary work for a number of private collections. She has been a lecturer at the University of California, Davis School of Veterinary Medicine since 1982 where she teaches marine mammal medicine and husbandry. She is presently the consultant veterinarian for Coyote Point Museum, and the Chief veterinarian for Six Flags Marine World in Vallejo, California.

The charts "Substitute Milk Formula For Opossum" and "Feeding Chart For The Modified Jurgelski Diet For Opossums" used by permission of Debbie Marcum.

© 2002 Iowa State University Press
A Blackwell Publishing Company
All rights reserved

Blackwell Publishing Professional
2121 State Avenue, Ames, Iowa 50014

Orders: 1-800-862-6657
Office: 1-515-292-0140
Fax: 1-515-292-3348
Web site: www.blackwellprofessional.com

Authorization to photocopy items for internal or personal use, or the internal or personal use of specific clients, is granted by Blackwell Publishing, provided that the base fee is paid directly to the Copyright Clearance Center, 222 Rosewood Drive, Danvers, MA 01923. For those organizations that have been granted a photocopy license by CCC, a separate system of payments has been arranged. The fee code for users of the Transactional Reporting Service is 978-0-8138-2683-7/2002.

First edition, 2002

Library of Congress Cataloging-in-Publication Data

Hand rearing wild and domestic mammals / edited by Laurie J. Gage.—1st ed.
  p. cm.
  ISBN-13: 978-0-8138-2683-7 (alk. paper)
  ISBN-10: 0-8138-2683-7 (alk. paper)
  1. Domestic animals.   2. Captive mammals.
3. Mammals. I. Gage, Laurie J.
    SF41+
                                        2002002888

Cover photo credits from top left and then clockwise:

Bottle feeding the walrus calf: Charlotte Fiorito, courtesy of Six Flags Marine World
Bottle feeding the tiger cubs: Darryl Bush, courtesy of Six Flags Marine World
Llama face: Lindsay Merrill Leonard, Rainbow Ridge Llama Ranch
Sloth infant: Luis Arroyo
Rhesus monkey infants: Vince Warren
Feeding the Somalian wild ass: Courtesy of San Diego Wild Animal Park
Infant squirrel nursing: Jackie Wollner, California Wildlife Center

The last digit is the print number: 9 8 7 6 5

To my teachers Mary, Murray, and Mishka

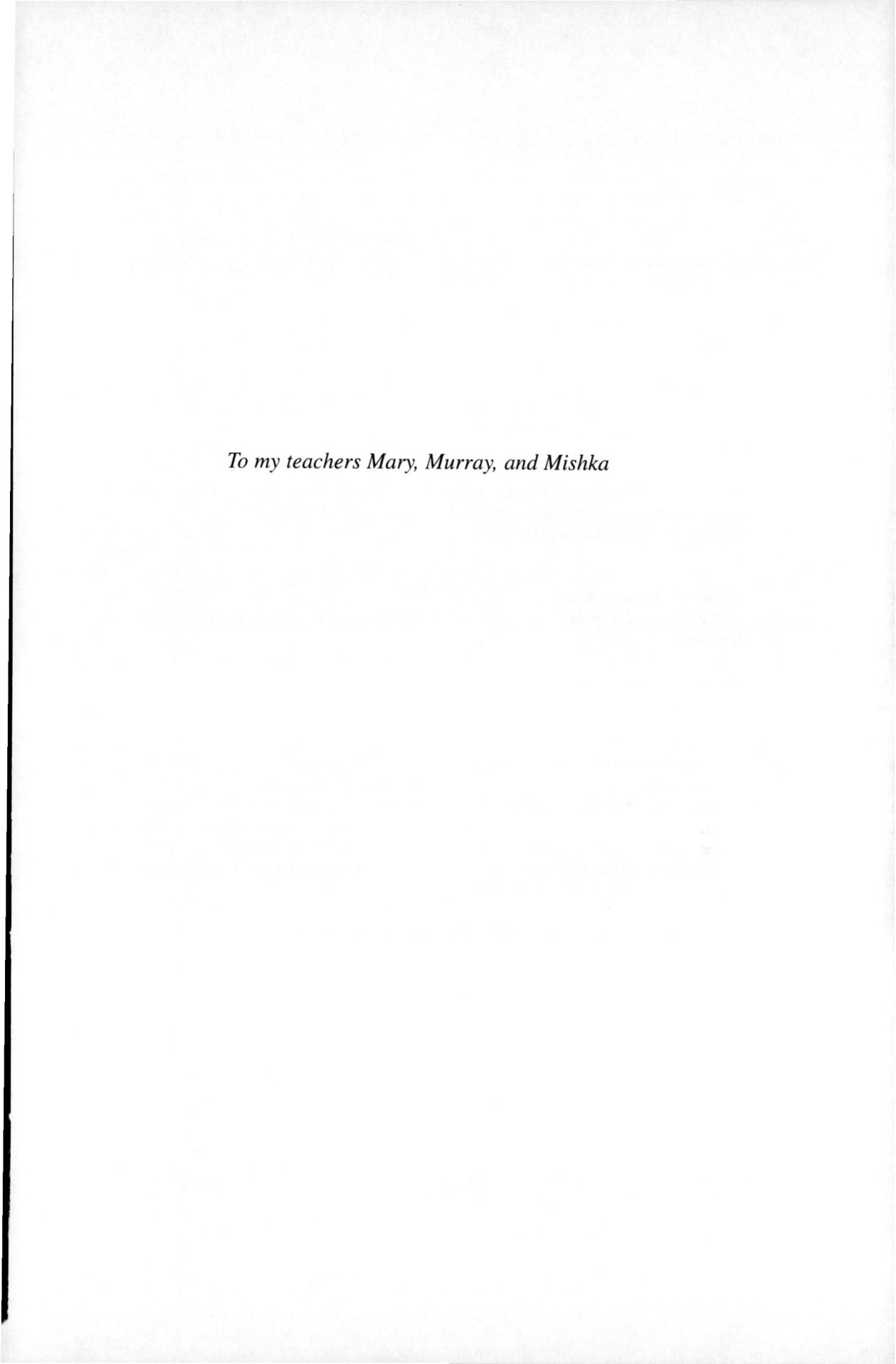

Contents

Contributors		ix
Preface		xiii
Acknowledgments		xv
Introduction		xvii

Part I Domestic Mammals

1. Orphan Rabbits — 5
   Karen Heller Taylor
2. Puppies — 13
   Valerie T. Barrette
3. Domestic Kittens — 19
   Laura Summers
4. Critically Ill and Orphaned Foals — 24
   K. Gary Magdesian
5. Pigs — 30
   Janet Fine and Rebecca Duerr
6. Goat Kids — 34
   Joan D. Rowe
7. South American Camelids — 39
   Robert J. Pollard and Susan D. Pollard

Part II Wildlife, Zoo, and Marine Mammals

8. Opossums — 45
   Paula Taylor
9. Sugar Gliders — 55
   Michele Barnes
10. Macropods — 63
    Rosemary Booth
11. Hedgehogs — 75
    Ian Robinson
12. Sloths — 81
    Judy Avey-Arroyo
13. Ground and Tree Squirrels — 90
    Dawn M. Smith
14. Insectivorous Bats — 96
    Susan M. Barnard
15. Lemurs — 104
    Cathy V. Williams

16	Tamarins	114
	Laurie Hrdlicka and Cynthia Stringfield	
17	Macaque Species	118
	Laura Summers, Laurie Brignolo, and Kari Christe	
18	Great Apes	125
	Dawn Strasser	
19	Harbor Seals and Northern Elephant Seals	132
	Rebecca Duerr	
20	Sea Lions and Fur Seals	143
	Laurie J. Gage	
21	Walrus Calves	150
	Laurie J. Gage and Terry S. Samansky	
22	Fox Kits	158
	Jennifer Convy, Darlene DeGhetto, and Sophia Papageorgiou	
23	Black Bear Cubs	170
	Sophia Papageorgiou, Darlene DeGhetto, and Jennifer Convy	
24	Polar Bears	181
	Gail Hedberg	
25	Raccoons	191
	Darlene DeGhetto, Sophia Papageorgiou, and Jennifer Convy	
26	Ferret Kits	203
	Vickie McKimmey	
27	Exotic Felids	207
	Gail Hedberg	
28	Elephants	221
	Karen A. Emanuelson and Colleen E. Kinzley	
29	Nondomestic Equids	229
	Terry Blakeslee and Jeffrey R. Zuba	
30	Rhinoceros	236
	Terry Blakeslee and Jeffrey R. Zuba	
31	Black-Tailed and White-Tailed Deer	244
	Sophia Papageorgiou, Darlene DeGhetto, and Jennifer Convy	
32	Exotic Ungulates	256
	Kelley Greene and Cynthia Stringfield	
	Appendix: Resources for Products Mentioned	263
	Index	267

Contributors

Judy Avey-Arroyo began working with sloths in Costa Rica in 1990. Finding no rescue centers for sloths, she developed a rescue/rehab/release protocol and opened an officially sanctioned rescue center in 1997. She has rescued, rehabilitated, and released injured adults and successfully released two hand-reared three-toed sloths using radiotelemetry.

Susan M. Barnard received her Bachelor of Science degree in 1983 from the University of the State of New York. She is assistant curator of herpetology at Zoo Atlanta, and executive director of Basically Bats, Inc. Barnard has served on the board of directors of the American Association of Zoo Keepers. She has authored numerous books and articles on aspects of reptilian husbandry, parasitology, and bat rehabilitation. As a licensed wildlife rehabilitator in the State of Georgia for over 20 years, Barnard pioneered bat rehabilitation in the United States. She makes routine television appearances and was featured in the National Geographic television special, "Keepers of the Wild."

Michele Barnes began her career as a wildlife attendant at Koala Country, Dreamworld, in 1991. A specialist with mammals, she has also cared for birds, reptiles, and amphibians. She has been successful in raising animals such as bats, bandicoots, phascogale, possums, macropods, and gliders. Barnes is life sciences coordinator at The Australian Wildlife Experience, Dreamworld.

Valerie T. Barrette has worked in the veterinary field since 1982 as an assistant and client educator. Her canine behavior counseling service, The Right Steps, specializes in puppies. She is a lecturer at the San Francisco SPCA Dog Training Academy and writes a column for the Association of Pet Dog Trainers' newsletter.

Terry Blakeslee became a keeper at the San Diego Wild Animal Park in 1972. As a member of the team of keepers at the Animal Care Center she has assisted in the hand rearing of approximately 2200 mammals, representing 116 species, mostly ungulates.

Rosemary Booth has worked as a veterinarian at Lone Pine Koala Sanctuary, Healesville Sanctuary, Melbourne Zoo, Currumbin Sanctuary, and the University of Queensland. Dr. Booth has broad experience in veterinary care and husbandry of Australian native species and has personally hand raised many Australian native species. She is an active lecturer and workshop host to volunteer wildlife carers, vets, and zookeepers. Dr. Booth obtained her veterinary degree in 1981 from the University of Queensland, and worked in private practice prior to her first zoo position.

Laurie Brignolo began working with infant monkeys as an undergraduate student. Dr. Brignolo has worked as a veterinarian at the California Regional Primate Research Center in Davis, California, for the last six years. She has monitored over five hundred nursery reared rhesus and cynomolgus macaque infants.

Kari Christe graduated from University of California, Davis, School of Veterinary Medicine, then completed a clinical residency at the California Regional Primate Research Center in 1998. She is a senior veterinarian at the center.

Jennifer Convy is wildlife rehabilitation manager at the PAWS Wildlife Department in Lynnwood, Washington.

Darlene DeGhetto received her DVM from Colorado State University in 1981. Dr. DeGhetto is presently employed by PAWS and has been a wildlife veterinarian since 1995. She has conducted research on marine mammals in Alaska, California, and Washington with the National Marines Fisheries Service, Alaska Department of Fish and Game and Washington Department of Wildlife; seabirds with U.S. Fish and Wildlife Service, Washington Department of Wildlife, and University of Washington; and wild ungulates and bears with Colorado Division of Wildlife.

Rebecca Duerr spent 14 years at the Marine Mammal Center in Sausalito, California, and worked extensively with many species of newborn marine mammals. In addition, she devoted many years to working in terrestrial wildlife rehabilitation facilities where she specializes in avian trauma care and hand-raising passerines for wild release.

Karen A. Emanuelson is director of veterinary services at the Oakland Zoo in Oakland, California. She assisted in the care of the small breeding herd of African elephants at the zoo included the hand raising of one male elephant calf, Kijana, in 1995–1996. Dr. Emanuelson was a private practitioner at Cottage Veterinary Hospital in Walnut Creek, California; taught in the Zoological Medicine Department at the University of California Davis; and interned with the Zoological Society of London, Whipsnade Park, United Kingdom.

Janet Fine operates the Piggypals' Fine Sanctuary in Marysville California, where she cares for many pigs including potbellies, farm pigs, Yorkshires and hand-raised feral pigs. In 2000, she was awarded the National Sanctuary Owner of the Year award by the Pigs As Pets Association of America.

Laurie J. Gage served as director of veterinary services concurrently at Marine World Africa USA and the Marine Mammal Center from 1980 to 1994. Dr. Gage continued to hold that title at Marine World Africa USA until 1998, when the park became Six Flags Marine World. She also has done consultant veterinary work for a number of private collections domestically and abroad. Since 1982 she has been a lecturer at the University of California, Davis, School of Veterinary Medicine, where she teaches marine mammal medicine and husbandry. She is the consultant veterinarian for Coyote Point Museum and chief veterinarian for Six Flags Marine World in Vallejo, California.

Kelley Greene became an animal keeper at the Los Angeles Zoo in 1983. Greene is a specialist in hand rearing exotic infants with particular interest in hoofstock. She has successfully raised gerenuk, bushbuck, duikers, and pronghorn. She is lead animal keeper in the Los Angeles Zoo's Children's Zoo.

Gail Hedberg received her professional training at Colorado Mountain College in Glenwood Springs, Colorado, and became a registered veterinary technician in California in 1977. For the past 25 years she has hand raised over 150 neonatal species. She has held positions at Marine World/Africa USA and works today at the San Francisco Zoological Gardens and various consulting situations.

Laurie Hrdlicka became an animal keeper at Los Angeles Zoo in April of 1979, and began handrearing infants in January of 1982. She currently works in the Animal Nursery hand rearing infants. She specializes in primates, carnivores, and marsupials.

Colleen E. Kinzley is general curator and elephant manager at the Oakland Zoo in Oakland, California, where she has worked since 1990. In 1995–1996, she was responsible for hand raising a male African elephant calf. She is the author of "The Elephant Hand-Raising Notebook." She has been animal keeper at the Brookfield Zoo and animal keeper at the Phoenix Zoo.

K. Gary Magdesian received his DVM from University of California, Davis, School of Veterinary Medicine in 1993. He interned at Texas A&M and then completed a residency in large animal internal medicine at UC Davis in 1997. Dr. Magdesian received board certification in internal medicine in 1997 and in emergency/critical care in 2000. He has been on the clinical faculty at UC Davis School of Veterinary Medicine since 1997.

Vickie McKimmey started breeding ferrets in 1990 and is the proprietor of Just a Business of Ferrets. She also does limited rescue and adoption of ferrets. McKimmey is past president of the American Ferret Association and is director for the association's Shows and Special Events Committee. She is a senior judge licensed with the AFA and has judged ferrets in the United States and in Japan.

Sophia Papageorgiou earned her bachelor of science degree in animal science and zoology from the University of California at Davis in 1980. She then earned a degree in exotic animal training and management from Moorpark College in Southern California. After graduating from Tufts University School of Veterinary Medicine in 1996, Dr. Papageorgiou completed a small animal internship in Tucson, Arizona, and a wildlife internship at PAWS Wildlife Center in Lynnwood, Washington.

Robert J. Pollard graduated from UC Davis School of Veterinary Medicine in 1970, after having been one of the first students in Dr. Murray Fowler's zoo and wildlife medicine class. He and his wife Suzi moved to Sonora, in the Sierra foothills, and started a small animal practice. As llamas became more popular in the area in 1983, Dr. Pollard used his wildlife medicine experience to work on llamas, and to help the new llama owners. He and his wife own 59 llamas, with almost a dozen other llamas visiting their Valley of the Llama Ranch for breeding, birthing, or medical care.

Susan D. Pollard works together with her husband Dr. Robert Pollard to care for their personal collection of 59 llamas, as well as privately owned llamas that visit their ranch for breeding, birthing or medical care. Suzi also raises orphan wildlife for the California Department of Fish and Game.

Joan D. Rowe is an associate professor in the Department of Population Health and Reproduction, School of Veterinary Medicine, University of California, Davis. She holds DVM, MPVM, and PhD degrees from the University of California, Davis. Dr. Rowe completed a residency in food animal reproduction and herd health at UC Davis, and is a Diplomate of the American College of Veterinary Preventive Medicine. Dr. Rowe is chief of the Food Animal Reproduction and Herd Health Service at the UCD Veterinary Medical Teaching Hospital. She is a licensed dairy goat judge and on the American Dairy Goat Association Board of Directors.

Ian Robinson is veterinary manager of the RSPCA Norfolk Wildlife Hospital, which rehabilitates native British wildlife and treats thousands of casualties per year. The commonest species admitted is the hedgehog. He qualified as a veterinarian in 1975 and holds the RCVS (Royal College of Veterinary Surgeons) certificate in zoological medicine.

Terry S. Samansky has worked with marine mammals for over two decades. He was directly involved in the successful hand raising of six orphaned walrus calves. Samansky holds a bachelor of arts degree in biology and chemistry from California State University at Sacramento and has held positions as keeper, rehabilitation specialist, trainer, curator, and director at facilities such as Marineland of California, Active Environments, Marine World Africa USA, and Six Flags Marine World. He has published numerous papers and articles, and is a lecturer and teacher on the subject of marine mammal biology, care and husbandry. He is a biological consultant operating the educational website DolphinTrainer.com.

Dawn M. Smith became a registered veterinary technician in 1982. She taught classes for Wildlife Rescue, Inc., and she was director of animal care at the Marine Mammal Center for ten years. In Portugal, she set up the sea otter and marine bird exhibits at the Oceanario de Lisboa. In Los Angeles county, she helped in the opening of the California Wildlife Center, where she is now a consultant. She is a member of the Mediterranean Monk Seal Recovery Team.

Dawn Strasser holds a BS in business management from College of Mount Saint Joseph. She has been at the Cincinnati Zoo since 1979 where she has worked with birds for five years before transferring to the animal nursery. She has been the head keeper for six years, and has raised numerous mammals.

Cynthia Stringfield worked as a veterinary technician raising numerous species and large numbers of exotic mammals at Marine World Africa USA in Redwood City and Vallejo, California, from 1982 to 1990. She received her DVM from the University of California, Davis, School of Veterinary Medicine in 1990. Dr. Stringfield interned in small animal surgery and emergency medicine at the California Animal Hospital in 1991, and has been a staff veterinarian at the Los Angeles Zoo since 1993.

Laura Summers began raising orphan kittens before entering veterinary school. At University of California, Davis, she helped raise orphan kittens taken in by the Feline Medicine Club. After working as a small animal private practitioner, Dr. Summers became a clinical veterinarian at the Oregon Regional Primate Research Center. She is currently a staff veterinarian at the California Regional Primate Research Center in Davis, California.

Karen Heller Taylor has been a laboratory animal veterinarian at North Carolina State University, College of Veterinary Medicine. She has worked with rabbits for many years as a laboratory animal veterinarian. She is a lecturer in the biology, care, and diseases of rabbits, and is a veterinarian in companion animal practice working with exotic pets and wildlife rehab.

Paula Taylor is a registered nurse with a degree from Golden West College in Huntington Beach, California. She has rehabilitated opossums since 1991. She has been a vice president and director of rehabilitation of the Opossum Society of the United States. She has published a manual and produced a video on opossum orphan care.

Cathy V. Williams is veterinarian for the Duke University Primate Center where she oversees medical care for 25 species of prosimian primates. Dr. Williams serves as the veterinary advisor for aye-ayes, sifakas, and bamboo lemurs to the Prosimian Taxon Advisory Group of the American Zoological Association, and is a representative on Duke University's Institutional Animal Care and Use Committee. She obtained her veterinary degree in 1985 from the University of California at Davis and completed an internship in small animal medicine and surgery at North Carolina State University College of Veterinary Medicine in 1986. She worked in private practice prior to joining Duke University in 1996.

Jeffery R. Zuba completed a zoo animal medicine residency at the Zoological Society of San Diego. Dr. Zuba was an assistant professor of zoo medicine at Colorado State University from 1990 to 1991. He is an associate veterinarian at the San Diego Wild Animal Park and has worked there as a clinical veterinarian for many years. In this capacity, he has taken part in the institution's well-known program of captive propagation of hoofstock, especially "megavertebrate" species. His special interest is neonatology, which comprises a great portion of his veterinary duties.

Preface

When I started my career working with wild and captive nondomestic animals in 1980, my only experience raising any sort of mammal was at the University of California at Davis while I was in veterinary school. There I helped to raise a litter of pigs, a couple of goats, and a calf.

I owe my first real "exotic animal" hand-rearing experience to Dr. Marty Dinnes, my first employer after I completed an internship in equine surgery at Washington State University. One afternoon while working at Marty's request on the set of the television show "Those Amazing Animals," I met Mary Fleming, the head veterinary technician from Marine World Africa USA. She had brought a baby baboon down for the show. At the end of the day, Marty arrived on the set. Mary had a plane to catch and was getting ready to go back to northern California. Marty announced that I (and not Mary) would be taking the infant baboon home with me. This came as a complete surprise, and I frantically took notes as Mary gave me instructions about feedings and offered husbandry tips including how to cut a hole in the disposable diapers to pull the tail through. And then she was gone. I still thought Marty was kidding—that he was really going to take the infant primate to his home. But it quickly became apparent that he meant for me to take the baby baboon. So I tucked little Jojo into his airline carrier, crammed it into the front seat of my Honda Prelude, and headed for my tiny trailer in Thousand Oaks.

And so my experience hand raising exotic animals had begun. I felt fortunate that Jojo thrived in spite of my lack of experience. He lived with me for a couple of months and then went on to a new home. I moved to the San Francisco Bay area to start my new position as Marine World Africa USA's first resident veterinarian.

I felt great excitement my first day on the job at Marine World as I approached the animal nursery, where I again met Mary who was now raising two black leopard cubs. What could be cuter than leopard cubs? Mary had allowed the cubs to run loose on the floor while she was cleaning their exhibit window. As I entered the nursery, one of the cubs, aptly named "Damien," bounded over to me and embedded his canine tooth into my kneecap. My appreciation of cute wild neonates grew from that point forward.

Over the years I helped Mary raise dozens of species of infants. It seemed we had occasion to hand rear infants representing almost every order of mammals. We raised hoofed stock, such as nilgai, blackbuck, eland, and a rhinoceros—not to mention countless sheep and goats. We even helped an infant giraffe to survive his first week of life until his mother finally took over. We had a blind female camel whose calves we hand reared each year. I observed and, many times, helped Mary and the veterinary technicians raise dozens of tiger cubs, lions, cheetahs, leopards, cougars, servals, and bobcats. We raised kit foxes, river otters, wallabies, opossums, squirrels, a sloth, a koala, a zebra, a binturong, and even a hyena. And I thought leopards bit hard.

Mary had a special love for primates, and she and the Marine World team raised five chimpanzees, two orangutans, and a gibbon. For years we had an infant primate of one species or another running around our veterinary clinic.

My first "solo" experience as "Mom" after Jojo happened a couple of years after I assumed the clinical veterinary position at the then California Marine Mammal Center in early 1981. I did this job while also maintaining my veterinary position at Marine World. A very ill northern fur seal had stranded with her tiny newborn pup. The mother died a few days after arriving at our center. The pup, who weighed barely 3 kg (7 lb), seemed healthy and very hungry. There were few volunteers back then, and no designated night crews, so I took the pup home with me. For lack of a better idea, I fed her our elephant seal formula, which was made with ground fish, whipping cream, and a number of other ingredients. I spent three days and nights encouraging the tiny pup to accept the bottle. Finally she figured it out, and began to thrive. I was flattered that she considered me to be Mom, and she vocalized in a special way whenever she saw me. I named her Mishka, and took her with me to work at Marine World each day where she had her own pool. At night she came home to my converted barn, which was located on an estate in Woodside.

Besides Mishka, I've had the opportunity to gain experience raising sea lions, harbor seals, elephant seals, walruses, a harbor porpoise, a Dall's porpoise, and two infant beaked whales. While the pinnipeds did very well, none of the infant cetaceans lived over a month. However, the experiences and challenges working with them were memorable.

While there are dozens of chapters about hand rearing many species of neonates in a variety of texts, there was no one single text that held practical information about how to hand rear the more common domestic, wildlife, and zoo species. The AZA *Infant Diet Care Manual* is an excellent resource, but does not cover hand rearing domestic mammals or some of the more common wildlife species. Also, it is not readily available to those outside of the zoo profession.

Two years ago, at the American Association of Zoo Veterinarians annual conference, I bounced around an idea about compiling a practical book on hand rearing mammals. My colleagues not only embraced the idea, but also contributed their expertise to my project. This book could not have been done without the contributions of many. The chapter authors have contributed wonderful insights on how to rear the many species covered here, and the staff and volunteers of numerous wildlife centers, zoos, marine mammal rehabilitation centers, and wild animal parks have enriched the body of knowledge contained on these pages.

Hand rearing mammals is probably more art than it is science. There is no "right way" to successfully raise any of the species represented in this text. In some cases, only one method of raising a species may be mentioned, even though many methods have proven to be successful by many different individuals. Each of the authors of this book has had extensive experience raising the species represented in his or her chapter. They have given their best tips on the science and also, more important, the art of hand rearing mammals.

Acknowledgments

This book is a result of the efforts of 34 authors, several of whom contributed to more than one chapter. They are an international group of veterinary technicians, wildlife rehabilitators, and veterinarians. I am very grateful for their efforts and hard work to produce chapters that will certainly enhance the knowledge of hand rearing the various mammals mentioned in this book. Special thanks to Rebecca Duerr, Dawn Smith, Dr. Murray Fowler, Debbie Marcum, Jane Ewer, and Dr. Laura Summers for their editorial assistance and encouragement. Thanks to Bob Wilson, Lindsay Leonard, Kent Hedberg, and Jackie Wollner for their photographic assistance.

Thanks to my husband, Kenji Ruymaker, for his support and help. Thanks also to the veterinary team at Six Flags Marine World—Eric Calvo, Lisa Counts, and Lee Munro—as well as former Marine World employees Andy Goldfarb and Mary Fleming for their expertise in raising infant wild animals.

Introduction

Hand-Rearing Wild and Domestic Mammals is designed to help veterinary practitioners, technicians, wildlife rehabilitators, and zoo personnel to raise healthy infant mammals. It is a practical guide with resources and information to help the reader achieve success with each hand-rearing project.

This book is organized into two parts: Domestic Mammals, and Wildlife, Zoo, and Marine Mammals. The species represented here are, for the most part, commonly encountered species presented for hand rearing to wildlife centers, zoo hospitals, and veterinary practices. The eminently qualified contributors were encouraged to include helpful tips and resource information along with their advice on choices of formulas and equipment. In most of the chapters, tried and true "made-from-scratch" recipes are included in addition to the commercial diet recommendations.

There are many ways to hand rear mammals, and certainly we cannot present all of them here. While each chapter of this book is designed to stand alone, it may be worthwhile for the reader to explore other chapters written about similar species to gain different points of view. For instance, a reader seeking advice on how to best hand raise a zebra foal may consider looking at both Chapter 29 on hand rearing nondomestic equids and Chapter 4 on critically ill and orphaned foals.

It is the hope of the authors of this book that the information presented here will help all readers to achieve optimal success in hand raising wild and domestic mammals that are placed in their care.

Hand-Rearing Wild and Domestic Mammals

Part I
Domestic Mammals

1 Orphan Rabbits
2 Puppies
3 Domestic Kittens
4 Critically Ill and Orphaned Foals
5 Pigs
6 Goat Kids
7 South American Camelids

1
Orphan Rabbits

Karen Heller Taylor

NATURAL HISTORY

This chapter discusses both domestic and wild orphan rabbits and hares. The term "rabbit" will signify either a rabbit (wild or domestic) or a hare. Specific differences will be noted.

The family Leporidae includes three major genera: *Lepus* (hares), *Sylvilagus* (e.g., cottontail), and *Oryctolagus* (e.g., domestic or European). Because they are prey animals, members of these genera tend to be more active at night (nocturnal) or at dawn and dusk (crepuscular). Females (does) are generally larger than the males (bucks). Offspring in the nest are called pups or bunnies. The act of giving birth is called kindling.

Offspring of the genus *Lepus* (hares) are born with fur and eyes open. Depending on the species, the hare breeds either year-round or biannually (spring and fall). The average birth weight is 110 grams. Weaning occurs at one week.

The eastern cottontail (*Sylvilagus floridanus*) is the most numerous species of this genus in North America. The cottontail breeds February to September. The young are born naked with average birth weight of 30–40 grams and eyes closed but open by seven to ten days. Weaning occurs at three to four weeks.

The genus *Oryctolagus* is more similar to *Sylvilagus* and reproduces year-round. The average birth weight depends on the breed but ranges between 30 and 80 grams. The young are born naked and eyes are closed. Eyes open at about ten days of age. Weaning occurs at four to six weeks.

RECORD KEEPING

To the person who raises a single animal, paperwork appears trivial, but to the rehabber or the veterinary practice that sees many orphans during a concentrated period, good records are vital to success. The most important aspect of record keeping is the tracking of body weight in preweanlings to determine gain or loss. Other information includes

Date of entry: Including information on the animal presenter (in case of zoonotic disease exposure and also helpful for release purposes)
Source: Physical location for wild animal or dam of domestic bunny
Age determination
Physical exam findings: On entry, including injuries, hydration status, and rectal temperature
Treatments: Fluids, antibiotics, other
Formula consumption
Urine and fecal production: At each feeding including fecal character (color and consistency)

EQUIPMENT

Equipment should be easily cleaned and disinfected. Low cost is also desirable for nonprofit facilities. The following items will be useful:

Rubber gloves: To prevent transmission of zoonotic disease and other diseases between different age and species groups
Gram scale (postal scale): To weigh the animal daily until weaned, then twice weekly until released. Use a lightweight box with a cover, a pillowcase, or a sock to contain high-spirited animals on the scale.
Enclosures: Need to be secure. A plastic or glass aquarium for animals less then one week old lined with newspaper and pine or aspen wood shavings is ideal. Because these animals are prey animals and nocturnal in activity, provide a burrow to reduce stress. Cardboard boxes with a cutout entry hole may be used but must be discarded when

soiled or between new animals. Plastic igloo-type burrows are available from many pet supply houses, which can be disinfected weekly or between animals. After 7 to 14 days, depending on species, the animal should be transferred to a wire cage to facilitate good air circulation and hygiene by allowing urine and feces to fall out the bottom. The wire openings should not be larger than 1 cm. Part of the surface area may be covered with straw and a burrow to provide a resting area. In the wild, a burrow is a small depression in the earth covered with dried vegetation or a nest within underlying brush. A burrow can be constructed from a clay pot turned on its side, upside-down plastic buckets with an entry hole cut out, or a small cardboard box.

Heat source: Electric heating pads should never cover the entire resting surface and should be set on the lowest setting to prevent skin burns and allow the animal to seek a cooler zone. Recirculating heat pads found in veterinary clinics are ideal, but are expensive. Hot-water bottles should be avoided because as they cool, they become a heat sink and actually pull body heat from the animal. Heat lamps may be used, but are hard to regulate. Like the electric heat pad, they should provide zones of coverage. If you place your hand on the enclosure floor under the heat lamp for a few minutes and your skin becomes uncomfortably hot, it is too hot for the animal and the lamp should be raised. Red heat-lamp bulbs are preferred to allow animals to sleep without the glare of white light.

Disinfectant: Household bleach at 1 oz per quart (33 ml per liter) mixed fresh works well and is inexpensive. Quaternary ammonia products or chlorine dioxide are recommended as well, but good ventilation and rinsing is required.

White vinegar: Rabbits produce alkaline urine with calcium crystals that form a scale on surfaces. Soaking in white vinegar before cleaning will help to remove scale.

Measuring devices such as spoons and cups

Syringes: 1, 3, and 5 cc Luer slip

Feeding tubes: 3–5 French, red rubber

CRITERIA FOR INTERVENTION

Most wild bunnies that are presented as orphans are probably not orphans. The general public is not educated about the life cycles of rabbits and does not understand that a doe does not sit on or attend her nest like a domestic dog or cat would do with a litter. Bunnies are quite small when they are weaned and unless the animal is obviously injured, it should be left alone. If a pet or lawn mower has disturbed a nest, the nest should be recovered and pets removed from the area. Since the doe will only return one to two times a day to the nest to feed and care for the young, the bedding may be replaced in a pattern (e.g., checkerboard) that can be visually rechecked for disturbance the following morning.

If a bunny is presented that is determined to be healthy and weaned, a reasonable attempt should be made to return it to its home environment. If this is not possible, the bunny should be released in a similar environment with the knowledge that regardless of the location, the animal is a prey species and will most likely be preyed upon at some point. The life span of an eastern cottontail in the wild is approximately one year. A licensed rehabber should be able to help with the release, and be knowledgeable about "safe" release sites.

Most states have laws against keeping native wildlife as pets even if the animal has a permanent injury that would preclude its release. People who are interested in rehabilitation of wildlife should check with their state wildlife office to determine what permits are necessary.

If the animal is determined to be a true preweanling and/or is injured, an experienced rehabber, veterinary technician, or veterinarian should assess the animal as soon as possible to determine if the animal can be reasonably treated for injuries and to provide supportive care.

Domestic rabbit neonates may require hand raising due to death of the dam, poor mothering ability that may occur with a doe with her first litter, or discovery of orphan feral bunnies. In this last instance, a domestic rabbit has been released by negligent owners or escaped after being bred and is termed feral. These does may not be capable of coping in the wild (especially during extreme weather) and are either killed or abandon their litter. If possible, in a breeding operation, cross-fostering (finding a surrogate doe) would be more economical.

ASSESSMENT OF THE NEONATE

Evaluate the bunny at entry to determine body temperature and evidence of life-threatening wounds. Puncture wounds from animal bites may be difficult to locate and are frequently fatal. Rabies virus infection should be considered in many geographical regions as a contaminant of bite wounds unless a vaccinated household pet is known to be the predator.

INITIAL CARE AND STABILIZATION

Neonatal mammals are very susceptible to hypothermia. The normal body temperature for most hares and rabbits is 100–103°F (37.8–39.4°C). If the bunny is chilled by 5–6°F (3–4°C), the quickest way to warm it is to submerge it (head above water) in a warm-water bath (100°F/37.8°C) and massage gently. Remove the animal within five minutes and continue to warm/dry it under a heat lamp or dryer taking extreme care not to burn it. Animals with severe hypothermia will probably not return to "normal" after warming. Rapid warming of these animals may result in fatal metabolic changes.

Keep in mind that warming the animal may exacerbate dehydration. Fluid therapy should be considered after warming. If the animal requires more than oral hydration, subcutaneous injections of a balanced electrolyte solution (lactated Ringer's or normal saline) for intravenous use can be used at a rate of 35–40 ml/kg/day. If the animal is weak and considered hypoglycemic, 2 1/2% dextrose in lactated Ringer's solution (LRS) may be substituted.

FORMULAS

Recipes for milk replacer formulas are in Table 1.1. Rabbit milk is generally high in fat and protein and low in carbohydrates. High-carbohydrate diets have a negative effect on the bacterial flora and motility of the rabbit gastrointestinal tract. The problem with milk analysis is that no good studies have been done to look at how milk composition changes over the lactation period except in domestic rabbits used for production. *Oryctolagus* milk solids are reported to range from a high of 30% down to 25% over the lactation period. *Sylvilagus* and *Lepus* are approximately 35% and 40%, respectively, but data are not available to determine how these numbers change during lactation.

Species-specific milk is considered to be best but is generally not an available option with rabbits. Milk replacement for orphan rabbits commonly utilizes a combination of Esbilac or KMR (Kitten Milk Replacer) and MultiMilk Esbilac is formulated for canine pups and has more fat but less carbohydrates and protein than KMR. KMR is formulated as a milk replacer for domestic felines, is higher in protein and carbohydrates than Esbilac, and therefore is not directly interchangeable with the Esbilac formula. The MultiMilk (or Milk Matrix 33/40) has the advantage of being able to increase the fat and protein when mixed with KMR or Esbilac without increasing the carbohydrates. All three products are manufactured by the same company and may be ordered. KMR and Esbilac are readily available from most pet stores and veterinarians. Heavy cream (36% milk fat, 0% carbohydrates) may be used to increase the milk fat of KMR or Esbilac formulas. Half-and-half should not be used because it will lower the protein and increase the carbohydrate content of the formula and may lead to digestive upset or poor weight gain.

Table 1.1. Recipes for Milk Replacer Formulas

Recipe I 6 parts Esbilac liquid 4 parts Multi Milk (powder) *(1.91 kcal/cc)*	*Recipe IV* 1 part Esbilac powder 1/4 part heavy cream 1 part water *(1.93 kcal/cc)*
Recipe II 1 part Esbilac powder 1 part Multi Milk powder 1 1/2 parts water *(2.01 kcal/cc)*	*Recipe V* 1 part evaporated milk 1 part water To each cup of this mixture add 1 egg yolk 1 tablespoon corn syrup
Recipe III 2 part KMR liquid 1 part Multi Milk powder *(1.73 kcal/cc)*	

Note: When mixing formulas a part equals a teaspoon or cup. For example, with Recipe I you would mix 6 teaspoons of Esbilac liquid and 4 teaspoons Multi Milk.
Sources: Recipes I–IV—Marcum (1998), Evans (1997); Recipe V—Cheeke (1987).

All formulas should be mixed in quantities that can be utilized within a two- to three-day period and be kept refrigerated. Only the amount of formula to be used at a single feeding should be removed and heated to reduce the probability of bacterial contamination and spoilage. Powdered formulas can be stored in airtight containers for up to six months and are generally more economical to use.

WHAT TO FEED INITIALLY

Once the bunny has been stabilized and is ready to be fed, it is best to start with an oral electrolyte solution. Gradually add in the milk replacer to avoid gastrointestinal upset. Rehydration should take place prior to starting the formula and should be corrected within a 24-hour period. A human oral electrolyte solution such as Pedialyte may be used to hydrate the animal and serve as its first meal. Calculate the fluid requirements for a 24-hour period and divide by the stomach volume limits to determine how many feedings need to take place (see below in Amounts to Feed). If hydration is corrected, mix formula and electrolyte solution 1:1 for the next meal. If the animal is doing well consider 100% formula. Depending on the degree of dehydration and the percentage of milk solids, the animal may take 24–48 hours to produce feces, but urine should be produced by the second feeding. The animal should also be content after it is fed and the abdomen should feel soft but full.

Neonatal rabbits, but not hares, require stimulation of the anogenital region to urinate and defecate. The doe will lick this region and frequently consumes the by-products. The rehabber must perform this stimulation task and can accomplish it by gently stroking this area with a warm moist cotton tip applicator or gauze. Remove urine and feces to maintain hygiene.

NURSING TECHNIQUES

Once the bunny is strong enough to nurse, syringe feeding is the method of choice. Excellent control of milk flow can be obtained with a 1 or 3 cc non-Luer lock (or slip tip) syringe placed in the corner of the rabbit's mouth. Placing a hand over the animal or laying a piece of cloth over the animal's head/eyes appears to increase the animal's comfort level and promote successful feedings.

Keep a warm moist clean cloth available to clean the bunny's face after nursing. Formula that is left to dry on the animal may cause hair loss and dermatitis.

Utensils that are used to feed the bunnies should not be shared between animals to reduce the chance of disease transmission. Between feedings, all utensils should be cleaned in hot soapy water, rinsed well, and allowed to dry. Dilute bleach (1 oz per quart of warm water) may be used as a disinfectant, but the utensils should be rinsed again before air-drying. Bleach will shorten the life span of the rubber plungers in the syringes.

TUBE FEEDING

If the animal has a poor suckling response, tube feeding is recommended for the first couple of feedings. A red rubber tube is attached to a 3 or 5 cc syringe. Starting with the tip of the catheter at the last rib, measure the tube against the side of the animal the distance from the last rib to the tip of the nose. Using indelible ink, mark the distance on the tube to the tip of the nose. This is the amount of tube to be passed into the animal's mouth and into the stomach. The syringe plunger is advanced until milk can be seen at the tip of the catheter (wipe off excess). Note that sufficient formula should be drawn up into the syringe to account for losses in the tube. It is also recommended to reduce the volume at each feeding by 25–30% when force-feeding and add an additional feeding to provide daily caloric requirements. With the animal restrained by the nondominant hand, the tube is passed into the back of the oral cavity and gently advanced in conjunction with swallowing. The length of tube if measured correctly can only be in the stomach as it would not be able to pass that distance if it were in the lungs unless it was advanced too roughly through the lungs and diaphragm. Administer the formula slowly, if you meet resistance, stop. The abdomen should be gently distended but not firm or hard.

FREQUENCY OF FEEDING

Does generally return to the nest to feed their young once a day to reduce the chance that a predator will follow her to the nest and prey upon her young. Because we are not feeding mother's milk, which resists spoilage in the stomach, it is best to divide the feedings into two to three a day to reduce bloat and be able to provide the estimated caloric requirements using artificial formula.

Once the bunny's eyes are open (or approximately seven days for hares) and the animal is nibbling on roughage, the number of feedings per day can be decreased. By two to three weeks of age (ten days for hares), one feeding should suffice and in another five to seven days, the animal should be weaned to solids completely. Allow an additional two weeks for domestic rabbits. Continue to weigh the animal every two to three days in case substantial weight loss is noted. If weight loss occurs, wait one to two additional days to decrease the number of feedings and make sure to reassess the overall health of the animal.

AMOUNTS TO FEED

The neonatal rabbit stomach can hold up to 100–125 ml per kg of body weight at each feeding. Depending on the caloric density of the formula, the animal should be fed one to four times over a 24-hour period.

Example: A 30-gram bunny should be able to handle up to 3–3.75 ml of formula per feeding.

$$30 \text{ g} \times 1 \text{ kg}/1000 \text{ g} \times 100\text{–}125 \text{ ml/kg}$$

To further expand the example, a 30-gram bunny would require

$$\{2 \times [70 \times (0.030 \text{ kg})^{0.75}]\} \text{ or } 10.1 \text{ kcal per day.}$$

Using a milk replacement formula that provides 2.01 kcal/ml, the bunny would need to be fed per day

$$10.1 \text{ kcal/day} \times 1 \text{ ml}/2.01 \text{ kcal} = 5 \text{ ml of formula}$$

Since this amount (5 ml) is greater than the amount the bunny's stomach can hold at one feeding, divide that number by two feedings per day and the bunny will need to be fed approximately 2.5 ml every 12 hours.

The amount to feed should be recalculated every two to three days. Construction of a feeding chart based on weight, kcal requirements, and use of a standard formula is helpful for quick reference of amounts to feed (see Table 1.2).

EXPECTED WEIGHT GAIN

Rate of gain is dependent on genus/species, adult target weight, genetics (domestic vs. wild), health of the neonate, and type of formula. For cottontails, weaning weight is somewhere between 150 and 200 grams depending on the age at weaning and successful transfer to adult diet (Fig. 1.1). Domestic rabbit weaning weights are very breed dependent since some meat breeds were founded specifically for high rate of gain. A domestic meat rabbit at 28-day weaning might weigh 550–650 grams and by day 70 reach 2.2–2.5 kg (deBlas and Wiseman 1998)!

Steady weight gain and good or average body-condition score are indicators of success. There may be instances when no weight gain is detected for 24–48 hours. This may be normal for the short term, but should not continue. Recalculate caloric requirements, assess the animal's health, or consider changing to a different formula in the future if you continue to have repeated problems with weight gains.

HOUSING

Orphan rabbits do not need to be maintained for long periods of time due to their short maturation time to weaning. Housing does not need to change drastically from that described above in Equipment.

In the first week of life neonatal bunnies are at greater risk of hypothermia due to their age and lack of hair coat. Temperature in the nest area should be maintained at 80–85°F (26.7–29.4°C) and by week three can be reduced to 70–75°F (21–23.9°C). Neonatal hares are not at risk for hypothermia because they are more precocious and able to regulate body temperature at a younger age than the rabbit species.

Wild rabbits and hares have a very strong flight instinct and once they are able to move around may rush around the enclosure and injure themselves in an attempt to escape. Some may even vocalize with fear. As mentioned in the previous description of equipment, these animals should be provided a burrow to reduce stress. Handling should be kept to a minimum to reduce taming down prior to release. When catching an animal to feed or treat, the handlers should be deliberate but gentle in their actions to avoid chasing the animal around the enclosure. Use of small washcloths to cover the animal before picking up may simulate a burrowlike atmosphere and reduce stress. For animals that are extremely difficult, lowering the light level in the room may facilitate capture.

Domestic rabbit orphans have been tamed down through generations of breeding and do not have as great a fear instinct as their wild counterparts. Regular and frequent handling will improve the pet quality of these animals.

TIPS FOR WEANING FROM FORMULA TO SOLID FOOD

If provided the right foodstuffs at the right age, rabbits wean readily. Within a few days of opening their eyes (or within five to seven days for hares), bunnies should be provided a selection of clean

Table 1.2 Sample Feeding Chart

Weight		Required kcal	Amount of formula in cc's per day*	Amount of formula in cc /feeding Feeding intervals in 24 hours			Stomach capacity: 100cc/kg**
grams	ounces			2X	3X	4X	
25	0.9	8.81	4.4	2.2	1.5	1.1	2.5
30	1.1	10.09	5.0	2.5	1.7	1.3	3.0
35	1.2	11.33	5.7	2.8	1.9	1.4	3.5
40	1.4	12.52	6.3	3.1	2.1	1.6	4.0
45	1.6	13.68	6.8	3.4	2.3	1.7	4.5
50	1.8	14.80	7.4	3.7	2.5	1.8	5.0
55	1.9	15.90	8.0	4.0	2.7	2.0	5.5
60	2.1	16.97	8.5	4.2	2.8	2.1	6.0
65	2.3	18.02	9.0	4.5	3.0	2.3	6.5
70	2.5	19.05	9.5	4.8	3.2	2.4	7.0
75	2.6	20.06	10.0	5.0	3.3	2.5	7.5
80	2.8	21.06	10.5	5.3	3.5	2.6	8.0
85	3.0	22.04	11.0	5.5	3.7	2.8	8.5
90	3.2	23.00	11.5	5.8	3.8	2.9	9.0
95	3.4	23.95	12.0	6.0	4.0	3.0	9.5
100	3.5	24.89	12.4	6.2	4.1	3.1	10.0

* Caloric density is assumed to be 2 kcal/cc for this example.
** The amount of formula at each feeding should not exceed 100–125 cc/kg body weight.

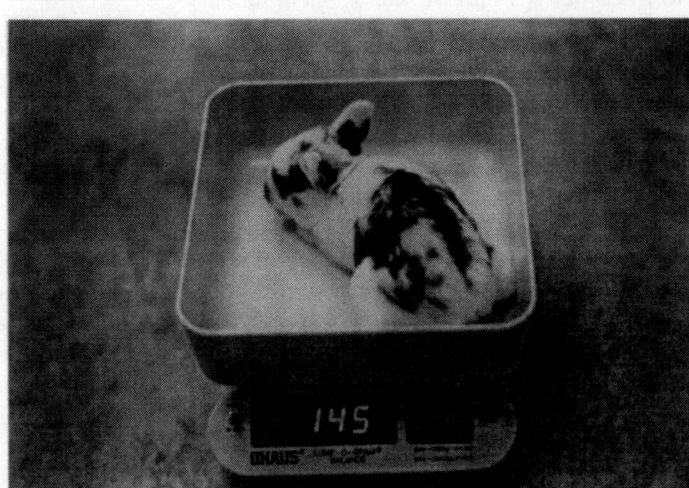

Figure 1.1. Bunny on a scale (photo by Laurie J. Gage).

leafy greens and good quality grass hay. Greens would include but are not limited to dark green lettuces, kale, broccoli, parsley, cilantro, other herbs, dandelion greens, and other greens (collards, mustard, turnip). Since these greens are not anchored in the ground by roots, it is recommended that the greens be chopped into smaller pieces initially to make them easier to consume by the young animal.

Fresh clean water should be provided daily as early as five days for hares. The water should be placed in a shallow heavy container. If the bunny is eating wet greens, water consumption will be minimal. If there are concerns over whether the animal is getting enough water, place the animal on white paper towels overnight to check for urine spots.

Hay may be obtained from many pet stores, horse farms, and even on-line. Some types of hays to consider are timothy, orchard grass, oat, and various prairie grasses. Commercial rabbit pellets may be used, but are not as readily accepted, are relatively high in carbohydrates, and even though labeled as high fiber do not contain long-stem fiber, which appears to be important for mechanically stimulating and maintaining good gastrointestinal health in the rabbit.

Fruits and vegetables high in natural sugars (e.g., apples and carrots) and processed cereals are not recommended and chronic feeding in domestic rabbits may lead to obesity and gastrointestinal motility disorders.

Rabbits utilize a process referred to as hindgut fermentation and are dependent on microbes in the cecum to break down fiber in the diet into a more nutritious product. The rabbit produces cecotrophs, which are large soft "feces," brown-green in color and sometimes mistaken for diarrhea in the rabbit. The rabbit stimulates the release of the cecotrophs from the cecum by licking its perineum and then consumes them. The cecotrophs provide water, vitamins, minerals, and protein to the rabbit diet. Feeding them to preweanling rabbits will help to seed the young rabbit's digestive tract with microbes that are beneficial to digestion. If older rabbits are available, check the wire bottom of the cage in the morning for left over cecotrophs (soft feces hanging from the wire or in the pan underneath) and dole them out to the preweanling bunnies two to three times a week until weaning.

COMMON MEDICAL PROBLEMS

Persons working with wildlife should be up to date on tetanus vaccinations and strongly consider rabies preexposure vaccination series.

Bite injuries and infection are frequently fatal in rabbits and hares. Wounds inflicted by the canine teeth of predators can cause deep underlying damage with minimal skin damage. Antibiotics are indicated when bite wounds are present. The microbial population of the rabbit gastrointestinal tract is particularly sensitive to certain antibiotics. Penicillin-type drugs like amoxicillin and lincosamides (e.g., clindamycin) cause fatal enteritis and colitis and should never be used orally in the rabbit. Quinolones (e.g., enrofloxacin), pediatric suspensions of trimethoprim and sulfa combinations, and chloramphenicol are good antibiotic choices. Concerns over joint problems in young growing animals receiving enrofloxacin do not appear to be a problem in young rabbits.

Wild rabbits and hares with fractures or eye injuries need to be critically evaluated on presentation to determine if they are suitable candidates for release. Euthanasia should be considered in animals with injuries that result in permanent impairment. While there are always exceptions, these animals do not make good pets. Domestic breeds of rabbits with the same injuries will generally adapt well to permanent impairment such as blindness and loss of limb because they do not succumb to the chronic stress of captivity that their wild cousins do.

Fly-strike occurs when adult flies lay eggs on an animal with an open wound, which is not cared for due to lack of medical attention or an inability of the animal to groom itself. The eggs hatch and the larvae feed on the decaying tissue and may invade body cavities. Start treatment by clipping the hair away from the wound and irrigating with sterile saline to remove diseased tissue. The larvae are quite resilient and physical removal is therefore the best way to get rid of them. Cuterebra can be a problem in rabbits that are housed out doors on the ground where feces are allowed to accumulate. These fly species lay eggs on the organic material. The hatched larvae enter the rabbit's body through natural openings and penetrate mucous membranes then travel through the body and exit through the skin to complete their life cycle. Removing the larvae, which can be visualized through the hole in the skin, with forceps, best treats this condition. Care should be taken not to crush the larva inside the animal. Ivermectin appears to be helpful in treating migrating forms of this "parasite" in areas where repeated infections are a problem. Prevention is through housing rabbits off the ground in raised hutches and maintaining hygiene.

Bloat and diarrhea in neonatal bunnies are usually due to a problem with feeding. Rapid formula introductions, acute changes in brands of formula, and incorrect mixing (too concentrated) are the most common mistakes. Feeding electrolyte solutions in lieu of formula for one to two feedings should help to alleviate problems and correct electrolyte imbalances due to the diarrhea. In some cases, simethicone suspension marketed for human infants may be used to treat bloat due to gas accumulation. When no other cause can be determined for loose stool or diarrhea, the pediatric suspension of trimethoprim and sulfa mentioned earlier may help to stabilize the gastrointestinal tract of the neonate.

Coccidiosis is a protozoan parasitic disease of the small intestine and liver of rabbits. The organism can cause fatal diarrhea in weanling domestic rabbits. Improved sanitation can reduce the incidence of clinical disease. Oral sulfa drugs used to treat coccidiosis in dogs and cats may be used to treat the diarrhea.

Rabies has not been reported with any significant frequency in wild rabbits and hares. As prey animals, they are probably killed by rabid predators and thus do not survive to support an infection that can be transmitted. In the last few years, an increased number of domestic pet rabbits have been diagnosed as rabies-virus positive. These rabbits were housed outdoors and the rabid predators probably did not have full access to them, so the rabbits were wounded and infected rather than killed (Karp 1999). Two cases from the same veterinary practice in Lillington, North Carolina, resulted in over 30 people receiving rabies postexposure treatment. People are infected with the rabies virus from contact with virus-laden body fluids like saliva through breaks in the skin when the animals are handled.

Tularemia is a bacterial disease caused by *Francisella tularensis*. Humans are infected through breaks in the skin by handling infected tissues from rabbits (and other wildlife). Humans have also been infected by arthropods (ticks) that have fed on infected wildlife. There are several forms of the disease, which can be fatal.

SOURCES OF PRODUCTS MENTIONED

Esbilac, KMR, Milk Matrix 33/40, and MultiMilk: PetAg Inc., 261 Keyes Ave., Hampshire, IL 60140; 1-800-323-0877, 1-800-323-6878; www.petag.com

Pedialyte: Ross Products Division, Abbott Laboratories, Columbus, OH 43215-1724; 1-800-986-8510; www.abbott.com, www.ross.com

REFERENCES

Brooks, Dale L. 1986. Rabbits, hares and pikas. In *Zoo and wild animal medicine*, edited by Murray E. Fowler. 2d ed. Philadelphia, PA: Saunders.

CDC. 1999. Human rabies prevention—United States, 1999: Recommendations of the Advisory Committee on Immunization Practices (ACIP). *MMWR*, 48(RR-1), 1–21.

Cheeke, Peter R. 1987. *Rabbit production*. 6th ed. Danville, IL: The Interstate.

de Blas, C., and J. Wiseman. 1998. The nutrition of the rabbit. New York: CABI.

Evans, Richard H. 1987. Rearing orphan wild mammals. In *Veterinary clinics of North America*, edited by Dennis F. Lawler and Emerson D. Colby. Volume 17(3). Philadelphia, PA: Saunders.

Karp, Beth E. 1999. Rabies in two privately owned domestic rabbits. *JAVMA* 215(12):1824–27.

Marcum, Debbie. 1998. Mammal rehabilitation: The basics. In *NWRA principles of wildlife rehabilitation*, edited by Adele T. Moore and Sally Joosten. St. Cloud, MN: National Wildlife Rehabilitators Association.

Sandford, J. C. 1996. *The domestic rabbit*. 5th ed. Cambridge, MA: Blackwell Science.

Weinberg, Arnold N., and David J. Weber. 1991. Animal associated human infections. In *Infectious disease clinics of North America*. Volume 5(1). Philadelphia, PA: Saunders.

2
Puppies

Valerie T. Barrette

NATURAL HISTORY

The scientific name of the dog is *Canis familiaris*. Average birth weight varies depending on breed: toy breeds are 100 to 400 grams, medium breeds are 200 to 300 grams, large breeds are 400 to 500 grams, and giant breeds can weigh in excess of 700 grams. Time to weaning is three to six weeks.

RECORD KEEPING

Keep a daily log of food intake, stool and urine production, consistency of stool, hydration, appetite, attitude, and weight.

EQUIPMENT

The following items should be on hand:

Nipples
Bottles 4–8 oz (120–240 ml)
Blender
Rubber catheters, size 5, 8, and 10 French
Catheter-tip syringes, sizes from 6 to 20 cc
Microwave or stove
Hot-water blanket, hot-water bottle, or rubber surgical gloves to fill with hot water
Scale (grams preferred)
Rectal thermometer

Nipples and bottles specifically for use with hand raising puppies or human baby bottles (4 to 8 oz) (120 to 240 ml) and nipples, depending on puppy size are acceptable. Nipples made for premature babies (obtained from a hospital) work very well.

A blender with an 8 oz (240 ml) jar attachment is helpful when raising tiny breed or single puppy litters.

CRITERIA FOR INTERVENTION

It is necessary to assist puppies that are unable to nurse adequately. This may be due to weakness, inability to compete, lack of bitch's milk supply, or lack of bitch's interest. In some cases, it may be possible to supplement the puppy and allow it to be cared for otherwise by the bitch. This is the preferred method and should be applied whenever possible. However, removing the puppy from the bitch and hand rearing it completely may sometimes be in the puppy's best interest. Healthy puppies that are receiving adequate nutrition will nurse vigorously, sleep soundly, and have a rounded, sleek appearance. Indications a puppy is not receiving adequate nutrition vary from constant crying and restlessness to extreme inactivity. There will also be a failure to achieve expected weight gain. Undernourished puppies may also have a "pinched" look to the hip area and a general unthrifty appearance.

ASSESSMENT OF THE NEONATE

Newborn puppies that are to be hand raised should receive a physical examination to assess respiration, pulse, and hydration and record temperature and body weight. When possible, a fecal examination for parasites should be performed. Normal temperature in newborns is about 96 to 97°F (35.5–36°C), and there will be incremental increases to 100°F (37.8°C) by four weeks of age. Age may be roughly determined by the appearance of the umbilicus. A fresh-appearing umbilicus indicates the puppy was born within the past 24 hours. The umbilicus will shrink and dry up within a day or two and typically falls off by the fourth day of age. Another helpful age assessment for young puppies is flexor/extensor tone. During the first four days of life, flexor tone is dominant. Holding the puppy by its head or scruff, it will curl its body inward. After four days, it will extend its head and appear to bend backward.

INITIAL CARE AND STABILIZATION OF THE NEONATE

Newborn or recently born puppies in need of intervention frequently present with hypothermia, hypoglycemia, and/or dehydration. No attempt should be made to feed milk replacement to a puppy whose temperature is below 95°F (35°C). Instead, a warmed mixture of half lactated Ringer's solution and half 5% dextrose should be administered subcutaneously at a rate of 1 ml/30 g (1 ml/oz) of body weight. Pedialyte or a similar nutrient-electrolyte solution should be administered orally to the hypoglycemic puppy at a rate of 1 ml/30 g (1 ml/oz) of body weight every 15–30 minutes until the puppy responds. Warming of the puppy should be accomplished slowly, over the course of one to three hours.

Puppies should not be warmed to the adult normal body temperature as their normal body temperature is several degrees lower. Puppies four weeks of age and younger have a normal body temperature of 96–97°F (35.5–36.1°C). Avoid warming them to the normal adult temperature of 100–102°F (37.8–38.9°C).

FORMULAS, SUPPLEMENTS, AND DAILY CALORIC REQUIREMENTS

Puppies require approximately 13–17 kcal of metabolizable energy per 100 grams of body weight per day. Commercial formulas typically provide 1 to 1.25 kcal/ml. The simplest formulas to use are commercially available powdered canine milk replacements. Esbilac (PetAg), Just Born (Farnam), and Mother's Helper (Lambert Kay) are the most commonly available products in the United States. Most of these products recommend a 1:2 (product to water) dilution of their formula. I have found that a dilution of 1:3 creates less potential for diarrhea or constipation. While commercial preparations are the preferred choice, when not available a homemade version may be prepared. Below is one example:

Puppy Milk Replacer Formula

Here is the recipe for puppy milk replacer formula:

300 ml (10 oz) goat's milk
177 ml (6 oz) boiled water
1 raw egg yolk (the yolk only, no white)
236 ml (1 cup) whole fat yogurt
30 ml (2 tablespoons) mayonnaise

Place all ingredients in a blender and mix until well blended. You may refrigerate the formula for four days, then discard it and make new formula.

If using commercially available milk replacements, chose one brand and use it throughout the hand-rearing process. Just as changes in solid food diets may cause digestive upset, so may changes in milk replacement. In addition, puppies become accustomed to the taste of the formula and may refuse an unfamiliar taste. It is important to make the formula in a consistent manner. A highly concentrated formula may cause digestive upset or inappetence. Formula that is too dilute may result in a frantic, hungry puppy that fails to thrive.

Many of the commercially available milk replacers now are made to mix easily and can be mixed by shaking in a jar. However, large quantities are more effectively mixed in a blender. It is recommended that formula be mixed in a blender well ahead of feeding, as the air bubbles generated may cause indigestion. Avoid overblending. Run the blender about ten seconds or less to combine the ingredients.

Formula should be heated to approximately 100°F (37.8°C) or near the puppy's body temperature. A microwave may be used, but care must be taken to not overheat the formula. Overheated formula may change in consistency and cause digestive upset. Thoroughly mix the formula to eliminate "hot spots," and always test the temperature by placing a few drops on the inside of your wrist.

Formula may be reheated if necessary during a feeding, but once heated, formula should not be refrigerated or reused later. Prepared formula should be discarded after 24 hours. Follow the manufacturer's directions for storage of the powder.

Bottles, nipples, and any other equipment used in the preparation of formula should be washed in hot, sudsy water and thoroughly rinsed after each use, to prevent bacterial growth. Formula should be stored in the refrigerator in a separate container. Storing formula in the same bottle used for feeding is not recommended.

WHAT TO FEED INITIALLY

Until the puppy's temperature is over 95°F (35°C), the only oral solution given should be plain Pedialyte (Ross) or other nutrient-electrolyte solution such as lactated Ringer's with 5% dextrose. In a pinch, 8 oz boiled water mixed with 1 tablespoon white Karo syrup (do not use honey) may be used. Once the rectal temperature is above 95°F, warmed, diluted formula (one part Pedialyte to one part milk replacement formula) may be started. Provided there is no gastrointestinal upset after two to three feedings, which is determined by stool consistency, and the puppy is able to maintain normal temperature, 100% formula may be fed.

NURSING TECHNIQUES

Unlike human babies, puppies should be fed while on their stomachs (Fig. 2.1). Feeding puppies on their backs puts them at an increased risk of aspirating the formula. It may take the puppy some time to acclimate and accept the nipple, especially if it is an older puppy that has had an opportunity to nurse from the dam. The different taste of the milk may also be a complicating factor. Have a variety of nipples on hand as puppies will frequently develop a preference for a particular nipple. I have had the best luck with nipples made expressly for premature human babies. These are not the nipples sold over the counter as preemie nipples, but are nipples obtained from a hospital. They are smaller and more pliable than store-bought nipples and I have found that puppies more readily accept them. Puppies may have a good suckle reflex for your finger, but fade off while on the bottle. Be persistent and patient. Slipping the bottle alongside your finger or placing formula on your finger may help start the process. Hold the bottle so that the puppy is not ingesting air. Do not squeeze the bottle. If the puppy seems to have difficulty getting milk from the nipple, the hole may be enlarged with a hot needle. However, check first to ensure the problem is not caused by a clot of formula or other obstruction. When held upside down, milk should drip at a slow rate from the nipple hole.

TUBE FEEDING

Tube feeding makes it possible to supplement a puppy too weak to suckle, or one who simply refuses the unfamiliar nipple and formula. Acclimating a puppy to the nipple is time-consuming, and having the option of tube feeding may relieve the caregiver of frustration, and give the puppy necessary nutrients. In general, feedings should be reduced in volume by 30% when tube feeding. While the formula will be delivered slowly it is not possible for the stomach to expand to accommodate a full meal. Regurgitation and the resultant aspiration of formula could be fatal. Tube-fed puppies will need to have more frequent feedings to overcome the deficit. For puppies that weigh less than 310 g (10 oz), a #5 French infant feeding tube should suffice. Puppies over 310 g (10 oz) will best be fed with a #8 to #10 French feeding tube. The tip of the tube should be placed just forward of the last rib, with the distance measured to the tip of the nose and marked on the tube in permanent marker. This measurement should be redone on a weekly basis for puppies who require long-term tube feeding. The appropriate amount of warmed formula should be drawn up into a syringe and the feeding tube attached. Do not warm the formula in the syringe as hot pockets of formula may occur and could cause internal tissue damage. Express formula through the tube to expel all of the air. Holding the puppy's head firmly in a normal position (not flexed up), gently pass the tube into the mouth and throat. Provided there is no resistance, continue to pass the tube until you reach the

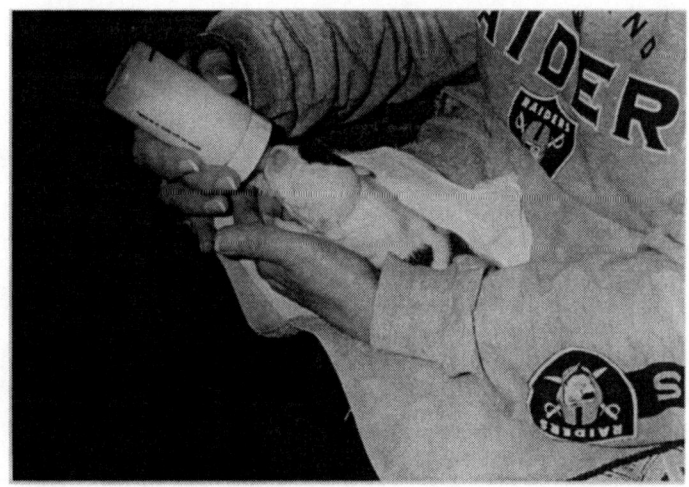

Figure 2.1. Two-week-old puppy nursing on a bottle (photo courtesy of Pat Wilson).

premeasured mark. Any resistance or obstruction should cause you to withdraw the tube and try again. Once properly passed, the formula should be administered slowly at a rate of 20 seconds per 10 ml. The puppy should be watched carefully for any signs of aspiration or regurgitation. If regurgitation results, abort the feeding until the next scheduled time and reduce the quantity.

It is important to note the possibility of delivering the formula to the lungs. This could be fatal to the puppy. Keeping the puppy's head level and slightly extended forward can help to direct the tube into the esophagus. One method to ensure proper placement is to insert the empty tube, unattached to the syringe, into the puppy's esophagus. Placing the end of the tube into a bowl of water can help to determine whether it is in the lungs or stomach, as a tube in the lungs will cause the water to bubble as the puppy breathes. Keep in mind that a small amount of bubbles will occur even if the tube is in the stomach, as the air in the tube is displaced. One drawback to this method is the ingestion of air into the puppy's stomach, as the syringe is attached to the empty tube and its contents delivered to the puppy. "Burping" the puppy in this case may be helpful. It can also be difficult for the single person who is tubing a wiggling puppy. However, if you are unsure of your tube-feeding skills, get help. Improper placement of the tube and delivering formula to the lungs could result in serious medical problems or even death. In the event the puppy does aspirate the formula, immediately withdraw the tube and suspend the puppy upside down in a gentle swinging motion, using gravity to help displace the liquid.

FREQUENCY OF FEEDING

For weak or compromised puppies, feeding may be necessary once every hour or two around the clock, until they are stabilized. For apparently healthy newborns, feeding should occur every two hours for the first few feedings. As they show evidence of gaining weight with no gastrointestinal upset, the amount of formula fed can be increased and the frequency of feeding reduced to every four to six hours. Bottle-fed puppies may start to refuse some feedings and increase their intake at other feedings. This is fine provided that the puppy's abdomen is not uncomfortably distended after feeding.

AMOUNTS TO FEED

On a daily basis, newborn puppies should receive approximately 25 to 30 ml per 120 g (4 oz) body weight. I have found that slightly underfeeding the puppies initially reduces the likelihood of digestive upset. If puppies are eating well and appear hungry, the feeding amounts may be gradually increased. Increasing the feeding amount too abruptly may cause problems with the puppy's digestive tract.

ELIMINATION

Newborn puppies must be stimulated to urinate and defecate. A moistened cotton ball, gauze, or washcloth gently massaging the anogenital region and abdomen simulates the mother's tongue action. This should be done at each feeding. Some puppies object vigorously to being stimulated, especially during defecation. These puppies may benefit from being stimulated prior to feeding, as their struggling on a full stomach can result in vomiting. The elimination reflex is present by three weeks of age, with some puppies exhibiting it much earlier. Care should be taken to stimulate around the sensitive anogenital area and not abrade it. The application of petroleum jelly after stimulation may help to reduce irritation.

EXPECTED WEIGHT GAIN

Weighing the puppies daily can help you spot the first sign of a puppy who is not thriving. For the first five months of life, puppies should gain 1 to 2 g/day/lb of anticipated adult weight (2 to 4 g/day/kg expected adult weight). For example, a male German shepherd's average adult weight would be 80 lb (36 kg). A male German shepherd puppy should gain 80 to 160 grams per day. While a puppy may not gain weight over a specific 24-hour period, weight loss or lack of weight gain within a 48-hour period should be reason for concern and intervention.

HOUSING

Newborn puppies are unable to regulate their body temperature for the first weeks of life. They require an ambient temperature of 86°F (30°C) to 90°F (32.2°C) for their first week, with gradual decreases over the following three weeks to 75°F (23.9°C). Newborn puppies should never be housed on heating pads. Neuromuscular reflexes are not present until seven days of age, and the puppy will not be able to withdraw and avoid a severe burn. Warm-water heating blankets and surgical gloves filled with water are good candidates for safely warming the puppy. The warm water gloves can be reheated in the microwave and reused repeatedly. Make sure there is plenty of bedding or toweling between the heat source and the puppy. It should be possible for the puppy to move away from the heat source if it chooses. Puppies should not be housed on newspaper or other slick surfaces. Instead they should be on a substrate that allows for good traction as they begin to support their weight and move about. Humidity should be maintained at approximately 55%. A damp towel partially draped over the nursery box works well, as does a cup of water in the close vicinity (out of range of the puppy). There is much controversy about whether a litter of puppies should be hand raised as a group or separately. One of the problems frequently encountered with puppies housed together is their tendency to nurse on each other. Besides the mess of puppies being stimulated to urinate and defecate in the nest and on each other, repeated sucking may result in actual damage to sensitive tissue. It is felt that until three weeks of age, puppies are relatively unaware of their environment. On the other hand, puppies hand reared by themselves have been known to suckle on their paws. Regardless of what the caregiver chooses to do, by three weeks of age the puppies should have regular contact with each other.

IMMUNE STATUS AND SPECIAL NEEDS

Puppies who have been unable to nurse from the bitch the first 24 hours after birth will not have received maternal antibodies. This means that they are at increased risk of disease and should be handled with extreme care. Precautions such as wearing specific clothing when caring for the puppy, washing and disinfecting of hands and all feeding materials, and keeping the puppy in an isolated area will keep risk of infection to a minimum.

TIME TO WEANING

Puppies may be weaned if necessary as soon as their eyes are open, although it is recommended to wait until three weeks of age. Once they are drinking and eating solid food well, supplemental feeding with formula may stop. The entire weaning process typically lasts until the fifth week.

TIPS FOR WEANING FROM FORMULA TO SOLID FOOD

There are many prepared weaning formulas available that can be mixed with the milk replacement. As the puppies learn to lap, the milk replacer can be reduced until the puppies are eating solid food. However, since the puppies will need to adjust to a new taste anyway, it may be more efficient to begin to use a mashed version of their future puppy food. Soaking dry puppy food in hot water until soft, and then mashing and mixing it with the milk replacer works well. Allowing the puppies to suck the mash off of your fingers can begin to acclimate them to the taste. Weaning is a messy business and puppies will frequently wear more of the food than they ingest at first. Using heavy casserole pans or pans manufactured expressly for feeding puppies will make it easier to do a group feed. I find it works the best to offer the mash just prior to a scheduled bottle feeding, this way puppies are motivated to try to eat, but don't lose out if they are slow learners. As the puppies become adept at lapping, use less milk replacer to create more solid food. At this point, water should be made available to the puppies. Over the next two weeks, the frequency of bottle feedings will be reduced to none, and less water will be added to their food until they are eating softened but formed kibble.

COMMON MEDICAL PROBLEMS

A chilled puppy will refuse to nurse and will quickly dehydrate and become hypoglycemic. This can be combated by administering equal parts of warmed 5% glucose and lactated Ringer's subcutaneously at a rate of 1 ml/30 g body weight (1 ml/oz). Warmed Pedialyte may be administered by gavage (tube fed) at a rate of 1 ml/30 g (oz) body weight every half hour until the puppy responds. The puppy should be warmed slowly over a one- to three-hour period. Too rapid warming can result in inadequate tissue oxygenation. Oxygen should be given if heart or respiratory rate is decreased. The normal newborn puppy's heart rate is 120–150 beats/min for the first 24 hours, while the respiratory rate is 8–18 breaths/min. After 24 hours, the heart rate increases to 220 beats/min and the respiratory rate increases to 15–35 breaths/min through five weeks of age.

Diarrhea or constipation is frequently a result of changes in the formula or incorrect feeding practices. Fecal analysis should be performed to rule out parasites. Formula that is too concentrated often results in constipation. Overfeeding may cause diarrhea in the neonate, as can bacterial overgrowth. Formula should be mixed in a consistent manner, with all feeding utensils kept scrupulously clean. Heated formula should not be stored and reheated, nor should formula be stored in the same bottle used for feeding. Mixed formula should be discarded after 24 hours.

SOCIALIZATION

Starting at three weeks, puppies should be handled more often than what is necessary for feeding and cleaning. Especially when keeping puppies separate or raising a single puppy, it is necessary for there to be some benign disruption in their lives. In a normal litter, puppies would be pushing for nipple access, climbing over and being climbed on by their littermates, and, in general, dealing with competition, frustration, and some stress. The hand raiser may need to simulate these circumstances. While it may seem counterintuitive, the quiet, stress-free "plastic bubble" environment is not the way to raise a normal puppy. While the critical socialization period lasts from three to twelve weeks of age, it is believed that it reaches a peak at 49 days. From this point on, human contact begins to have increasingly less of an impact on socialization. From 21 days to 49 days of age, we have the chance to make the greatest impact on how puppies will relate to humans. In addition, every effort should be made to give the single puppy an opportunity to interact with its own species during this critical time.

SOURCES OF PRODUCTS MENTIONED

Farnam Companies, Inc., Phoenix, AZ 85067-4820; 1-800-234-2269; www.farnampet.com

Lambert Kay, 1-609-951-4700
PetAg Inc., 261 Keyes Ave., Hampshire, IL 60140; 1-800-323-0877, 1-800-323-6878; www.petag.com

Ross Products Division, Abbott Laboratories, Columbus, OH 43215-1724; 1-800-986-8510; www.abbott.com, www.ross.com

REFERENCES

Hoskins, Johnny D. 1990. *Veterinary pediatrics.* Philadelphia, PA: Saunders.

Lewis, Lon D., and Mark L. Morris, Jr. 1984. *Small animal clinical nutrition.* Chapter 3. Topeka, KS: Mark Morris Associates.

Rutherford, Clarice, and David Neil. 1992. *How to raise a puppy you can live with.* Loveland, CO: Alpine Publications.

Veterinary clinics of North America. February 1978. *Canine pediatrics.* Volume 8 (1). Philadelphia, PA: Saunders.

3
Domestic Kittens

Laura Summers

NATURAL HISTORY

The scientific name of the cat is *Felis domesticus domesticus*. Average birth weight is 100 grams. Birthing takes place spring to summer (all year round in tropical climates). Time to weaning is three and a half to four weeks.

RECORD KEEPING

Kittens should be weighed daily for one to two weeks, then every two to three days until they are three to four weeks old. For those under two weeks of age, an intake log should also be kept, which includes the time of feeding and the amount fed.

NURSING TECHNIQUES

Kittens will naturally be competitive with each other for a nipple. If you are raising a litter, it is wise to move the kitten being fed away from the others to keep competition to a minimum. Simply bring the kitten up to your lap for a turn at the bottle. Keep the kitten in a natural position with its feet in your lap; do not turn the kitten on its back for feeding (see Fig. 3.1). In the beginning, hold the kitten's head gently with your thumb and forefinger. With the other hand, open the mouth and insert the nipple. Using the hand holding the kitten's head, gently keep it from turning its head and losing the nipple. Squeeze the bottle just enough so a drop of formula is on the tip of the nipple. Generally there will be some chewing on the nipple and some frustration on the part of the kitten and the handler. Be patient! Once the kitten learns the routine, it will begin latching on to the nipple when you touch it to the kitten's mouth. It is natural for kittens to want to knead with their paws while nursing. Once the kitten is nursing consistently, you should be able to hold the bottle and the upper part of the kitten with one hand, allowing the kitten to knead on your hand. As the kitten nurses formula from the bottle, you will need to allow air into the bottle to prevent a vacuum from forming. This can be accomplished by loosening the bottle top slightly to allow air to enter the bottle, or by periodically removing the nipple from the kitten's mouth. In the beginning, this will not be an issue, as the kitten will not eat very much. However, as the kittens get older and are eating more, they will become upset if you attempt to take the bottle away from them before they have finished their meal. Therefore, getting used to loosening the top just enough to let in air is the preferred method.

Allow each kitten to nurse until it refuses the bottle, feed kittens in sequence until all kittens are fed. It is wise to offer everyone "seconds," as some will eat more at the second offering.

The preferred bottle type is the PetAg Nurser, specially sized for kittens and small mammals (see Fig. 3.1). If this is not available, a 3 cc syringe will work for feeding. However, this does not allow the kitten to suckle properly, and if the formula is given too quickly, the kitten may aspirate formula.

After each nursing session, all kittens need to be stimulated to urinate and defecate. Use soft, dry, absorbent material (tissue or cotton balls) and gently rub the genital area (see Fig. 3.2). Kittens will usually urinate after each feeding and defecate once or twice each day.

Most kittens will learn to nurse from the bottle. However, if you have a particularly weak kitten or one who does not have a strong suckle reflex, you may need to begin tube feeding. Use a #5 French red rubber catheter and measure from the mouth to the last rib. Mark the tube with an indelible marker. Once again, keep the kitten in a natural position and

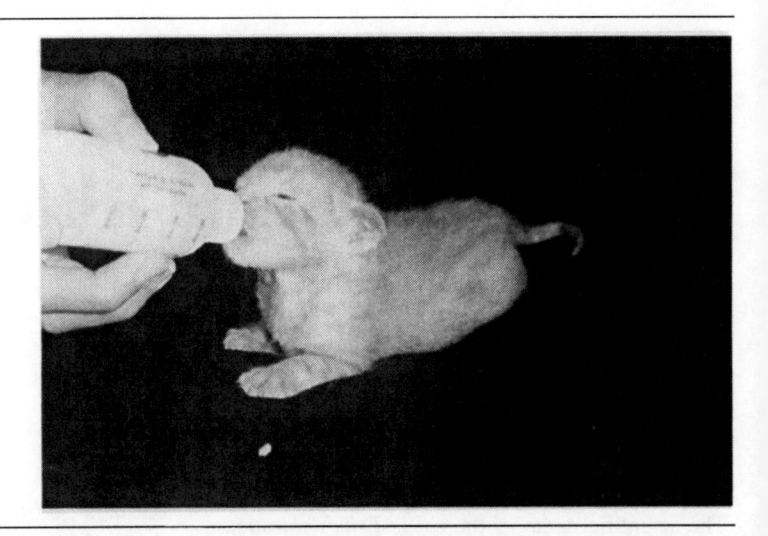

Figure 3.1. Young kitten nursing on a PetAg nurser.

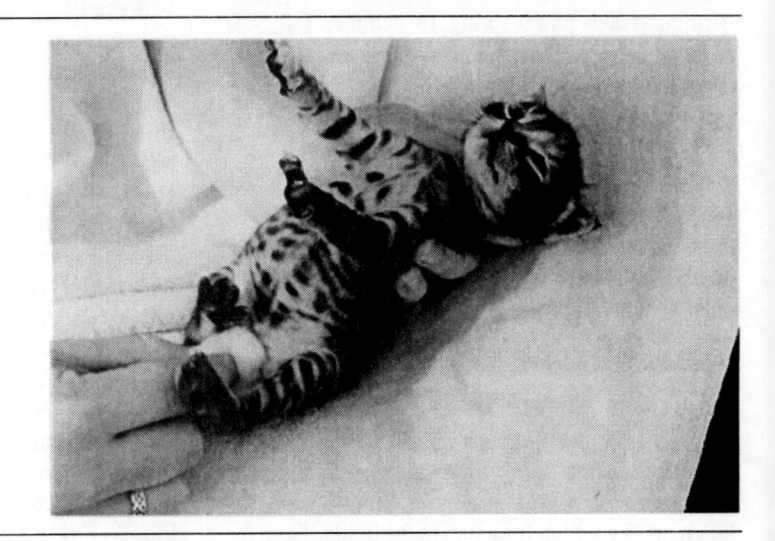

Figure 3.2. Stimulating a kitten to urinate and defecate.

pass the tube through the mouth and into the stomach. You may do this by gently sliding the blunt tip into the kitten's mouth and advance it slowly into the stomach. If the kitten begins to gag or the tube does not advance easily, remove the tube and start over. Kittens that are being tube fed are usually only a few days old and will require about 2–3 ml of formula per feeding. To remove the tube, crimp the end to prevent leakage of fluid while the tube is in the esophagus and gently pull the tube from the kitten's mouth. Kittens should be encouraged to nurse after tube feeding and they will eventually get used to nursing from the bottle. It may be tempting to tube feed late-night feedings instead of allowing the kitten to nurse. Avoid this. Kittens need to suckle and it is undesirable for them to receive their full feeding in just a few seconds.

AMOUNTS TO FEED

Kittens less than one week of age will generally eat 13 ml of formula per 100 g (3.5 oz) body weight per day. This should be divided up into several feedings of 1.25 to 2 ml per feeding spaced two to three hours apart during the day, and three to four hours apart at night. From one to two weeks, they will generally eat 17 mls of formula/100 g body weight per day and can be fed every three to four hours. From three to four weeks, feed 20 ml of formula/100 g body weight per day divided into feedings every four to six hours. From week four to five, feed 22 ml of formula/100 g body weight per day, again divided into feedings every four to six hours. After feeding, the abdomen should be enlarged but not distended. Note: It is better to underfeed rather than overfeed during the first few weeks of life to avoid gastrointestinal disturbances.

FORMULAS

Fortunately, there is a variety of commercial kitten formulas readily available in pet food stores. The most widely used formula is Kitten Milk Replacer (KMR; PetAg). This formula comes in a powdered and reconstituted (canned) form. When raising a litter, it is most practical and economical to use the powdered form; however, the reconstituted form may be used if needed. Use the following guidelines for mixing:

Powdered KMR formula:
  For kittens less than two weeks old, mix one part powder to two parts water. For kittens over two weeks, mix two parts powder to three parts water.
Reconstituted KMR formula:
  For kittens less than two weeks, mix one part reconstituted formula to one part water. For kittens over two weeks, mix two parts reconstituted formula to one part water.

These dilutions reflect a higher water content than the directions commonly printed on the packaging. I have found that additional water improves the formula consistency and reduces GI upset in kittens.

Powdered formula may be mixed in a blender or by hand. If a blender is used, mix only for a few seconds and allow the formula to settle for at least 30 minutes prior to feeding. (This will reduce the number of air bubbles in the formula.) The formula should be heated to about 100°F (37.8°C) before feeding. At this temperature, the formula should be warm but not hot when a small drop is placed on the inside of your wrist. The formula/water mixture may be kept refrigerated between feedings. Discard any unused formula after 24 hours. If you are using reconstituted formula from a can, discard it after it has been open for 24 hours.

If in an emergency situation you cannot obtain a commercial kitten formula, you may use the following recipe to make a kitten formula from scratch: Blend 0.5 cups whole milk, 1 egg yolk, 1 drop multiple vitamin infant vitamins, 3 $CaCO_3$ (Tums) tablets. Blend for one minute then strain through a kitchen strainer. Feed the same amounts as outlined for the commercial formula.

EXPECTED WEIGHT GAIN

Normal kittens weigh about 100 g (3.5 oz) at birth and will gain 7 to 10 g/day. Most kittens gain weight daily. If a kitten is not gaining weight, or eating well, its clinical condition must be taken into account. For example, if a kitten misses a single meal or does not gain weight for a single day but is active and alert, there is usually no need for concern. If a kitten misses a meal or does not gain weight AND is quiet and less active, then supportive care (SQ fluids and tube feeding) as well as investigation into an underlying cause is warranted. It is not uncommon for a weight plateau to occur when weaning to solid food.

HOUSING

For the first week of life kittens are unable to regulate their own body temperature. From birth to seven days, kittens should be kept at an ambient temperature of 86–90°F (30–32.2°C). Over the next few weeks, as the kittens' ability to self-regulate body temperature improves, the ambient temperature may gradually be decreased to 75°F (23.8°C). Humidity should be maintained at 55–60%. The area they are kept in initially should be quiet and free of drafts. A small-sized, portable animal crate works well to house the kittens. Line the bottom with a clean towel; a fleece on top of the towel is helpful to provide additional padding and to wick away any moisture. A towel over the top of the crate will make the crate dark and secure. Additional heat may be provided by placing warm-water bottles in the crate, or by placing half of the crate over an electrical heating pad set on "low." (Remember—warm-water bottles become cold-water bottles and will need to be rewarmed at each feeding; and electrical heating pads may overheat easily.) Take a moment at each feeding to feel inside the crate to be sure that the temperature is comfortable.

Because of the frequency of feedings of newborns, the litter will on occasion have to travel with the foster parent. For traveling, the crate is fairly easy to transport. An alternative temporary house is a flat-bottomed duffel bag. Line the bottom with a towel and fleece and you are ready to go. If the bag has side pockets, this is the perfect place to store supplies such as cotton balls, formula, and bottles. The duffel bag affords the foster parent some additional privacy since everyone will want to stop and poke their fingers into a crate full of kittens, however, someone carrying a duffel bag generally goes unnoticed.

After three weeks of age, the kittens will become more explorative of their environment and will need more space. At this time, a large-animal crate is an ideal house; alternatively, space may be blocked off in a bathroom or kitchen. At this age they are beginning to urinate and defecate on their own and it is advisable to house the kittens on an easily cleaned surface.

CLEANING AND CARE

With any litter, cleanliness is of paramount importance to a successful outcome. Budgeting your time for feeding as well as cleaning will pay off in the long run.

Be sure to clean the nipple of the bottle with dishwashing soap after each feeding and rinse well with hot water. Bottles should be cleaned in the same way ideally after every feed but at least once daily. A bottle brush will aid in scrubbing the inside of the bottle. Once a week, bottles and nipples should be boiled for ten minutes.

Animals that are stimulated to urinate and defecate after feedings are less likely to have accidents in their "den." Kittens for the first three to four weeks will need to be stimulated after feeding to urinate and defecate. If care is given to do a thorough job after feeding, fecal and urine messes can be kept to a minimum. It is much easier to clean messes as they occur (i.e., when the kitten is stimulated) than it is to bathe a litter of kittens that defecated in their den. However, accidents will invariably occur. When this happens change all the soiled bedding immediately. If any kittens have urine or feces on their fur, they can be gently bathed with dilute, mild pet shampoo and dried with a hair dryer set on low.

IMMUNE STATUS AND SPECIAL NEEDS

Kittens may be orphaned at various stages of kittenhood. Those that have nursed from the queen have an added advantage of receiving colostrum. However, even if kittens have not received this first milk they will often still thrive. It may be assumed that kittens within a litter have all been exposed to the same pathogens and can be cohoused and nursed from the same bottle without consequence. Care must be taken to avoid cross contamination if you are burdened with more than one litter to hand raise at the same time. If this is the case, it is wise to dedicate housing space and equipment to each litter separately. Adult cats should always be housed away from litters of young kittens.

Feline leukemia virus (Felv) and feline immunodeficiency virus (FIV) may be transmitted in utero or by nursing from mother to offspring. All kittens should be tested at eight weeks of age for these viruses. Kittens should not be exposed to other noninfected cats until they have tested negative for these viruses.

TIME TO WEANING

Weaning may begin at three and a half to four weeks of age. If you don't know the age of a litter for sure, weaning age will correlate with the time you begin to see teeth erupting. The weaning process may be difficult but even the most stubborn kittens should be eating commercial kitten food by the time they are six weeks old.

TIPS FOR WEANING FROM FORMULA TO SOLID FOOD

While there are several ways to accomplish weaning, the easiest is to begin by making a 50/50 mix of formula and warm, canned kitten food. Hills Science Diet or Iams Growth Formula work well. Place the food in a shallow dish and allow the kittens to explore this new experience. The kittens will at first prefer to walk through the new food so it is advisable to put a towel down under the food container. You can help by placing a very small amount of food into the kittens' mouths. As the kittens get used to eating the new food, the amount of formula may be gradually reduced until they are eating only canned food. Once they are eating canned food, the transition to dry kibble is usually uncomplicated. Leave a small bowl of fresh kibble available and they will begin eating the kibble between the meals that you provide for them.

At about the same time that kittens are learning to eat commercial food they will begin to use a litter box. Provide a low-sided container (such as a pie pan or Styrofoam meat packaging pan) filled about half-full with general-purpose kitty litter or shredded paper. Clumping litter is not recommended since many kittens will try to eat the litter when they first encounter it. It may be helpful to gently stimulate the kittens to urinate and defecate while they are standing in the litter pan. This will help them to get the idea, however most kittens will naturally begin to use a litter box if one is provided for them.

COMMON MEDICAL PROBLEMS

When you first acquire an orphan kitten, it will often be dehydrated and/or emaciated from lack of nutrition. Since IV access is not always possible in a newborn, giving isotonic crystalloids (preferably lactated Ringer's solution) intraperitoneally is the most effective way to rehydrate a severely dehydrated kitten. Fluids may also be given subcutaneously if the kitten's hydration status is only mildly compromised. It may be difficult to assess hydration status in a newborn kitten; however, there are some reliable methods. Check the mucous membrane moisture; the gums should be moist, not dry. Examine the skin turgor by gently tenting the skin over the kitten's shoulders: it should snap down almost immediately.

Fleas are often seen on kittens that have been recently abandoned or orphaned. If possible, it is best to avoid using pesticides on newborn kittens. If the problem is minor (one or two fleas) simply use a fine-toothed "flea comb" to remove fleas manually and change the bedding daily. However, often the parasite load is too great to handle with the manual removal of the fleas. The kittens may become anemic very quickly if a large number of fleas are allowed to remain on the animal. In these cases, the animal should be bathed with a diluted pyrethrin-based shampoo approved for kittens to aid in flea removal. An alternative to bathing is to apply a very small amount (one drop) of imidocloprid (Advantage, manufactured by Bayer, sold only through veterinarians) to the skin at the base of the skull of each kitten. The fleas will begin to die almost immediately and can be removed using the flea comb.

Kittens are susceptible to and commonly acquire upper respiratory infections. These infections are caused by feline viruses that can subsequently lead to secondary bacterial infections. It is important to keep the nasal passages clear of mucus. This may be done by gently swabbing the kitten's nose to keep it clean. It is also helpful to bring the kitten into a bathroom filled with steam to help relieve congestion. If the mucus secretions are green or yellow, or if the kitten's body temp is greater than 103°F (39.4°C), then antibiotics for the bacterial infection are indicated. These infections generally respond well to antibiotics such as amoxicillin (Amoxi-drops) or amoxicillin with clavulenic acid (Clavamox). Both are sold through veterinarians or human pharmacies and are manufactured by Pfizer.

It is not uncommon for orphan kittens to suckle the genital areas of their littermates. This may lead to a serious health problem for the victim. Urinary strictures will form from excessive irritation; this is especially a problem for male kittens. To identify the problem, look for a kitten with red or inflamed genitals when stimulating the kittens to urinate/defecate. Also watch for a kitten that routinely has urine or feces on its head and seems to spend a lot of time "rooting" after feedings. The only way to handle this situation is to house the kittens in different areas.

Some newborn kittens develop diarrhea especially when they are first fed kitten formula. When this happens, it is important to keep the animal well hydrated. If an animal is having diarrhea for 12 to 24 hours, begin diluting the prepared formula with an additional amount of water. Mix one part prepared formula to one part water. As the diarrhea resolves, gradually decrease the additional water until the original formula is being fed. If kittens are over four weeks of age when they develop diarrhea, intestinal parasites should be suspected. Ascarids (roundworms) are the most common pathogen and are readily identified microscopically when doing a fecal parasite examination. Pyrantel or fenbendazole are appropriate anthelmintics to use to treat parasites in kittens.

ACKNOWLEDGMENTS

Special thanks to the Cornell University, College of Veterinary Medicine and the University of California-Davis, School of Veterinary Medicine, Feline Medicine Club.

SOURCES OF PRODUCTS MENTIONED

Most supplies may be purchased at any pet food supply store. Bottles and formula may be purchased on line at www.petag.com.

PetAg Inc., 261 Keyes Ave., Hampshire, IL 60140; 1-800-323-0877, 1-800-323-6878; www.petag.com

Pfizer Animal Health, Exton, PA 19341; 1-800-733-5500

REFERENCES

Hoskins, Johnny D. 1990. *Veterinary pediatrics.* Philadelphia, PA: Saunders.

4
Critically Ill and Orphaned Foals

K. Gary Magdesian

NATURAL HISTORY

The scientific name of the horse is *Equus caballus*. Average birth weight is 45–50 kg for light-breed horses (Thoroughbred, Quarter Horses, etc.). Births are seasonal and take place January 1 to July 1 for performance, racing, and show breeds in the United States. Mares will naturally foal through the spring and summer months. Gestational length averages 330 to 345 days, with a range of 320–365 days. Miniature breeds have a more variable gestation, and often foal earlier than 320 days. Time to weaning is three to six months of age.

RECORD KEEPING

Keep a daily log of food intake, fecal and urine production, fecal consistency, hydration, body weight, and behavioral notes including attitude and appetite. Keep a record of vaccination and deworming schedule.

EQUIPMENT

The following items should be on hand: Human baby bottles, lamb or human Gerber NUK nipples, microwave or other method of heating formula, 60-cc catheter-tip syringes, stomach tubes/infant feeding tubes.

The nasogastric tube that I use most often is a 12 French, 45 in (114 cm) polyurethane human feeding tube (Ross). This is a very soft, pliable tube with a small diameter that is nonirritating to the pharynx, esophagus, and stomach. It is radiopaque for confirmation of placement.

Other tubes that can be utilized for indwelling nasogastric feedings include the following:

Harris flush or enema tube (#24 French;, 60 in, seamless; Professional Medical Products, Inc.)—good for ease of placement but stiffer, larger size, and not ideal for long-term use
Kaslow Stomach Tube (#18 French 30 in; Baxter)
Infant Feeding Tube (#8 French; 42 in; Mallinckrodt)—soft, small, gentle on tissues but at a disadvantage for placement

If these are unavailable, then a soft, rubber, stallion urinary catheter may be used.

Whenever nasogastric (NG) tubes are placed for long-term use, consideration as to size and consistency (stiffness) of the tube should be made. Small diameter (12 French), soft (such as polyurethane) tubes may be left in the stomach, as esophageal reflux is rarely associated with these tubes. If large-bore, rigid tubes are used, they should be passed to the level of the distal esophagus to avoid disrupting the esophageal sphincter. Such placement prevents reflux around the tube at the cardia. Pharyngeal irritation and edema will be minimized with smaller gauge tubes. Correct placement of smaller NG tubes, those that cannot be palpated in the esophagus readily, can be confirmed with radiographs.

CRITERIA FOR INTERVENTION

Orphaned foals require hand rearing, with feeding and socialization activities being assumed by a human caretaker. Other foals requiring intervention include premature foals and foals with systemic illnesses, such as sepsis, hypoxemia, and enterocolitis, that preclude them from normal nursing behavior. In addition, hypogalactia, or inadequate milk production by the mare, is another criterion for intervention. Grafting foals onto nurse mares, if available, is the ideal management solution for orphan foals. Grafting can be facilitated by sedating the mare, placing the mare's placental membranes (if available) or urine on the orphan, restraining the mare in stocks or chutes, and using aromatic decongestants on the mare's nostrils. Close observation of the pair is essential until the mare accepts the foal.

Foals with adequate nutrition will be active and playful, and gain weight daily. Those with inadequate intakes will often show milk staining of the muzzle and face, due to the dripping of milk from a nonnursed, full udder. Mares with low milk production will have foals that nurse incessantly due to hunger.

Other early warning flags for intervention include pre-, intra-, and postpartum abnormalities of the dam or foal of any type. Resultant foals should be considered "high-risk" foals in terms of their potential to develop sepsis or hypoxic encephalopathy. These early indicators include historical information regarding the dam during pregnancy and parturition. A history of systemic illness in the dam, premature lactation (often an indicator of placentitis or placental separation), or dystocia warrants close examination of the neonate along with proactive antibiotic administration. Premature placental separation ("red bag") and meconium staining of the foal are also examples of high-risk criteria. Delays in rising or nursing are also indications for intervention.

ASSESSMENT OF THE NEONATE

Postpartum evaluation of a neonatal foal should include taking vital signs and monitoring behavioral responses. Immediately postfoaling, the foal should have a heart rate greater than 60 bpm, respiratory rate greater than 60 for the first 30 minutes, then the rate should be down to 30–40 bpm. It should be sitting sternal and respond to nasal stimulation with a cough or sneeze. Body temperature of the neonatal foal is normally 99–101.8°F (37.2–38.8°C). The foal should rise and nurse within one and two hours of birth, respectively. Subsequent to this, the foal should be nursing four to seven times per hour. Passage of meconium should occur within three hours of birth, otherwise one to two Fleet enemas may be gently administered (maximum of two in order to avoid hyperphosphatemia). If constipation is unresolved, soapy water or acetylcysteine retention enemas should be administered. Mean time to first urination is 8.5 hours. Constant straining to urinate may indicate asphyxiated-bladder syndrome or ruptured bladder. Evaluation of relative gestational maturity should be done. Premature foals and foals that are small for gestational age should have their cuboidal bones (carpal and tarsal) radiographed to evaluate for degree of ossification.

The umbilicus should be evaluated for size, patency, and infection. Dipping the umbilicus in 1:4 chlorhexidine (Nolvasan) solution:water should be performed immediately postfoaling, and then every 6–12 hours for 48 hours. Tincture of iodine solutions should not be utilized, as they may increase the risk of infection and complications such as patent urachus.

The foal should be weighed daily and its hydration status monitored. Blood should be drawn for a complete blood count, serum chemistry profile, blood glucose, and blood gas for any foal deemed "high-risk." Tetanus antitoxin (1500 units) should be administered subcutaneously to the foal if the mare was not boostered with a toxoid in the last four to eight weeks of gestation. A selenium/vitamin E injection (1 mg of selenium per 100 lb body weight IM) should be administered to foals in geographic areas potentially deficient in selenium, as well as to foals having been subjected to hypoxic injury. Oral vitamin E (200 IU daily) should be administered in regions known to be deficient in vitamin E and selenium.

INITIAL CARE/STABILIZATION

Hypothermia, hypoglycemia, dehydration, and bacteremia (translocation from gut) are the immediate concerns for an orphaned or high-risk neonatal foal. The foal should be kept in a clean, dry, well-ventilated environment, with heating pads or heat lamps available. Hypoglycemia and dehydration can be addressed or avoided through the provision of colostrum or milk administered via bottle, pan, or nasogastric (NG) tube. Feeding through a NG tube should be performed if the foal is weak or at risk of aspiration. Hypoglycemia or dehydration should be treated with 5–10% dextrose in a crystalloid such as lactated Ringer's solution or physiologic saline. Bacteremia can be minimized or prevented through the early use of broad-spectrum antimicrobials such as amikacin or gentamicin and penicillin, ceftiofur, or third-generation cephalosporin. Renal function should be monitored in foals receiving aminoglycoside antibiotics, such as amikacin or gentamicin.

FORMULAS, SUPPLEMENTS, AND DAILY CALORIC REQUIREMENTS

Foals can be successfully raised on a variety of formulas. The immediate goal should be directed at provision of passive transfer in the foal that is less than 24 hours of age. The gastrointestinal (GI) tract of the newborn foal is capable of macromolecular absorption, in order to allow for uptake of intact immunoglobulins. The newborn foal is devoid of IgG. Early administration of colostrum is recommended to allow for early gut maturation and closure, in order to minimize uptake of bacterial agents by the GI epithelium. For orphaned foals, banked colostrum (frozen for less than one year) should be used. Colostrum with an adequate concentration of immunoglobulins (greater than 6 g/dl) should have a specific gravity of 1.06 or greater. Alternatives to mare colostrum include bovine or caprine colostrum, plasma administered orally, or colostral substitutes (commercial concentrated immunoglobulin products such as Seramune [Sera]), although these have disadvantages of reduced specificity for equine pathogens, immunoglobulins with shorter half-lives, and reduced concentrations of immunoglobulin. One to 1.5 liters of colostrum should be administered by feeding 8 oz hourly for the first six to ten hours.

Once the provision of passive transfer has been ensured the foal can be fed a variety of formulas, including mare's milk if available. If equine milk is unavailable, I prefer to use a 50:50 mixture of mare's milk replacer and goat milk. Foals have been raised successfully on goat milk alone, however this may lead to metabolic acidosis and constipation. Milk replacer, on the other hand, can lead to loose stool or diarrhea. In addition, goat milk enhances palatability. A variety of milk replacers is available. Some of them are listed here.

1. Foal-Lac (PetAg)
2. Mare's Match (Land O' Lakes)
3. Acidified cold ad libitum formula (Buckeye Mare's Milk Plus)
4. Homemade formulas (Madigan 1997):
    a. 24 oz cow milk
       12 oz saturated lime water
       4 tsp dextrose (not table sugar)
    b. 4 oz evaporated milk
       4 oz warm water
       1 tsp white corn syrup
    c. 8 oz 2% cow milk
       1 tsp white corn syrup

The milk substitute should closely approximate mare's milk: approximately 0.5 kcal/ml as fed, 22% crude protein (dry matter), 15% crude fat (dm), less than 0.5% crude fiber (dm), and 11% total solids (as fed). Mare's milk has less fat, slightly less protein, and more carbohydrate than do cow's or goat's milk.

Ensure that milk substitutes are mixed according to directions, and are not either too dilute or concentrated. Temperature of the formula is important to ensure acceptance, especially when first introducing it to the foal. Avoid overheating the formula. Bottles, nipples, and buckets should be cleaned, disinfected, and dried after each use, and uneaten formula should be discarded. Unheated formula should be refrigerated and discarded after 24 hours.

Orphan foals can be bottle or bucket/pan fed. I prefer the latter, as there is less risk of aspiration. This method aids in disassociating feeding from the handler, which is advantageous from a behavioral standpoint. If the foal is bottle fed, a lamb nipple should be used. The hole should not be large enough to allow milk to spontaneously run from the nipple; rather, the foal should have to suckle in order to release the milk.

NURSING TECHNIQUES

Healthy neonatal foals require little nursing care other than frequent feeding and a clean environment. Most newborns will accept a bottle readily, however foals that have been nursing their dams will take longer to suckle from a bottle. Pan feeding of orphans is a safer method of feeding, but may take longer for the foal to accept. Teaching a foal to feed from a bucket or pan requires persistence. The foal should not be fed for two to four hours, and then its muzzle can be plunged into the pan of milk by the handler. This will encourage a suckle and subsequent drinking. This must be repeated every one to two hours until the foal begins drinking. If bottles are to be used, lamb nipples or NUK human nipples (Gerber) will mimic the shape of a mare's nipple. The hole in the nipple should be of a sufficiently small size that milk does not stream out.

Foals that are recumbent due to prematurity, sepsis, or hypoxic encephalopathy will require an extensive amount of nursing care. They must be kept clean and dry, in a well-ventilated but warm environment. Mattresses, blankets, and fleeces work well, along with diaper-padding to absorb urine. The foal should be turned every one to two hours to prevent the development of decubital ulcers. The eyes should be monitored for corneal ulceration and be well lubricated with artificial tears. Urine and fecal output should be monitored. Recumbent foals, especially those with hypoxic insult, may require urinary catheterization because of an inability to urinate. Limbs should be passively flexed and extended as part of physical therapy.

TUBE FEEDING

Some foals have reduced mentation or weakness and cannot suckle. These foals require frequent feeding of small volumes. They should be monitored for gastric reflux prior to feeding. Foals should be in sternal recumbency, with their heads in an upright position, or standing when tube fed, in order to prevent reflux. See above for types of nasogastric tubes and radiographic confirmation of placement. The tube is held in place with sutures at the nares. Many of the smaller tubes are more readily swallowed and placed if a wire stilet is used. The wire should be well lubricated prior to insertion into the tube to allow for removal. Large tubes should be left in the distal esophagus, while smaller tubes are advanced into the stomach. Small diameter polyurethane tubes are ideal for long-term use. If more than 60 ml of reflux is obtained, food should be withheld for that period. If reflux continues for more than a few hours, parenteral nutrition should be implemented.

FREQUENCY OF FEEDING

Newborn foals should be fed every two hours. The frequency can be decreased to every four hours after five days of age, and then gradually down to every six hours by ten days of age in healthy foals. As the frequency of feedings is decreased, the volume of each meal is increased, in order to obtain the desired daily intake.

AMOUNTS TO FEED

A normal, healthy foal will ingest 20–28% of its body weight per day in milk. The energy requirement for foals is 120–150 kcal/kg/day. In order to avoid complications associated with milk substitutes, including enteritis, reflux, ileus, and distention, the amount fed should be between 10 and 15% of the body weight per day initially. Weak or sick foals should be fed 8–10% of their body weight on day one, and this can be gradually increased (see Table 4.1).

The minimum maintenance caloric needs for maintenance of body weight are 50–60 kcal/kg/day, and would be met by 10% of a foal's body weight. Foals not tolerating enteral nutrition due to prematurity or hypoxic/ischemic injury to the gastrointestinal tract, or those with ileus should be placed on total parenteral nutrition. However, a small amount of oral intake is critical to normal intestinal development. Enterocytes derive growth factors and

Table 4.1. Amount to Feed Weak or Sick Foals

Age (days)	% of body weight per day
1	8–10
2	12
3–5	15
6–8	18
9–11	20
12–14	20–25

nutrition from enteral nutrients. Therefore, such foals should be fed small volumes (50–60 ml every two hours) for this reason. Total parenteral nutrition consists of a provision of all nutritional requirements through an intravenous formula consisting of dextrose, amino acids, lipids, electrolytes, vitamins, and minerals.

Once foals are a few days old, they may develop interest in solid feeds. Fresh leafy alfalfa, grass, and grain should be offered. In addition, Foal Lac pellets can be provided free choice. Fresh water should be made available, but the foal should not be allowed to drink large quantities in place of milk. Orphan foals should be allowed access to fresh feces from a healthy adult horse, as coprophagia is a normal behavioral activity allowing for inoculation of gastrointestinal flora.

EXPECTED WEIGHT GAIN

Accurate daily weighing is very important. Foals of light breeds (Thoroughbred, Quarter Horse, Warmblood) should gain 1–1.5 kg per day. Draft foals should gain 1.4–1.5 kg/day. In one study, Thoroughbred foals gained an average of 110 kg during the first three months and 75 kg during the second three months of life.

HOUSING

Orphaned foals are ideally housed in a draft-free, well-bedded, and warm environment. Ventilation should be adequate to prevent respiratory problems. Deep straw bedding or shavings (if older than one day of age) are suitable bedding materials. Heat lamps can be provided in one corner of the stall, should the ambient temperature drop below 59°F (15°C). As noted above, the foal should have access to hay, creep feed, milk-substitute pellets, water, and fresh feces from an adult animal. Companionship can be provided with another foal, a goat, or an older, gentle pony. This will allow for socialization of the foal, in order to prevent undesirable aggressive behavior from developing toward the handler. Once the foal has adjusted to the milk-substitute diet, it should be allowed free exercise by daily turnout into a pasture or paddock.

IMMUNE STATUS AND SPECIAL NEEDS

Foals are completely dependent on colostrum as an immunoglobulin source, because of the epitheliochorial nature of the mare's placenta. Every effort should be made to provide the foal with 1–1.5 liters of high quality (specific gravity greater than 1.060) colostrum over the first four to eight hours. Colostrum also provides for lactoferrin, complement, and lysozyme, and helps to regulate cell-mediated immunity, activates polymorphonuclear leukocytes, and may decrease intestinal colonization by infectious agents. It also promotes intestinal maturation and "closure" of intestinal absorption of macromolecules. Early administration is thus key to minimizing the opportunity for bacteria to gain systemic access. Alternatives to mare colostrum include bovine or caprine colostrum (4 liters over 20–24 hours), or colostrum substitutes, but are not ideal. Oral plasma may be utilized. If the foal is over 16–24 hours, then 1–2 liters of equine plasma should be administered intravenously, as the gastrointestinal uptake of intact immunoglobulins occurs decrementally over the first 24 hours. Anywhere from 8 to 24 hours after the administration of colostrum or an alternative, the foal's immunoglobulin status should be addressed. Passive immunity status can be evaluated through commercial immunoassays (SNAP Foal IgG Test—IDEXX), zinc sulfate turbidity tests, as well as radial immunodiffusion techniques. Plasma should be administered if the concentration of immunoglobulins is less than 800 mg/dl. Orphan foals are considered at high risk for sepsis, especially if they did not receive colostrum. Any such foal should be administered broad spectrum antibiotics such as ceftiofur or a combination of penicillin and gentamicin or amikacin prophylactically for the first three days of life.

TIME TO WEANING

Foals can be weaned from milk replacers when two to four months old, depending on the amount of solid feed being ingested. Milk replacer pellets (Foal-Lac) should be offered.

TIPS FOR WEANING FROM FORMULA TO SOLID FOOD

Alfalfa hay, grass, grain, or a complete pelleted foal diet, and milk replacer pellets should be made available to the foal during the first few days of life. Access to fresh feces from an adult horse will encourage coprophagia and inoculation of gastrointestinal microflora. Grazing may be imitated from other horses or a companion goat.

COMMON MEDICAL PROBLEMS

Gastrointestinal problems such as diarrhea, constipation, ileus, gastric reflux, and gas distention are common with milk substitutes or replacers. Foals with a systemic inflammatory response syndrome such as sepsis, or those with hypoxic injury (part of "neonatal maladjustment syndrome"), may have ileus manifested as reflux, mild colic, and bloat. These foals should be treated by temporary discontinuation of oral feeding.

If intolerance of enteral feeding is persistent (more than four to six hours), then parenteral nutrition at a veterinary clinic should be instituted.

Diarrhea may result from milk replacers as well as enteritis associated with pathogens, including *Clostridium perfringens, C. difficile*, Rotavirus, *Cryptosporidium*, Corona virus, *Salmonella*, and *Strongyloides westeri*. Clostridial enteritis should be treated with metronidazole (10 mg/kg PO BID-TID). These cases are marked by gas distention, colic, and diarrhea ranging from loose to hemorrhagic and watery. Foals less than five days of age are most susceptible. The other forms of enteritis are treated with supportive care, intravenous fluid therapy, and antibiotics to prevent bacteremia. Enterocolitis should be suspected if the foal is febrile and colicky, and develops leukopenia.

Diarrhea caused by milk replacers does not lead to fever, severe colic, or changes in the CBC. Loose stool is often the result of lactose intolerance or overfeeding. If this is the case, the amount fed should be reduced to 10–15% of body weight per day, with very gradual reintroduction of the desired volume. Lactase enzyme (Lactaid—McNeil; or Lac-Dose—Rugby), 6000 units PO, every three to four hours, may be administered along with the milk feedings. Keep in mind that even orphaned foals will develop "foal heat" diarrhea at six to ten days of age. The term "foal heat" is a misnomer, as the diarrhea is currently believed to occur as a result of flora changes associated with ingestion of feedstuffs from the environment. These foals remain bright and alert, and require no therapy.

Constipation may result from persistent meconium impactions, dehydration, pica, or goat milk. This can be treated by adding mineral oil (50–100 cc twice a day) to the formula until the constipation resolves. Pica can lead to severe impactions and colic, and thus the foal should be monitored closely for excessive ingestion of feedstuffs or bedding during the first few days of life. If goat milk is causing constipation it should be replaced in part by milk replacer. Meconium impactions may be treated with Fleet or soapy water enemas. These should not be used more than two times each, as Fleet enemas can lead to hyperphosphatemia, and water enemas may lead to hyponatremia. If the impaction persists, saline can be used in place of water. Acetylcysteine enemas are very effective at resolving meconium impactions. A solution of 4% acetylcysteine in water (40 ml of the 20% Mucomyst solution to 160 ml of water) is administered as a retention enema with a 30 French Foley catheter (Sherwood). A total of 120–240 ml (4–8 oz) is used and is maintained for 40 to 60 minutes using the 30-cc balloon on the end of the Foley catheter while the foal is sedated.

Another common medical problem of foals is septicemia. The hallmarks include scleral injection, mucous membrane hemorrhages, obtundation, dehydration, anorexia, increased heart rate, fever or hypothermia, respiratory distress, diarrhea, and enlarged joints. Sepsis should be treated as a medical emergency under the care of a veterinarian. Broad spectrum antibiotics and supportive care are the mainstays of therapy.

Hypoxic-ischemic encephalopathy (HIE), also known as "neonatal maladjustment syndrome," is an ill-defined neurological disorder of newborns manifested by a number of neurological signs. The cause is believed to be at least in part due to hypoxic injury to the central nervous system prepartum, during parturition, or postpartum. Clinical signs include wandering, seizures, abnormal vocalizations, lethargy, loss of affinity for the dam or handler, and virtually any other neurological sign. These foals should also be treated aggressively and promptly. Treatment includes the use of mannitol, vitamin E, and intensive care including oxygen, IV fluids, antibiotics, and pressure support. The prognosis for return to normal neurological function is good with appropriate medical care.

Other disorders that the neonate should be monitored for include uroperitoneum and neonatal isoerythrolysis. Uroperitoneum is usually the result of a ruptured bladder, but can also occur secondary to urachal, ureteral, or renal rents. The clinical signs associated with uroperitoneum include abdominal distention, lethargy, anorexia, and repeated stranguria. Neonatal isoerythrolysis is an alloimmune hemolytic anemia caused by anti-RBC antibodies in the colostrum. This is treated with blood transfusions (washed dam's red blood cells are ideal), oxygen therapy, and IV fluid therapy. Clinical signs include jaundice, tachypnea, tachycardia, pallor, and lethargy.

SOURCES OF PRODUCTS MENTIONED

Baxter Healthcare Corp., Deerfield, IL 60015

Buckeye Feeds, Dalton, OH; 1-800-321-0412

Gerber Products Company, c/o Consumer Affairs, 445 State Street, Fremont, MI 49413-0001; 1-800-443-7237; www.gerber.com

IDEXX Corp., Westbrook, ME 04092

Land O'Lakes, Webster City, IA; 1-800-328-4155

McNeil Consumers Health Care, Ft. Washington, PA; 1-800-522-8243

Mallinckrodt Medical, Inc., Mallinckrodt Anesthesia Division, St. Louis, MO 63042

PetAg, 30 W. 432 Rt. 20, Elgen, IL 60120; 1-800-332-0877, 1-800-323-6878; www.petag.com

Professional Medical Products, Inc., Ocala, FL 32670

Ross Products Division, Abbott Laboratories, Columbus, OH 43215-1724; 1-800-986-8510; www.abbott.com, www.ross.com

Rugby Laboratories, Inc. Norcross, GA 30071

Sera, Inc., Shawnee Mission, KS; 1-913-541-1307

Sherwood Medical, St. Louis, MO 83103; obtained from Kendall Corp., 1-800-962-9888

REFERENCES

Buechner-Maxwell, V. A. 1998. Enteral feeding of sick newborn foals. *Compendium on Continuing Education for the Practicing Veterinarian* 2:222–27.

Madigan, J. E. 1997. *Manual of equine neonatal medicine*. 3d ed. Woodland, CA: Live Oak Publishing.

Massey, R. E. 1991. Feeding and socializing orphaned foals. *Equine Practice* 5:518–26.

Wilson, J. H. 1987. Feeding considerations for neonatal foals. In *Proceedings of the American Association of Equine Practitioners* 33:823–29.

5
Pigs

Janet Fine and Rebecca Duerr

NATURAL HISTORY

The term "pig" encompasses a wide range of species, from domestic farm breeds and potbellied pigs to wild Red River hogs and peccaries. However, all of these animals bear enough similarities that using the potbellied pig and farm pigs as models, as we will here, is appropriate (see Fig. 5.1).

Pigs are artiodactyls (even number of toes) belonging to the taxonomic group Suina. This includes the families Suidae (pigs and warthogs), Tayassuidae (peccaries), and Hippopotamidae (hippopotami). The European wild swine is classified as *Sus scrofa*, the Southeast Asian wild swine as *Sus vittatus*. North American feral pigs are a mix of European wild boar and domestic farm pig genes. In California, feral piglets may show the brown and yellow striping of the wild boar and the white or spotted markings of the farm pig within the same litter. Pigs are characterized by a simple stomach, omnivorous diet, and relatively unspecialized teeth. They give birth to litters of varying size, and the young are quite precocial; some will literally hit the ground running when born. Farm pigs are born at one to two kilograms (2–4 pounds). North American feral piglets have been hand raised with great success to become tame pets.

EQUIPMENT

Pigs will usually suckle from a bottle readily, and nipples designed for calves or sheep work well. Any small soft nipple, including human infant nipples (0–3-month) may be used with success. We prefer to use Pritchard flutter valve nipples, which are widely available at livestock feed stores and lambing supply companies. These are small red nipples with a ball bearing inside, and are designed to fit over a soda bottle or other similarly sized bottle top. As for any baby mammal, one needs to have a method of heating formula, such as a microwave or hot-water bath, and appropriate containers and a whisk for mixing powdered milk replacers.

CRITERIA FOR INTERVENTION

As pigs may have large litters, there is often a runt that is smaller and weaker than its siblings. Piglets are often very possessive of the particular nipple they suckle from, and thus the runt may not be able to get enough suckling time. Any piglet who appears unable to compete with its siblings, or who is lethargic and unable to keep up should be offered supplemental feedings. The decision of whether to pull the baby completely from the group or to merely separate it a few times a day for a feeding will be based on the situation at hand.

ASSESSMENT OF THE NEONATE

Each new piglet should receive a complete medical examination upon admission. Piglets presented as orphans from a wild situation may be severely dehydrated, emaciated, injured, or heavily parasitized. Upon intake, these animals should be rehydrated with subcutaneous fluids such as lactated Ringer's solution at 100 ml/kg/day. Subcutaneous drips work well for debilitated, immobile piglets. Pedialyte (Ross) or similar oral rehydration fluid should be offered as well. Wild-rescued piglets should be treated with a puppy or kitten flea and tick powder or spray. Wild pigs may carry ticks that transmit Lyme disease, so any ticks should be removed promptly. Pigs do not generally have fleas, but may be infested with lice and mites (mange). Fly eggs should be removed promptly, and may be found in

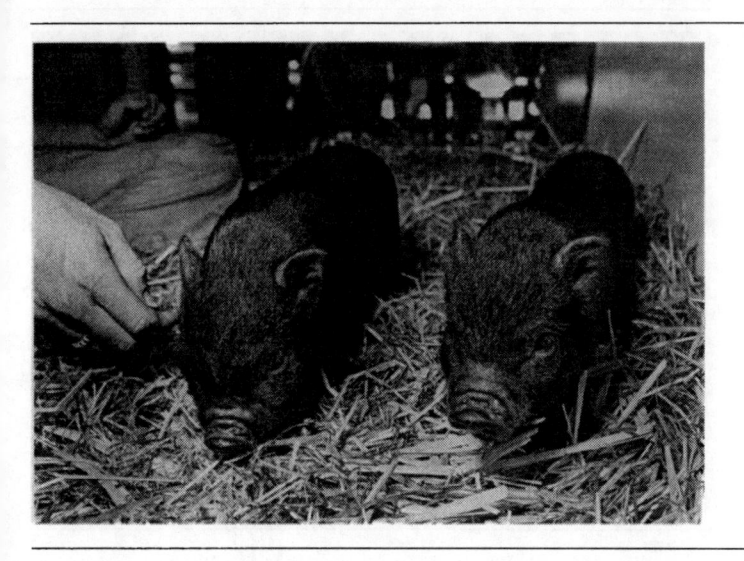

Figure 5.1. Two young potbellied pigs.

the mouth, nose, ears, anogenital region, around the eyes, or elsewhere. Fine-toothed combs may be of assistance when removing external parasites. Deworming medication such as fenbendazole should be administered, as determined by the veterinarian. Adequate ventilation is important when treating any baby animal with pesticides, especially if the infant is depressed.

INITIAL CARE

Baby pigs should be kept warm but not too hot. They will display shivering when too cold or panting when too hot. Pigs do not often display sensitivity to humidity. Small newborns may be kept in a 90°F (32°C) brooder for the first few days, then moved to larger housing. Heat lamps or hot pads may be used, but the animals should have an unheated area of the container available, as pigs are prone to hyperthermia.

Oral hydration with Pedialyte or other rehydration fluids should continue until the baby is well hydrated and urine is normal. This may be unnecessary in piglets that are pulled from a litter at the first sign of trouble, or may need to last 24 hours or more in a wild-rescued or debilitated animal.

Some babies will present with smelly, loose stools, and this may be treated with Biosol (Upjohn) at 1 tsp/100 lb (0.11 ml/kg). Biosol is a neomycin sulfate antibiotic for treating *E. coli*-related intestinal difficulties.

FORMULAS AND SUPPLEMENTS

My first choice for milk replacement in pigs is LitterMilk, a powdered pig milk product made by Land O' Lakes. This formula, however, is manufactured with oxytetracycline and neomycin added, so may not be appropriate in some circumstances. Another excellent formula for piglets is Just Born Milk Replacer for Puppies (Farnam), which is available through many pet supply companies. Goat's milk has also been used with success, and I prefer to use canned or powdered goat's milk for convenience.

Pigs do not usually require supplementary vitamins or minerals. Occasionally, a piglet will be anemic and will be prescribed iron supplements. Also, a weak lethargic piglet down on its knees may be deficient in selenium. This may be corrected with the administration of Bo-Se (Schering-Plough).

FEEDING

Once the piglet is well hydrated, it may be started on milk replacement formula at 3.5–5% body weight (1 ml per oz [30 g] body weight) delivered via bottle with nipple (Fig. 5.2). Piglets should be encouraged to accept feeding from a pan as soon as possible. Many farm pig breeds will take to pan feeding very quickly, but potbellied pigs will often not accept pan feeding until a few weeks of age. Newborns should be fed every two hours, with the feed interval lengthening to four hours by the time the piglet is two to three weeks old. Also, by ten days to two weeks of age, the middle of the night feedings may be skipped, and the baby is fine to fast six to eight hours while resting.

Tube feeding is not recommended for piglets. Their throats are very small and the animals always fight a tremendous amount. Tube feeding pigs,

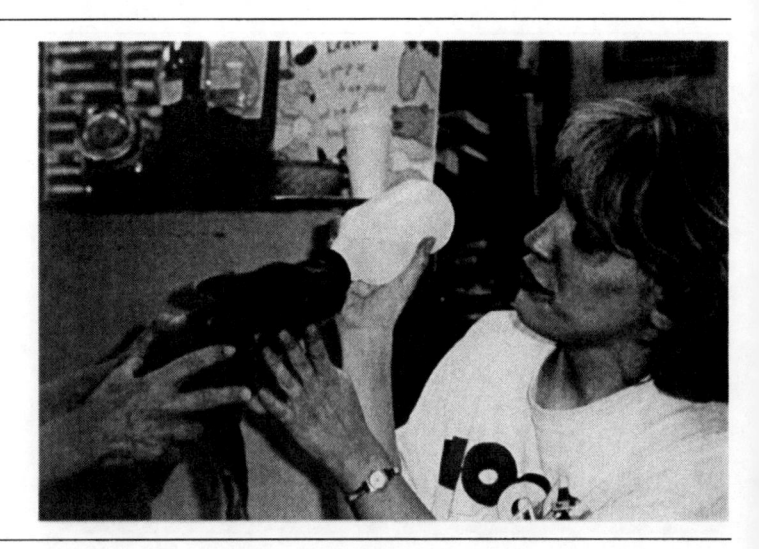

Figure 5.2. Bottle-feeding a wild piglet (photo courtesy of Teri Furey).

unlike many other mammals, can be a nightmare for all concerned. Piglets that will not take formula from a bottle or pan should be examined for congenital defects of the mouth. It is recommended that babies with cleft palate be euthanized if they are unable to suckle, due to the difficulties involved with tube feeding.

EXPECTED WEIGHT GAIN

Piglets in good condition should look rounded rather than sunken in the belly, and be vigorous and frisky in demeanor. Pigs born at 1 kg may gain up to 4 kg in the first three weeks of life. It can be quite a challenge to get healthy piglets to hold still long enough to obtain an accurate weight; hence, visual and tactile estimates of progress may be the best choice. Holding the piglet and weighing oneself may be the most effective way of getting a reasonably accurate weight regularly.

HOUSING

Newborns may be housed in a ten-gallon 90°F (32°C) brooder if they are small, weak, and immobile. The temperature and the animal's condition should be closely monitored to avoid overheating.

Small active piglets may be housed in human children's playpens, with a selection of bedding, such as clean towels, in one area. A soft fuzzy blanket will allow the baby to adjust its temperature by burrowing into the blanket as it wishes. Supplemental heat may be supplied to the playpen in the form of a heat lamp or heating pads, and again, the piglets must be able to move away from the heat source. The playpen should be placed out of drafty areas. By the time the piglets are over one month of age, they usually do not require supplemental heat unless they are being housed in an unheated structure in more extreme climates. Nighttime heat sources may be necessary in some locales.

TIPS FOR WEANING

Farm pig breeds usually take to drinking formula from a pan quite easily, while potbellied pigs often will become amenable to pan feeding after they are a few weeks old. The main disadvantage to pan feeding is less control over the amount fed, especially if using a group feeding dish. Successfully switching the piglets onto pan feeding makes weaning much easier, however, as one can begin introducing solid foods directly to the formula in the pan. Solid foods may be introduced as early as two weeks, however, even if the piglet is eating a significant amount of solid food on its own, formula feeding should continue as scheduled until the animal is six to eight weeks old. Solid foods to offer include vegetables and a quality commercial baby pig starter, initially offered soaked in formula. Brands that do not include alfalfa are preferred. Fruit has been known to cause diarrhea, so should be offered in limited quantities. If a piglet is resistant to pan feeding, weaning may begin by introducing human baby rice cereal into the formula in the bottle, then thickening it with more rice cereal to feed with a spoon. Once the animal is eating formula from a spoon, one may gradually switch to a handheld bowl, then place the bowl on the ground, and finally phase into offering pig chow from a pan. Clean fresh water must be available to pigs of all ages at all times.

COMMON MEDICAL PROBLEMS

Pigs are subject to the usual maladies of newborn mammals such as diarrhea and constipation. Dehydration should be dealt with as discussed in Initial Care above, and this will usually resolve constipation. Farm pigs, especially Yorkshires, display a number of inbreeding-related genetic problems. Cleft palate is encountered in many breeds of pig, and euthanasia is recommended if the piglet is unable to suckle. Some piglets are born with heart defects and/or liver shunts, an abnormality of the hepatic vasculature that allows blood to bypass the liver. Infections with the bacterium *Erysipelothrix rhusiopathiae* may also be a problem, and an affected animal may present with inappetence, high temperatures, lethargy, and sloughing skin lesions. Pigs over three months old and less than three years of age are at greatest risk for erysipelas infections. Pigs are vulnerable to many domestic livestock diseases such as hoof and mouth disease, and the veterinarian should determine a vaccination schedule, as determined by risk factors in the geographic area.

OTHER CONSIDERATIONS

Male piglets should be castrated quite young or removed from the litter, as they may impregnate their mothers at four to eight weeks of age. Altered males are at risk for urinary calculi, which may cause difficulties urinating or more serious blockages. Minimizing the feeding of alfalfa, either as hay or as an ingredient in pelleted formulations, may reduce this problem. It is rare for female pigs to have this problem, but it does happen. Female pigs should be spayed at 10–16 weeks. Females may become pregnant as early as four months of age.

A veterinarian who has experience working with pigs should regularly evaluate the health of the animals, perform any needed surgeries (e.g., alteration), and provide a vaccination schedule. Castrating potbellied pigs may be problematic if it is done as if the potbellies were farm pigs, so a veterinarian familiar with potbellied pigs is preferred.

FURTHER INFORMATION

The internet has a number of excellent resources for pig-related information. The Duchess Fund maintains a site dedicated to the dissemination of information on pig diseases, nutrition, behavior, and other topics. This site is at www.duchessfund.org. The National Committees on Potbellied Pigs also has an informative website at http://www.ncopp.com, and posts numerous full-text articles written by veterinarians or state agricultural extension services on such topics as brucellosis, erysipelas, and other health concerns. The American Association of Swine Veterinarians (AASV) has an abstract list on its website covering pig livestock production, which includes citations to many pig-related scientific publications. This site may be found at http://www.aasp.org.

SOURCES OF PRODUCTS MENTIONED

Farnam Companies, Inc., Phoenix, AZ 85067-4820; 1-800-234-2269; www.farnampet.com

Land O'Lakes, St. Paul, MN; 1-800-328-4155

Ross Products Division, Abbott Laboratories, Columbus, OH 43215-1724; 1-800-986-8510; www.abbott.com, www.ross.com

Schering-Plough Animal Health Corp., Union, NJ 07083

Upjohn Pharmaceuticals, Kalamazoo, MI

6
Goat Kids

Joan D. Rowe

NATURAL HISTORY

Goats are classified in the family Bovidae, suborder Ruminantia, order Artiodactyla (Fig. 6.1). Goats are divided into two genera: *Capra* (60 chromosomes) and *Hemitragus* (tahr, with 48 chromosomes). The genus *Capra* is divided into five species: *C. ibex* (ibex), *C. pyrenaica* (Spanish ibex or Spanish wild goat), *C. caucasia* (tur), *C. falconeri* (markhor), and *C. hircus* (bezoar or pasan). Domestic goat is *C. hircus aegagrus*. The Rocky mountain goat is actually a goatlike antelope, *Oreamnos americanus*.

Breeds of domestic goat commonly found in the United States include those used for milk, meat, fiber, and pleasure/companionship. Dairy (standard size) breeds include Alpine, LaMancha, Nubian, Oberhasli, Saanen, and Toggenburg. Meat breeds/types include Boer, Kiko, and Spanish goats; fiber breeds include Cashmere and Angora (mohair). Miniature or dwarf breeds include Pygmy (companion) and Nigerian Dwarf (milk). Many breeds are used for companionship, packing, and harness/cart pulling.

Goats are extremely social and adapt well to diverse husbandry situations. While goats do well reared away from other goats, it is best, if possible, to rear kids in groups of two or more. Littermates and kids reared together form bonds that last throughout their life in the herd. The capricious nature of goats makes them a pleasure to work with and well suited to families with children.

RECORD KEEPING

Kids should be examined for body condition, if possible, at birth, and for the presence of congenital defects such as pseudohermaphroditism (intersex), teat anomalies, cryptorchidism (retained testicles), atresia ani, cleft palate, jaw defects, or congenital goiter (thyroid enlargement). The placenta should

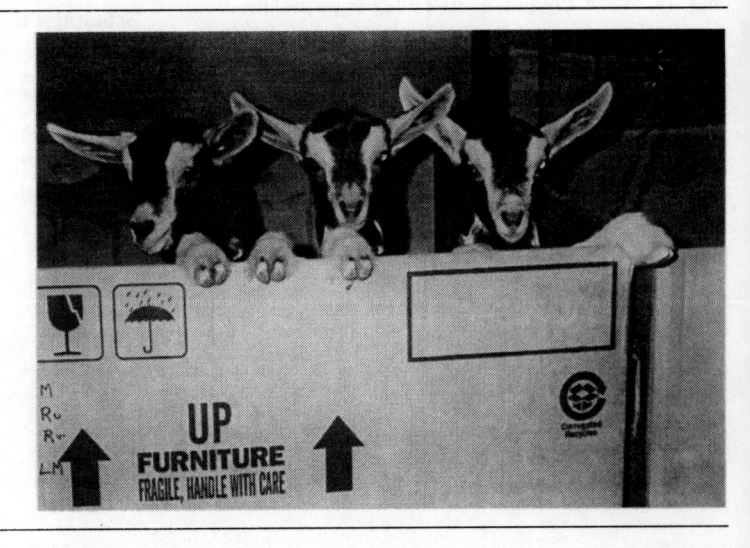

Figure 6.1. Kids playing in a box.

be examined at birth. Abnormal placental appearance may be an indicator of in utero infection.

Normal body temperature for a kid is 102–103.5°F (38.9–39.7°C). Rectal temperature and fecal consistency should be monitored on weak or otherwise high risk kids. Elevation of temperature above 103.5°F (39.7°C) would be cause for concern. Recording voluntary feed intake, fecal consistency and body weight on a routine basis will aid in early detection of infection, digestive upsets, or poor growth.

FORMULA

Goat kids are born without maternal transfer of immunity, therefore colostrum is essential for the passive transfer of antibodies to the kid. Colostrum, the doe's first milk, is rich in antibodies, energy, and vitamins, and has a laxative effect. Kids should receive adequate quantities (at least 40 ml/kg bodyweight [BW]) of high-quality colostrum within the first few hours of life to assure adequate passive transfer of immunoglobulins. Cow or goat colostrum may be used for kids. Colostrum may be frozen and stored for up to one year. Heat-treating colostrum for one hour at 131°F (55°C) will reduce the risk of disease transmission to kids.

Goat kids may be raised on whole goat milk, whole cow milk, or high-quality goat, calf, or lamb milk replacers. Kids are generally fed from nipple bottles or buckets with multiple nipples. Weaning is recommended at two to three months of age. Dam-raised kids raised for meat may be weaned at a later age. Pasteurized goat's milk or cow's milk should be fed for at least the first two to four weeks of life.

Pasteurizing milk at 165°F (74°C) for 15 seconds will prevent the transmission of milk-borne diseases such as caprine arthritis-encephalitis virus and mycoplasma infections. If milk replacers are used, high-fat, low-lactose, high-protein, and low-fiber milk replacers are preferred. High-lactose milk replacers may cause digestive upsets. Mixing milk replacers (one half reconstituted milk replacer, one half whole milk) seems to minimize problems associated with milk replacers and increase their palatability.

The amount to feed will vary, but many kids voluntarily consume a total daily milk intake of 10–15% body weight. Many kids are successfully raised on twice-daily feedings, but three-time daily feedings are preferred for the first month of life. Weak or sick kids may require smaller but more frequent feedings. Overfeeding may result in diarrhea or enterotoxemia.

Fresh water and free choice high-quality hay (for example, alfalfa) should be available by at least two weeks of age. A 16–18% protein kid or calf starter grain also should be made available according to manufacturer's directions. Further information on kid nutrition and management is available elsewhere (Smith and Sherman 1994).

NURSING TECHNIQUES

A sucking reflex may be stimulated by stroking the kid's face between the eye and the muzzle (Fig. 6.2). Weak or reluctant kids may also respond with nursing behavior to the warmth of a human cheek placed against their face and nose during attempts to bottle feed kids. Be sure that the colostrum is warm

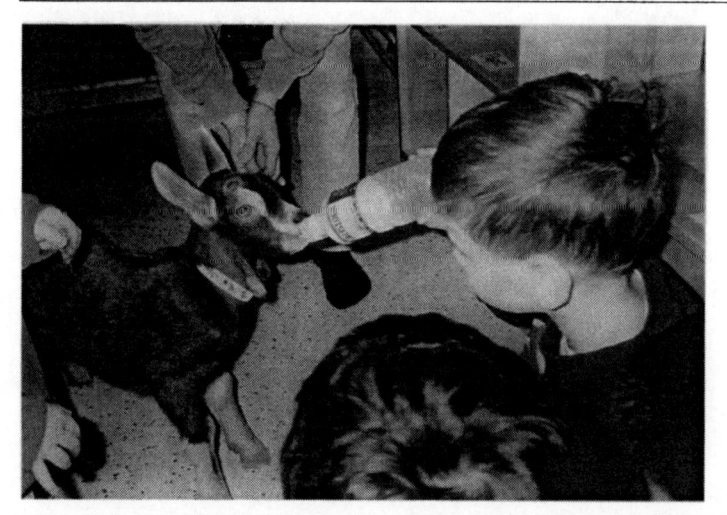

Figure 6.2. Bottle-feeding kid with latex nipple and soda bottle. Note paper collar for temporary identification.

throughout attempts at feeding, and the kids are warm and dry when being fed. Many inexperienced feeders give up trying to bottle feed kids if the kid fails to suckle readily in a short time. Patient extended efforts to encourage nursing at the first feeding often preclude the need for tube feeding and reduce the time needed to train kids to bottle-feed.

Soft latex or rubber lamb nipples are available from many suppliers (see Sources of Products Mentioned at the end of this chapter). For weak or small kids, I prefer the smaller nipples with a non-return valve. Lamb nipples attach to standard soda or water bottles. Firmer rubber nipples are useful for older kids; group feeding systems for up to ten kids from a single bucket are available. All feeding equipment should be sanitized between feedings to reduce the incidence of diarrhea. Self-feeding systems can be devised with a nipple, tubing, and bucket or reservoir, but care must be taken to avoid spoilage of milk.

TUBE FEEDING

Weak kids that fail to suckle within the first few hours of life may by given colostrum by using an 18 French soft rubber catheter as a stomach tube and the barrel of a 60-ml catheter-tip syringe as a reservoir for gravity flow. (These are available as a complete kit from goat supply houses.) The tube is measured and marked to a point from the mouth to just behind the kid's last rib; the tube is passed gently down the esophagus to that point. The tube should be palpable beside (i.e., not within) the trachea if it is properly positioned. Care should be taken not to overfill the stomach of a newborn kid.

Extra time spent to stimulate the suckle reflex of a weak kid often eliminates the need for tube feeding.

EXPECTED WEIGHT GAIN

Breed, litter size, gestation length, and gender of kid affect body weight at birth. Expected weight gains for kids varies by breed and management, but routine charting of weight allows the charting of a growth curve. Kids not conforming to normal growth curve may have inadequate nutrition or subclinical parasitism or other disease.

HOUSING

Large cardboard boxes with clean bedding material (e.g., straw) work well for hand rearing goat kids in small groups through the first two weeks of life (Fig. 6.3). They provide a clean, draft-free environment with enough confinement to minimize loss of body heat. Heat lamps may be used for supplemental heat, but care must be taken not to overheat the kid. It is desirable to place heat lamps on one side of an enclosure to allow the kid a choice of whether to use supplemental heat. Disposable boxes are a useful means of preventing buildup and spread of enteric pathogens. Kids can be kept in these boxes for about two weeks (past the time of greatest susceptibility to infectious neonatal diarrheas), after which the box may be destroyed and kids moved to larger and more permanent housing.

Temporary outdoor housing for young kids may be constructed from portable wire panels. An 8-ft by 16-ft (2.4-m by 4.8-m) enclosure can be easily constructed from three of these 16-ft hog panels. A large portable dog kennel can serve as temporary

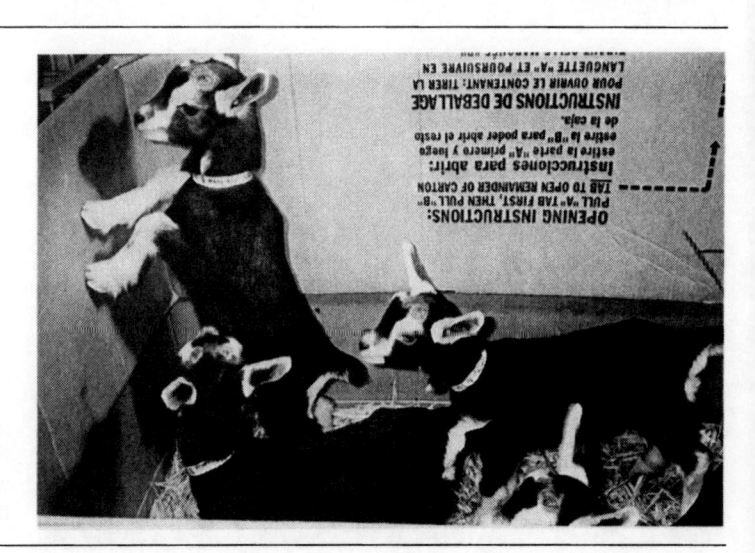

Figure 6.3. Cardboard boxes provide clean comfortable housing for neonatal kids. Heat lamp may be used for additional warmth.

shelter/sleeping area within the enclosure. Basic housing needs are minimal. Care should be taken to protect kids from predators. Higher (60 in or 152 cm) panels are recommended if dogs and other predators are a concern. Kids will play on boxes, tables, or spools provided for them to jump on.

In herds where kids are dam reared, the doe and kids must have access to draft-free shelter from environmental extremes to minimize risk of hypothermia, heat stress, or pneumonia. Young kids naturally seek out protected "hiding" places where they spend many hours sleeping away from their dam, with the dam returning to nurse her kids for brief periods. Herd owners may provide small boxes in pastures for kids to use. Restricting does to a small pasture or paddock during kidding and for a few days may be helpful in assuring strong maternal bonding.

Goats tend to jump in or on equipment located inside their pens. Avoiding fecal contamination of feed and water by having containers and feeders located on the outside of the pen or by utilizing feeding equipment designed to decrease the ability to climb on it will minimize exposure to coccidia oocysts. Housing adult goats separately from kids will also help to minimize risk of parasite and pathogen exposure.

IMMUNE STATUS AND SPECIAL NEEDS

Colostral Antibodies

As stated earlier, kids are dependent on colostrum for the transfer of maternal antibodies. Kids deprived of colostrum are at much higher risk of succumbing to opportunistic infections. In extreme cases and where medically available, plasma transfusion may be used to compensate for failure of passive transfer of antibodies. Artificial colostrum supplements may provide some benefit, but are not a replacement for adequate colostral intake.

Umbilical Cord

The navels of newborn kids should be inspected for hemorrhage or herniation, and the umbilical stump disinfected with tincture of iodine (2% or 7%) or chlorhexidine (1:4 dilution of concentrate). Continued treatment of navel for several days is preferred.

Tetanus Antitoxin (and Toxoid Vaccination)

Tetanus vaccination of does in late gestation is recommended to provide antibodies against tetanus in colostrum. Kids not likely to have received adequate colostral protection should receive 500 IU of tetanus antitoxin before disbudding or castration. Kids should receive a tetanus toxoid vaccination series beginning at four weeks of age.

Disbudding

If disbudding, or removal of horns, is desired, kids should be disbudded as soon as the horn bud can be distinctly palpated, usually at five to seven days of age. Swiss-breed kids may have palpable horn buds at a few days of age, while Nubian kids may take up to two weeks to develop distinctly palpable horn buds. Identification of the characteristic swirls of hair and visualization of the differentiated tissue of the horn bud before disbudding will help to avoid accidental "disbudding" of naturally polled (hornless) kids. Early disbudding of kids with a disbudding iron is much less stressful and far more humane than surgical removal of horns at a later age.

Tattooing

Goats can be permanently identified early in life by means of a tattoo applied in either the ears or the tail web (in the small-eared LaMancha). Necessary equipment and instructions are available from Caprine Supply, Nasco, and the American Dairy Goat Association (see below).

Castration

If males are not to be kept for breeding, it is recommended that they be castrated before puberty (development of odor and onset of sexual behavior), which usually occurs by five to seven months of age. Castration within the first month of life is less stressful than later castration, but may be associated with smaller urethral diameter and thus predispose to urethral calculi.

TIPS FOR WEANING FROM FORMULA TO SOLID FOOD

Although weaning schemes may call for weaning as early as two months of age, domestic goats grow well and achieve rapid growth when weaned at three months of age. Delay of weaning beyond that time is acceptable, but care should be taken to monitor body condition for obesity if solids intake is high and weaning occurs late.

If high-quality alfalfa hay and a commercial starter grain are available, milk can be gradually decreased over a one- to two-week period. In a group rearing situation, special care should be taken to observe and record feed intake to assure that all kids in a group have adequate feed intake, and smaller animals are separated from a group if needed.

COMMON MEDICAL PROBLEMS

In the first few days of life, kids are at greatest risk of hypothermia, hypoglycemia, and neonatal diarrheas. Hypoglycemic kids may be treated with warmed oral or intraperitoneal glucose solution. *E. coli* infections commonly occur in kids less than five days of age. Cryptosporidiosis and floppy kid syndrome are most commonly seen in kids from three to ten days of age. Clinical signs of white muscle disease (selenium deficiency), copper deficiency, *Pasteurella haemolytica* pneumonia, mycoplasmosis, and coccidiosis frequently begin to occur at between two and four weeks of age. Additional information on kid diseases is available in Rowe and East (1997) or Smith and Sherman (1994).

Coccidiosis is a common protozoal disease causing poor growth rates, diarrhea, and, if severe, death in kids over three weeks of age. Coccidiocidal sulfa drugs (e.g., sulfadimethoxine) or cocciostatic feed supplements (e.g., deccoquinate or lasalocid) may be used, in addition to management practices minimizing fecal contamination of feed, to control coccidiosis in kids.

All kids should be vaccinated for tetanus and enterotoxemia (*Clostridium perfringens* Type C and D; overeating disease). This is available as a combination vaccine and requires at least two initial doses starting at one month of age followed by annual boosters.

REINTRODUCTION TO THE HERD

This chapter addresses the needs of kids that will be reintroduced into domestic herds after weaning. For meat-and fiber-producing goats on range or where hand rearing is otherwise not desired (for example, if the goal is to reintroduce the kid to its dam after a short period of medical care or supplemental feeding), care must be taken to minimize human bonding and allow the doe to maintain her maternal bond to the kid. This can be done by housing the doe and kid together in confinement, holding the kid up to the teat of the doe to encourage nursing, and supplementing the diet only as absolutely needed to properly nourish the kid. A kid can easily become dependent, prefer bottle-feeding, and fail to maintain bonds with its dam.

SOURCES OF PRODUCTS MENTIONED

Selected websites for information and/or goat supplies include:

American Dairy Goat Association: www.adga.org

Caprine Supply: www.caprinesupply.com. Caprine Supply is a mail-order house for goat supplies. Its website includes an online catalog for supplies, articles on many aspects of goat management, and links to a large number of organizations for meat, dairy, and companion/utility goat breeds and breeders.

Goat care practices: www.vetmed.ucdavis.edu/vetext/INF-GO). *Goat care practices* text

Nasco Supply: www.nascofa.com. Nasco Supply is a mail-order house for general livestock and farm supplies, including goat equipment.

National Goat Handbook: www.inform.umd.edu/EdRes/Topic/AgrEnv/ndd/goat/

University of California at Irvine, 4-H Goat Information website: www.ics.uci.edu/~pazzani/4H/Goats

REFERENCES

Mason, I. L. 1981. Wild goats and their domestication. In *Goat production*, edited by C. Gall. New York: Academic Press.

Rowe, Joan Dean, and Nancy E. East. 1997. Postpartum care of the doe and kid. In *Current therapy in large animal theriogenology*, edited by Robert S. Youngquist. Philadelphia, PA: Saunders.

Smith, Mary C., and David M. Sherman. 1994. *Goat medicine*. Philadelphia: Lea & Febiger.

Stull, Carolyn, ed. 2000. *Goat care practices*. Veterinary Medicine Extension, Davis: University of California School of Veterinary Medicine; www.vetmed.ucdavis.edu/vetext/INF-GO

7
South American Camelids

Robert J. Pollard and Susan D. Pollard

NATURAL HISTORY

The South American camelids we will discuss here are the llama (*Llama glama*), alpaca (*L. pacos*), guanaco (*L. guanicoe*), and vicuna (*Vicugna vicugna*). The birth weight of the llama is 6–18 kg, the alpaca is 6–9 kg, the guanaco is 8–15 kg, and the vicuna is 4–6 kg.

Guanaco and vicuna are the wild relatives of the domesticated llama and alpaca. While intervention with guanaco and vicuna crias (Spanish for baby animal) would be rare, it would follow the guidelines of a small alpaca cria (Fig. 7.1).

The birth season may be year round for these animals. The time to weaning is four to six months.

RECORD KEEPING

Keep a daily log of body weight and milk supplement intake.

EQUIPMENT

The following items should be on hand: human baby bottles (8 oz/ 240 ml), artificial lambs' nipples, 12-oz (360-ml) glass soda pop or beer bottle, microwave or other method of heating milk, #18 French rubber catheter, 60-cc catheter-tip syringes, scales accurate to 4 oz (125 g).

CRITERIA FOR INTERVENTION

It is necessary to hand rear orphan crias and to supplement premature nonambulatory or rejected crias as well as nursing crias that do not maintain an adequate weight gain. The dense fiber covering on newborn llama and alpaca crias hides their body condition very well so the only true assessment is daily weighing.

INITIAL CARE AND STABILIZATION

Most crias are born late in the morning to midafternoon as is typical in the Altiplano in the Andes. Birth at other times is usually due to a malposition dystocia or a compromised cria (infection or twisted umbilical cord). Measures taken at birth should

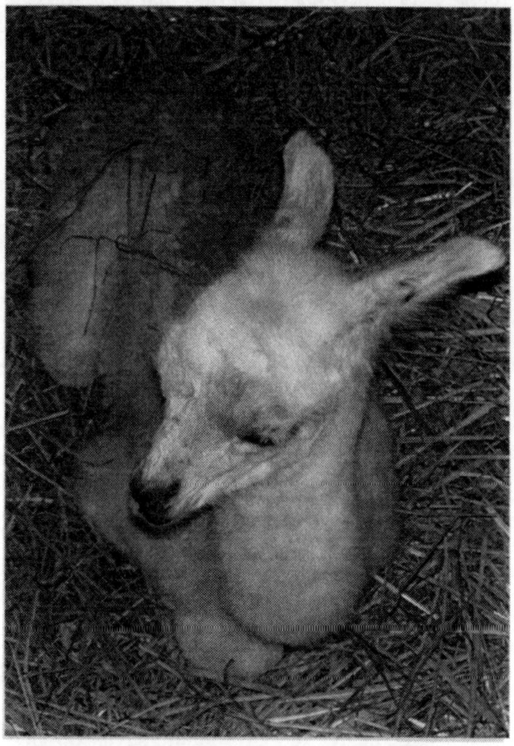

Figure 7.1. White llama cria (photo by Lindsay Merrill Leonard, Rainbow Ridge Llama Ranch).

include dipping the umbilical stump in 7% iodine, Nolvasan solution (0.5%; Fort Dodge), or even 85% isopropyl alcohol. Dipping several times is recommended. Newborns may be hypothermic even on warm days if the delivery is prolonged, so vigorous rubbing with dry towels or drying with a human hot air hair dryers may be used to "fluff" dry the wet fiber. Body temperature should stay in the 99–101°F (37.2–38.3°C) range.

Failure of passive immunoglobulins transfer (FPT) because of insufficient colostrum may lead to fatal septicemia. Causes may include the mother's poor immune status or premature birth, which may not allow enough time for the mother to produce sufficient amounts of colostrum. Weak, cold, or premature crias may fail to nurse enough colostrum in the first 24 hours; which is the critical time when IgGs can be absorbed across the gut lining.

Signs of a premature or dysmature (full term of 335–365 days but underdeveloped) birth included unerupted lower central incisor, ears that flop down instead of the normal upright position when dry, rubbery toenail slipper covering that fails to come off easily, and the adherence of the epidermal membrane to mucous membrane attachments at the lips, anus, vulva, and prepuce.

Causes of premature births include maternal stress (prolonged transport), being chased, high heat index causing overheating, or lack of enough micronutrients such as selenium.

Failure of passive immune transfer (FPT) is much better understood now because of the large North American domestic population of llamas (143,145 reported by the International Llama Registry in April 2001) and alpacas (32,195 reported by the Alpaca Registry, Inc., in April 2001). The high monetary value of these animals has led to maximum effort in saving crias. Dr. Murray E. Fowler's book *Medicine and surgery of South American camelids* (1998) has a good review of early life-saving options that include oral supplementation in the first 24 hours with good-quality colostrum from South American camelids, goats, or cattle.

Testing for FPT used to depend on the cria having a total serum protein level at 24 hours old of 4 g/dl or greater. A total protein of less than 4 g/dl suggested some degree of FPT and an increased risk of infection in the next three weeks before the cria becomes immune competent and starts producing its own IgG.

Since 1991 a radial immunodiffusion (RID) test plate has been available (Triple J Farms) that allows accurate measurement of camelid IgG levels. This RID plate is now the gold standard used by many commercial veterinary diagnostic laboratories as well as teaching hospitals at universities. Serum levels above 800 mg/dl of IgG on the Triple J Farm RID are considered well protected, levels of 400–800 mg/dl are suspect, and any level below 400 mg/dl is considered as FPT with a high risk of infection in the first three weeks of life.

WHAT TO FEED INITIALLY

The intake goal in the first 24 hours is 10% of the newborn cria's weight of colostrum given in six to eight small feedings. An example would be to feed a 10 kg newborn cria 1000 ml of formula divided into eight 125 ml feeds. Compared to true ruminants, South American camelids have a small capacity udder where normal healthy crias nurse 1–2 oz (30–60 ml) every hour or so. This results in very small production when the mother is hand milked for colostrum (along with the challenge of very small 0.5-in [1-cm] teats). Supplies of colostrum from local healthy goats is frequently collected ahead of the need and frozen in 4-oz or 120-ml (one feeding) containers. If less than a sufficient amount of fresh or frozen colostrum is available, the balance of the 10% body-weight goal is made up with goat's milk, cow's milk, or commercial milk replacers. Sheep colostrum is not recommended because it is 17.7% fat, while the llama colostrum is only 0.95% fat. Before feeding, all colostrum should be warmed to body temperature by a warm-water bath, not a microwave oven.

Colostrum and/or milk is fed to crias by either having them suckle from a rubber or latex nipple on a bottle or by stomach tube through an 18 French (6-mm) 16-in rubber tube (Kendall). Crias strong enough to suckle will usually accept the latex nipple on a human baby bottle especially if a few drops of corn syrup (Karo) are used as an initial inducement. Crias unable to suckle the whole meal are tube fed the remaining formula. Most crias increase nursing time and amount at a rapid rate. Poor nursers need regular reinforcement to increase sucking reflex, neck strength and endurance so if they are rebonded to their own mother or adopted mother, the transfer is easier.

Choice of nipples is either a rubber lamb's nipple on a clean used soda pop bottle or a latex human nipple on a plastic baby bottle. Nipples should be washed several times in hot water to remove the rubber/latex taste as well as to soften them. Before use the opening in the nipple is adjusted to the strength of the cria with weaker crias needing a large cross "x" cut in it and stronger more vigorous crias needing a smaller opening so as to not suck so much that they choke. It is desirable to keep a selection of well-washed nipples with different-sized openings on hand so that the correct one can be used as the cria gains nursing strength and skill. The normal nursing position is the head vertical with the bottle at the top similar to the crias' natural nursing behavior. As with using any milk products, cleaning equipment between use is important and includes removing any soap residues.

NURSING TECHNIQUES AND TUBE FEEDING

Crias not strong enough to suckle or that fail to finish nursing a bottle will need to be tube fed. Inserting the tube usually takes less than five minutes and is safer if two people use a team approach (Fig. 7.2). The cria is put in a kush position, upright on its sternum with the front legs folded back at the carpal joints and hind legs folded forward from the hocks. The restrainer straddles the cria kneeling over it but being careful not to sit on it with full weight. The restrainer's left hand holds the cria's throat under the jaw while the right hand introduces the 18 French rubber tube into the right side of the cria's mouth behind any incisors (lower only). The head is held level or slightly flexed as the tube is advanced to the rear of the mouth, eliciting the swallowing reflex. As the tube is pushed down the esophagus, its passage may be felt by the left hand on the left side of the trachea. A cria whose head is held too high vertically or who has the tube passed too quickly before a swallowing reflex is elicited might allow the tube to enter the trachea. There could be fatal results if milk is introduced into the lungs. The 16-inch tube is advanced until 4 inches remain out of the cria's mouth and must be held tightly under all circumstances or the consequence of a swallowed tube will have to be dealt with. It is important for the tube to only extend down to mid-neck so that milk flows properly from the esophagus past the first chamber by way of a groove that directs liquids to the third chamber for correct digestion.

The second person, our "feeder," using a 60-cc syringe pushes 60 ml (2 oz) of colostrum/milk into the tube being held by the restrainer. The feeder either refills the 60-cc syringe or picks up the second prefilled syringe, attaches it to the feeding tube, and slowly pushes in the second 60 ml. Crias larger than 10 kg are initially fed three or four meals of 120 ml. Then the feeding is gradually increased to one-eighth of the total daily goal of 10% of the cria's body weight. Meals should be no less than two hours or more than four hours apart, so with good planning only one middle-of-the-night (2 to 3 A.M.) feeding will be necessary for the first week if tubing or bottle-feeding is needed that long.

FREQUENCY OF FEEDING

Newborns should have eight feedings per day. Decrease the number of feedings per day starting on day ten. Ultimately, it is only necessary to feed four

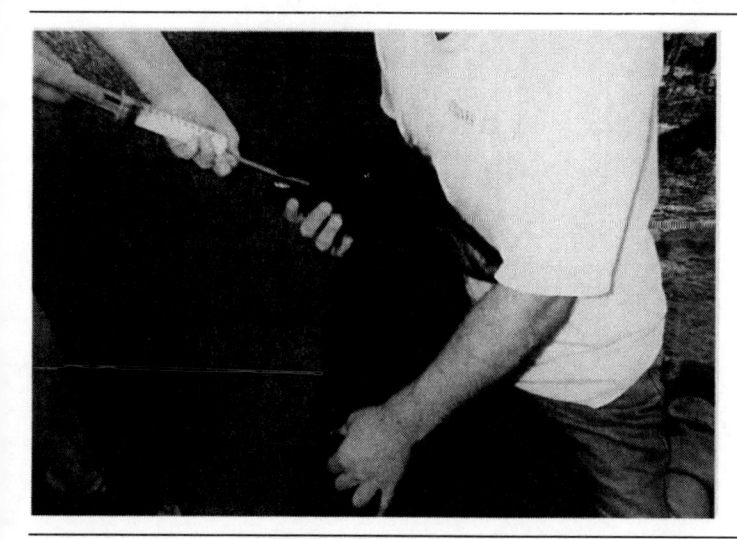

Figure 7.2. Tube feeding a cria.

times per day, but increase the volume of milk per feeding to sustain proper weight gain.

EXPECTED WEIGHT GAIN

A llama cria should gain 0.5 pound (225 g) per day the first week and then should gain one pound (450 g) per day. Alpaca crias will gain half the weight expected of a llama cria.

HOUSING

The orphaned crias should be kept in a warm environment until it has stabilized. Use rags or straw for bedding, not shavings. Some owners have constructed small blankets with Velcro fasteners to protect weak crias from cold weather.

TIME TO WEANING

Crias will start nibbling at solid food by two weeks of age. A premature cria or septicemic cria will be delayed in starting on solid food. The compartmented stomach of a neonate functions as a simple stomach until the organisms of digestion become established. Continue providing milk or milk substitutes until adequate intake of solid food occurs. Provide access to a leafy, high-quality grass or alfalfa hay. Some caregivers provide a little sweet feed (grain with molasses) or Calf Manna (Manna Pro).

Some normal crias wean themselves by two months of age, orphaned animals usually appear dependent on supplemental feeding for a longer time.

COMMON MEDICAL PROBLEMS

As in all species, if the cria fails to breathe, action must be taken, such as vigorous rubbing, compression of the chest, or mouth-to-nose resuscitation. Also, hypothermia can be detected by taking a rectal body temperature.

Common problems seen immediately following birth or within the first few days include retained meconium (constipation), diarrhea, and umbilical infection. Congenital defects that may interfere with sustaining life include nasal obstruction (choanal atresia), lack of an anus (atresia ani), twisted face (wry face), or urine flowing from the umbilicus (patent urachus).

SOURCES OF PRODUCTS MENTIONED

Fort Dodge Animal Health, 9401 Indian Creek Parkway, Suite 1500, Building 40, Overland Park, KS 66210; 1-800-477-1365 or 1-913-664-7000

Kendall Company, Mansfield, MA 02048; 1-800-962-9888

Manna Pro, St. Louis, MO; 1-800-690-9908; www.mannapro.com

Triple J Farms, 777 Jorgensen Place, Bellingham, WA 98226; 1-360-398-9512. Contact for current availability and prices.

REFERENCES AND READING

Fowler, M. E. 1998. Neonatology. In *Medicine and surgery of South American camelids*, edited by Murray Fowler. 2d ed. Ames: Iowa State University Press.

Smith, B. B., K. I. Timm, and P. O. Long. *Llama and alpaca neonatal care*. Originally published by Clay Press, Jackson, CA. Now distributed by B. B. Smith.

Part II
Wildlife, Zoo, and Marine Mammals

8 Opossums
9 Sugar Gliders
10 Macropods
11 Hedgehogs
12 Sloths
13 Ground and Tree Squirrels
14 Insectivorous Bats
15 Lemurs
16 Tamarins
17 Macaque Species
18 Great Apes
19 Harbor Seals and Northern Elephant Seals
20 Sea Lions and Fur Seals
21 Walrus Calves
22 Fox Kits
23 Black Bear Cubs
24 Polar Bears
25 Raccoons
26 Ferret Kits
27 Exotic Felids
28 Elephants
29 Nondomestic Equids
30 Rhinoceros
31 Black-Tailed and White-Tailed Deer
32 Exotic Ungulates

8
Opossums

Paula Taylor

NATURAL HISTORY

Virginia opossums (*Didelphis virginiana virginiana*) are marsupials whose distribution is throughout North and Central America. The Virginia opossum in North America typically breeds in the winter, with the young leaving the pouch in the spring at approximately 70 days of age. They produce an average of seven young in a single litter.

OPOSSUM ORPHAN CARE

Those of us who have been involved in the care of orphaned or injured opossums have found methods that work for us (Fig. 8.1). Although there is often more than one way to rehabilitate an animal successfully, it is easy to fall into the trap that "our way is the only way." Yet, when a method works, it is hard to argue with that success. Techniques constantly change and it is suggested you follow these basic guidelines while working with the Opossum Society of the United States (OSUS). The goal is to meet the physical and behavioral needs of the animals in order to ensure they are equipped for survival in their natural environment.

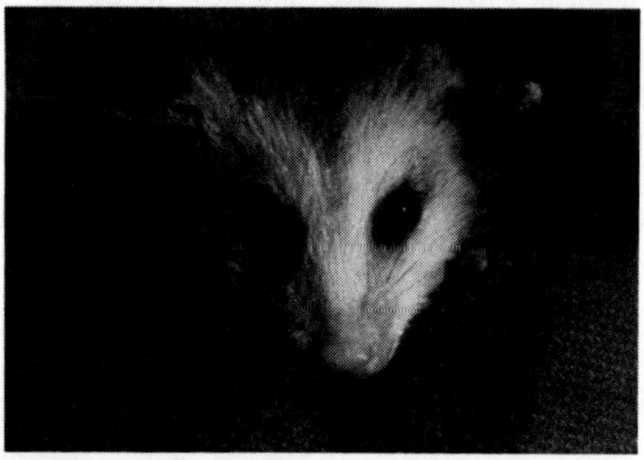

CRITERIA FOR INTERVENTION

When receiving a call asking you to care for orphaned opossums, it is imperative to collect as much information as possible in order to adequately prepare for the arrival of the animals. First, obtain the name, address, and telephone number of the caller. Ask where the animal was found, when it was rescued, and if any food or fluids have been given. Inquire about possible injuries to determine if it might be necessary for you to seek veterinary assistance. Find out the size of the animal by asking what its length is from tip of nose to base of tail. If the infant is small, ask if it is warm or cold. If cold, tell the person how to warm it while it is being transported to you. For example, the individual could fill a hot water bottle or plastic container with hot water, wrap it in toweling so the temperature of the outside fabric approximates human body temperature. Ask the person to wrap the opossum in a soft fabric such as flannel or cotton knit, place it next to the toweling-wrapped container, and place everything in a box. Stress the use of ravel-free fabric in order to avoid injuring the animals.

Any person who handles a nondomesticated animal should be warned to take precautions from injury or disease. Occasionally, infant rats or other rodents are brought in and misidentified as infant opossums. All wild mammals can bite, scratch, defecate and infect an existing wound with bacteria that are a potential zoonotic concern to humans. While opossums are relatively benign animals, no one should assume that they are free from risks when handling them.

Figure 8.1. Infant opossum (photo by Jackie Wollner, California Wildlife Center).

INITIAL CARE

Wash your hands with antibacterial soap prior to and after handling the infants. If you receive small, cold opossums, it is imperative that they be warmed for up to two hours before giving rehydrating fluids. Carefully check the temperature of the top towel to ensure that it is no higher than 95°F (35°C). Do not try to warm the infants too quickly, as you could burn them or cause them to go into shock. Check for injuries. If any serious injuries are found, seek veterinary assistance.

Before feeding the opossums, weigh each one on an accurate gram scale. This will determine the amount of formula needed to meet each infant's caloric requirements. If the animals are tiny, weigh them together and divide the total weight by the total number of animals in order to obtain an average weight. Check the Feeding Chart included in Table 8.1. Infants generally need to be fed four to five times a day, depending upon how much they weigh and the formula that is used.

FEEDING AND FORMULAS

Stimulation to Expel Waste

Prior to feeding it is important to manually stimulate the infants to urinate and defecate. Use a warm, damp cotton ball, facial tissue, or cotton tipped swabs to gently stroke the perineal area from front to back. Turn as it becomes soiled. Make sure that the stomach is not bloated (taut) before feeding. If you are caring for a litter of seven or more, do not be alarmed if no urine is expelled from one of the animals, as they sometimes stimulate each other to urinate through touching.

Occasionally, when an infant demonstrates a lack of interest in eating or is fidgety, stimulation will help it relax and cooperate. As the infant grows, it will usually let the caregiver know by its actions when stimulation is no longer needed. You may also see stool and/or urine in the cage. They are well furred at this time. Remember to wash your hands with an antibacterial soap after assisting the animals.

TUBE FEEDING

The most effective and efficient method of feeding infant opossums formula and oral rehydrating fluid is by tube feeding. Once you have learned how to tube feed, you can feed with more accuracy and can care for more animals. You should watch someone skilled at tube feeding before you attempt to do it yourself. Consult your vet or an experienced orphan caregiver who can teach you and monitor your progress until you gain confidence.

It is much faster to tube feed unweaned opossums than to use other feeding methods. Accurate weight must be obtained before starting and checked every two to three days thereafter. This enables you to check the Feeding Chart in Table 8.1 to determine the proper amount to feed and to keep accurate records of each animal's growth. The amount fed should fill the stomach comfortably.

Overfeeding may cause diarrhea or stomach paralysis. Pay close attention to the fullness of the stomach before, during, and after feeding. It should be soft to the touch and gently rounded, not hard and taut like a drum.

Sometimes you will be able to see the whiteness of the milk as it enters the stomach. Feeding intervals are generally four to five times per day. Middle-of-the-night feedings may be necessary for severely dehydrated infants and for those with medical problems. A "pinkie" opossum, one that has no pigment and weighs less than 20 grams, is difficult to hand rear without a surrogate lactating female. Caring for them is labor-intensive and often results in failure. It is usually best for all concerned to have these infants euthanized.

Measuring and Inserting the Feeding Tube

Wash your hands thoroughly with antibacterial soap before you begin tube feeding. Use a soft rubber #3 1/2 French feeding tube (Kendall) to feed unweaned infants that weigh up to 35 grams. A #5 French feeding tube can be used to feed those that weigh from approximately 36 grams to 60 grams, but some people find the #3 1/2 French feeding tube easier to get down the throat and more comfortable for the animal.

Measure the tube for proper placement. Lay the animal on its back and take the tip of the tube and measure the distance from the end of the sternum (chest bone) to the tip of the nose. Be sure to hold the head straight back in line with the body. At the tip of the nose, wrap a piece of masking tape tightly around the tube. The tape will serve as a marker to prevent you from inserting the tube too far and puncturing the stomach wall or not far enough and possibly entering the lungs. If you enter the lungs rather than the stomach, you risk drowning the infant or contaminating its lungs with formula. This will lead to pneumonia and death. Second, you could puncture any of the animal's very fragile membranes. To avoid these problems, always measure the proper placement and mark the tube with tape. If the tape is not touching the infant's mouth when it is inserted, you may be in the lungs. Do not ever force the tube. It should go easily to the stomach if it is in the esophagus. Withdraw the tube and start again. By being gentle and taking your time, you can avoid problems. Recheck the measurement every few days and mark the tube with new tape as each animal grows.

Attach the tube to a 1-cc or 3-cc syringe and fill it with formula that has been warmed to the opossum's body temperature. Heat only enough formula for that feeding. Hold the syringe vertically and tap the side until all air bubbles are at the top. Push the plunger on the syringe to release the air and pass the formula into the tube. Make sure that all the air bubbles have been expelled. If necessary, draw more fluid or formula into the tube so that the syringe contains the proper amount to feed the animal.

Hold the opossum with its back in the palm of your hand. Right-handed individuals should hold it in their left hand and left-handed individuals in their right. Grip the head firmly with the thumb, index finger, and middle finger. The middle finger will also hold the animal's legs down so that it will not be able to pull on the tube. An alternative method is to hold the infant in a standing position on a flat, nonslick surface. If you are right-handed, put your left hand around its body near the base of the head. Position your thumb and forefinger on either side of the mouth under the jaw. Keep the head and tube straight during feeding.

Wipe any formula from the tip of the tube. Moisten the tip with water. Hold the tube near the tip and gently insert it into the front of the mouth, over the tongue, in line with the throat. To avoid insertion into the lungs, keep the head straight and do not extend it when inserting the tube. It may be necessary to use a twisting motion to get the tip over the tongue (or you may need to remoisten the tip with water). Gently slide the tube forward until the tape is against the mouth. Hold the tube in place and keep the mouth completely closed. Slowly insert the formula, making sure to check the fullness of the stomach. Never force the tube. It should go down the throat easily. If it does not or if the tube appears to stop, pull back slightly, twist, and try again. If the tube comes out of the mouth, remoisten with water and start again. Feed slowly, stopping after each 0.5 ml (cc) and check the stomach during feeding.

After feeding, place the opossums that have been fed in a separate pouch. Two small buckets, each containing a T-shirt, may be placed on a double-size heating pad. All the babies are put in one bucket and as each is fed, it is transferred to the other bucket. This keeps any animal from being fed twice. If an infant has a problem, mark the ears (or tail, if ears are turning black) with a colored nontoxic marker so that you can identify that animal. To avoid cross contamination, feed the marked infant last. It might be necessary to remove this animal from the litter. For even greater accuracy, you can mark each animal's tail with a different color nontoxic marker in order to avoid feeding an opossum twice and to accurately monitor each individual's growth. After feeding, flush the syringe and tube at least six times with very hot water. Allow the equipment to air dry.

Many rehabbers successfully boil their tubes for fifteen minutes daily to sterilize, but I have had tubes permanently curl when boiled. It is important to boil any tube that is used on a sick animal or throw it away so that healthy animals are not infected.

SYRINGE FEEDING

An alternative method of feeding is syringe feeding, which utilizes a 1-cc to a 3-cc syringe (or larger, if the litter is large) and a Tomcat catheter or IV catheter without the needle, (available from veterinarians). Shorten the Tomcat catheter so that the tip is still small in diameter, but not so long that it is awkward. File the tip of the Tomcat catheter until all the edges are smooth to the touch. Also, remember that these devices are meant for oral use and are not safe for tube feeding.

Prior to feeding, it is necessary to rehydrate the opossums. Have lactated Ringer's solution, Pedialyte (Ross), or Gatorade (diluted 1:5 parts water) available, which has been warmed to the opossum's body temperature (95°F–97°F or 35°C–36°C). We prefer lactated Ringer's or Pedialyte, but in an emergency Gatorade may be used.

If none of these are available, you can make an emergency rehydrating solution by combining 1 quart (948 cc) hot water, 1 tablespoon (15 cc) sugar, and 1 teaspoon (5 cc) salt. Cool to body temperature before feeding and store in the refrigerator.

A syringe of lactated Ringer's or Pedialyte may be warmed in a container of hot water or in a microwave on low power. Rehydrate the opossums at least three times with any of the above rehydrating

Table 8.1. Substitute Milk Formula For Opossum

VIRGINIA OPOSSUM MILK					
	%SOLIDS	%FAT	%PRO	%CARBO	KCALS/CC
Barker, et. al.	23.2	11.3	8.4	1.6	1.42
Jenness and Sloan	24.4	7.0	4.8	4.1	0.99

SUBSTITUTE FORMULA

	%SOLIDS	%FAT	%PRO	%CARBO	KCALS/CC
Esbilac® powder and Multi-Milk® powder	21.7	10.5	7.3	2.3	1.33

MIXING INSTRUCTIONS

1 part Esbilac® or Zoologic® Milk Matrix 33/40 (powder)
1/2 part Multi-Milk® or Zoologic® Milk Matrix 30/55 (powder)
2 parts water

- Mix by volume (i.e., teaspoon, tablespoon, cup, etc.)
- If water quality is poor, use distilled water
- Values shown are wet matter basis (% of mixed formula)
- Esbilac®, Multi-Milk®, and Zoologic® Milk Matrix powders are mfd. by PetAg, Inc. (1-800-323-0877 for product questions)

FEEDING CHART

BODY WEIGHT		DAILY CALORIC REQUIREMENT	AMOUNT TO FEED IN CC (To convert cc to oz., divide by 28.35)			
OUNCES	GRAMS	KCALS/DAY	4X/DAY	5X/DAY	6X/DAY	
0.35	10.00	4.42	****	****	****	
0.53	15.00	5.99	****	****	****	
0.71	20.00	7.43	****	****	1.12	
0.88	25.00	8.78	****	****	1.32	
1.06	30.00	10.07	****	****	1.51	
1.23	35.00	11.30	****	****	1.70	
1.41	40.00	12.49	****	****	1.88	
1.59	45.00	13.64	****	2.35	2.05	
1.76	50.00	14.77	****	2.56	2.22	
1.94	55.00	15.86	****	2.78	2.39	
2.12	60.00	16.93	****	2.98	2.55	
2.29	65.00	17.98	****	3.18	2.70	
2.47	70.00	19.00	****	3.38	2.86	
2.65	75.00	20.01	****	3.57	3.01	
2.82	80.00	21.01	****	3.76	3.16	
3.00	85.00	21.98	****	3.95	3.31	
3.17	90.00	22.95	****	4.13	3.45	
3.35	95.00	23.90	****	4.31	3.59	
3.53	100.00	24.83	****	4.49	3.73	
				4.67		

Weigh the animal periodically. Based on the feeding interval used, feed the corresponding amount. The amount to feed is at least 2 times the basal energy requirement daily (generally during a 16- to 18-hour period). For marsupials, this is approximated by the formula KCALS required = $2.85 \times (49 \times$ body wt in $kg^{0.75})$. **** indicates that minimum caloric requirements cannot be met with this feeding frequency.

CC per feeding are based on the fact that the stomach capacity of marsupials will hold a comfortable maximum of 50 to 66 cc per kg of body weight (5% to 7%). The stomach may hold more, but distension problems are likely if this range is exceeded. This chart is based on 60 cc per kg of body weight. THE CHART IS A GUIDELINE, NOT AN ABSOLUTE.

Infant opossums are generally able to lap by 45 to 50 g (1.6 to 1.8 oz). This species suckles in the pouch of the female. In captivity, the animal should be taken from the bedding area and placed in front of a shallow container of warm formula every 3 to 4 hours during the day and evening until it is routinely eating on its own. Formula can also be left out during the day if it is replaced frequently. Supplemental tube feeding may be necessary. Opossums can generally be weaned by 100 g/3.5 oz. They can be released when they are self-feeding, acclimated to the outdoors, and are approximately 5 months old (approximately 681 g/1-1/2 lbs, measuring 10" to 12" from tip of nose to base of tail).

Barker, P.R., et al. 1967. Marsupial biomodule evaluation study. Life Sciences Operations, Space and Information Systems Division, North American Aviation, Inc., El Segundo, CA.
Evans, R.H. 1982. Verbal and written communications.
_____. 1987. Rearing orphaned wild mammals. The Veterinary Clinics of North America: Small Animal Practice, 17(3):755-783.
Fowler, M.E. 1979. Care of orphaned wild animals. The Veterinary Clinics of North America: Small Animal Practice, 9(3):448-471.
Hainsworth, F.R. 1981. Animal Physiology Adaptations in Function. Addison-Wesley Publishing Co., Reading, MA.
Jenness, R. and R.E. Sloan. 1970. The composition of milks of various species: a review. Dairy Science Abstracts, 32(10): 599-612.
Copyright © 1988 by Debbie Marcum; revised 1997 Opossum—Chart 02

agents to cleanse their digestive tract and prepare them for the introduction to formula.

After a minimum of three feedings of rehydration solution (more if an infant is dehydrated), formula should be introduced gradually as follows:

3/4 part rehydrating solution + 1/4 part formula
1/2 part rehydrating solution + 1/2 part formula
1/4 part rehydrating solution + 3/4 part formula

When introducing formula, start with three-fourths part rehydrating solution and one-fourth part formula. Give three to six times before advancing to the next dilution. It is better to go slowly in order to prevent digestive problems. Progress to one-half part rehydrating solution and one-half part Esbilac formula (PetAg) and give at least three times before advancing to the next dilution (see Table 8.1). Monitor how well the infant tolerates the formula. Progress to one-fourth part rehydrating solution and three-fourths part formula and give at least three times. Finally, progress to full-strength formula. Whenever you change to a new formula, you should follow the above rehydrating method of introducing fluids and formula in order to prevent diarrhea or other digestive problems.

When syringe feeding an infant, wrap it in a soft ravel-free cloth with its front legs in or out (whatever is comfortable for the animal). Feed the formula one drop at a time. You can gauge the approximate amount fed by the amount in the syringe. Go slowly. It will take ten minutes or longer to feed each animal. You do not want formula coming out of the nose. If it comes out the nose, blot, hold the animal upside down, and gently pat it between the shoulder blades. Sometimes more formula will be expelled. If this occurs, blot it immediately. Check the infant's stomach to see if it is gently rounded, not taut. Flush the syringe and tip at least six times with hot water.

If you have a single opossum and cannot locate a litter to place it with, it is essential that you hold and stroke the animal for at least a few minutes after feeding. This will replicate the stimulation provided by the litter and the nurturing that is essential to thriving. You should also place a small stuffed animal in the pouch or bedding with the baby for additional comfort and security. Remember to remove any hazardous pieces from the stuffed animal.

When comparing syringe feeding with tube feeding, it is important to remember that tube feeding is much faster, more accurate, more efficient, and less stressful for the animal, despite any apprehension associated with tubing. The time factor will enable you to care for more infants in much less time, and it is often the difference between an opossum that merely survives and one that thrives.

LITTER TRAINING

Litter trays should be introduced when the opossum's eyes have opened, and it is beginning to walk well. Some examples of litter trays are plastic flowerpot saucers that are filled with natural clay cat litter or Teflon-coated cookie sheets filled with clay litter or lined with newspaper and topped with paper towels. The paper towels absorb urine quickly. To litter train, stimulate the infant over the litter tray. When cleaning the litter tray, leave one stool in it. Opossums quickly learn to eliminate in the litter tray.

TIME TO WEANING

When infants have their eyes open and are not too wobbly (generally 45 g or more), they can be taught to lap the formula. Lapping is not a natural feeding routine for them, so they must be encouraged. At this point, it is suggested that soft, quilted-type paper towels be placed on top of the newspaper in the feeding area of the cage. This will enable the animal to stand and grip more easily.

Fill a shallow jar lid to the rim with formula (see Fig. 8.2). More than one lid or larger lids may be needed depending on the number of animals. When necessary, a tiny drop of Karo light syrup can be added to the formula prior to heating to encourage self-feeding. Dip your finger in the formula and

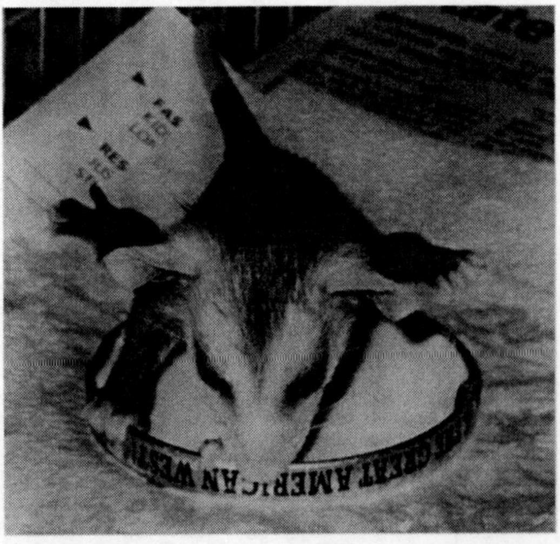

Figure 8.2. Opossum infant feeding from lid.

wipe it around the edge of the rim to attract the animals. Gently touch the mouth of each opossum to the formula. After they attempt to self-feed, it may be necessary for you to supplement the infants with additional formula. Check each stomach for fullness. Extend the time between feedings, and put the infants in front of the lids often. Do not assume that all of the infants are coming out of the nest area to eat. Keep shallow lids of warm formula in the cage.

Change the formula frequently to ensure freshness. You might find it easier to use a small plastic spoon and put it in the formula. Tip it slightly to the infant's mouth to encourage it to lap.

When the opossums are lapping regularly on their own and hand feeding has been reduced to once or twice a day or discontinued when they weigh 60 g or more, the formula needs to be thickened by adding ground or whole Purina Kitten Chow ("Original Formula" only) that has been mixed with water. This mixture will be called "chow-pudding." Grind dry Purina Kitten Chow (Purina) in a blender or food processor. Add a sufficient amount of water to give the chow a puddinglike consistency. Allow the pudding to set in the refrigerator for approximately ten minutes and check. It absorbs water faster when refrigerated. The whole consistency changes (there should not be any hard chunks). More water or more chow may be added to get the desired consistency. Store the chow-pudding in an airtight container in the refrigerator. Thicken the formula with a small amount of chow-pudding mix (it should resemble formula that has small particles of Kitten Chow throughout). As the animals become accustomed to the taste, increase the amount of chow-pudding. Provide a lid of whole dry Purina Kitten Chow and another lid of Kitten Chow that has been soaked in water five to ten minutes (in whole form). Some animals eat the softer chow more readily. A shallow container of water should be available at all times.

MODIFIED-JURGELSKI DIET

By the time the opossums weigh 80–100 g, introduce the Modified-Jurgelski Diet. This diet consists of one part ground, raw beef liver and nine parts Purina Kitten Chow-pudding (see Table 8.2). The amount of liver is not discretionary. These are precise measurements. Altering the amount of liver or using another brand of kitten food has and will cause metabolic bone problems.

The Modified-Jurgelski Diet can be refrigerated for up to three days. Then it should be discarded. The liver can be frozen in small containers, if tightly wrapped, for up to one month. Offer the Modified-Jurgelski Diet every evening. This is not optional! Some animals take longer than others to acquire a taste for this diet. If they refuse to eat it after several days, offer crickets that have not been contaminated with any insecticides, and are high in protein. After eating crickets for several days, they will most likely eat the liver chow. When all of the opossums that are being housed together are consistently eating the Modified-Jurgelski Diet, gradually add small quantities of various fresh fruits and vegetables (add one item at a time). Cut into bite-size pieces prior to offering them to the youngsters. It is important that the animals are eating the Modified-Jurgelski Diet, which is the balanced dietary staple and constitutes 90% of the total diet, before they get fruits and vegetables, which should total only 10% of the total diet.

DISINFECTING BEDDING, CAGES, AND DISHES

Good hygiene is essential to your health and that of the opossums in your care. After feeding, wash all utensils in a solution consisting of 3 tablespoons (15 ml) liquid bleach to a dishpan of hot, soapy water. Rinse thoroughly. A dishwasher may be used for crock bowls, plastic lids, and jars. It would also be advisable to wash animal dishes in a container separate from your own dishes. Wash all bedding in hot water with the appropriate amount of detergent and 1/2 cup (120 ml) liquid bleach with each load. A small amount of unscented liquid fabric softener may also be used. Use a brush to clean the cages with a solution of 1 tablespoon (15 ml) liquid bleach to 1 cup (240 ml) hot water. Rinse well and allow to dry completely in the sun. The cages should be cleaned thoroughly after each litter's use.

HOUSING

Housing for infants that have some gray pigment along the backbone, or scant fur, or infants whose eyes are closed should consist of a sturdy box or aquarium that is at least 18 inches (46 cm) high. An aquarium is preferred, as humidity is much easier to control. Always place a heating pad under the container, not in it, and make sure it is only under a portion of the "nest" area. It is usually set on "low" when there is a towel under the aquarium. "Medium" setting might be needed for wood or other containers. When using an aquarium, soak a terry-cloth towel in hot water, wring it out, and

Table 8.2. Feeding Chart For The Modified Jurgelski Diet For Opossums (Purina® Kitten Chow®, Water, Raw Beef Liver, Calcium Carbonate)

INSTRUCTIONS

Diet: Mixture of 1 part ground, raw beef liver and 9 parts Kitten Chow®/water mixture, all by volume (i.e., tsp, tbsp, cup, or parts of any of these). Soak Kitten Chow® in enough water to create a pudding-like consistency. Combine 1 part ground, raw beef liver with 9 parts Kitten Chow®/water mixture. The amount of liver is not discretionary. Pulverize Caltrate® 600 tablets (or use a calcium carbonate powder which specifies on the label that it contains 700 to 800 mg of calcium per tsp), and add 1/4 tsp per cup of Kitten Chow®/water/liver mixture. No other supplemental vitamins or minerals should be used with this diet unless recommended by a veterinarian for a specific medical condition.

	%SOLIDS	%FAT	%PRO	%CARBO	KCALS/TBSP
Diet Composition	33.2%	3.3%	13.9%	11.2%	21.2

FEEDING CHART

BODY WEIGHT		DAILY BASAL ENERGY REQUIREMENT	AMOUNT TO FEED PER DAY	
			2 TIMES BASAL REQUIREMENT (1 tbsp = 3 tsp)	2-1/2 TIMES BASAL REQUIREMENT (1 tbsp = 3 tsp)
OUNCES	GRAMS	(KCALS/DAY)	(To convert to cups: 4 tbsp = 1/4 cup)	
2.5	70.0	9.5	1 tbsp + 0 tsp	1 tbsp + 0 tsp
2.8	80.0	10.5	1 tbsp + 0 tsp	1 tbsp + 1 tsp
3.2	90.0	11.5	1 tbsp + 0 tsp	1 tbsp + 1 tsp
3.5	100.0	12.5	1 tbsp + 0 tsp	1 tbsp + 2 tsp
3.9	110.0	13.4	1 tbsp + 1 tsp	1 tbsp + 2 tsp
4.2	120.0	14.3	1 tbsp + 1 tsp	1 tbsp + 2 tsp
4.6	130.0	15.2	1 tbsp + 1 tsp	1 tbsp + 2 tsp
4.9	140.0	16.0	1 tbsp + 1 tsp	2 tbsp + 0 tsp
5.3	150.0	16.9	1 tbsp + 1 tsp	2 tbsp + 0 tsp
7.1	200.0	21.0	2 tbsp + 0 tsp	2 tbsp + 1 tsp
7.9	225.0	22.9	2 tbsp + 0 tsp	2 tbsp + 2 tsp
9.7	275.0	26.6	2 tbsp + 1 tsp	3 tbsp + 0 tsp
11.5	325.0	30.2	2 tbsp + 2 tsp	3 tbsp + 2 tsp
13.2	375.0	33.6	3 tbsp + 0 tsp	4 tbsp + 0 tsp
14.1	400.0	35.2	3 tbsp + 1 tsp	4 tbsp + 0 tsp
15.9	450.0	38.5	3 tbsp + 2 tsp	4 tbsp + 2 tsp
17.6	500.0	41.7	4 tbsp + 0 tsp	5 tbsp + 0 tsp
19.4	550.0	44.8	4 tbsp + 0 tsp	5 tbsp + 1 tsp
21.2	600.0	47.8	4 tbsp + 1 tsp	5 tbsp + 2 tsp
22.9	650.0	50.7	4 tbsp + 2 tsp	6 tbsp + 0 tsp
24.7	700.0	53.6	5 tbsp + 0 tsp	6 tbsp + 1 tsp
26.5	750.0	56.5	5 tbsp + 1 tsp	6 tbsp + 2 tsp
28.2	800.0	59.3	5 tbsp + 1 tsp	7 tbsp + 0 tsp
30.0	850.0	62.0	5 tbsp + 2 tsp	7 tbsp + 1 tsp
33.5	950.0	67.4	6 tbsp + 1 tsp	8 tbsp + 0 tsp
37.0	1050.0	72.7	6 tbsp + 2 tsp	8 tbsp + 2 tsp

Notes:
Weigh the animal periodically. Based on its weight, feed the corresponding amount shown. For more than one opossum, multiply the amount to feed by the total number of animals. THIS CHART IS A GUIDELINE, NOT AN ABSOLUTE. The daily basal energy requirement represents the energy required by the animal for basic bodily functions (i.e., respiration, circulation, glandular function, peristalsis, temperature regulation) when in a resting and a thermal neutral state. Infant mammals require 2 to 4 times the basal energy requirement daily (Evans, 1987). This chart includes calculations for both 2 and 2-1/2 times the basal energy requirement.
Copyright © 1992 by Debbie Marcum; revised 1996

place it on the bottom of the aquarium. Cover with layers of bedding. To maintain humidity, cover the aquarium with a wet towel. The towels must be resoaked as needed. A hygrometer is generally used to monitor the humidity. Place several layers of receiving blankets, T-shirts, or sweatshirts without frays over the pad to avoid burning or overheating the infants. When using a box or any other container for infants, a tall plastic container partially filled with water should be securely taped to the box in the farthest corner away from the bedding. This will prevent spilling and provide the necessary humidity. Cover and punch holes in the lid to maintain the humidity inside.

Cut a sleeve from a sweatshirt and close it at one end by rolling it or sewing it closed. This sleeve will be the "holding pouch" for the infants. Once the animals have been placed inside, fold the other end of the sleeve underneath to prevent them from scattering. For practical purposes, this setup is called a "pouch," since it simulates the mother's pouch where she carries her young. Examples of other pouches include flannel pillowcases (turned inside out with the opening tucked underneath) and various sizes of pillowcase-type pouches that are made from flannel and have Velcro closures across the opening. Always put a small stuffed animal (after removing any hazardous plastic pieces, such as the eyes) in the pouch. This enables the opossums to get away from each other if they want and appears to provide security. Always make sure that a single infant has a stuffed animal for companionship. Have at least two pouches ready for the incoming orphans, and make sure the heating pad is turned on ahead of time in order to warm the bedding. The temperature underneath the pouch should be checked with an oral or rectal thermometer and should not exceed 95°F (35°C).

Cage Setup

For infants that have their eyes open and are walking, a cage that has grids of 1/2 in × 1 in (1.3 cm × 2.5 cm) can be used to prevent the animals from escaping. A rule of thumb for caging is use mesh that is small enough: If the head can go through, the body will follow!

Keep the cage clean and dry. Line the floor with newspaper to prevent damage to tender feet. For bedding, use infant blankets, sweatshirts, or T-shirts, and layer the fabric so that the animals can crawl under some of the bedding. Terry-cloth towels are never used as bedding for any species because of dangers from the loops and raveling. It is easy for an animal to strangle, lose toenails, or have threads wrap around its digits, causing damage. *Always* have a small shallow dish of fresh formula in the cage as soon as the opossum's eyes open. Remember to change the formula every two to four hours, especially during warm weather.

It is advisable to group the animals before or shortly after their eyes have opened. The larger they are, the more potential there is for problems to occur. Never house infants together that are not the same size, as cannibalism may occur. Never house a wounded or ill animal with other opossums because of the species' tendency toward cannibalism.

As the infants grow, they need to be transferred to larger outdoor cages (Table 8.3). Den boxes with bedding should be placed off the floor. Equip the cage with hollow logs and secure branches for climbing. Cover at least one-third of the cage to provide the animals with shade and privacy. Outdoor cages need fiberglass or metal roofs and tarps that can be dropped in inclement weather. If the cages are small, they can be completely covered with a tarp when necessary. It is important not to overcrowd opossums. As the animals grow, they must be moved into larger cages or litters must be divided. The cages must have adequate floor space.

When the opossums are thermoregulating (able to maintain body temperature), self-feeding, and 5–6 in (12.7–15 cm) in body length, they need to be housed outside. Transfer them out when the weather is warm and sunny. Once outside, it is important that healthy animals stay outside, regardless of the weather. When the animals are weaned, limit your contact to feeding and cage cleaning in order to prepare them for release. Your goal is to make them forage for food and to be wary of humans. Do not pet the animals. Scatter food around the cage at dusk before they awaken. Since opossums are nocturnal, you want them to look for food only after dark. Do not leave lights on around the cages. You do not want them to be attracted to lights.

Keep dogs and cats away from the cages. If the opossums have no fear of dogs and cats, they may lose their natural wariness of other animals, which could be fatal to them after their release. If the opossums seem overly friendly to you and come out to greet you, try to arrange to transfer them to someone else. A move to an unfamiliar location will generally elicit a more intense wariness of their surroundings.

RELEASE

Opossums should be released when they weigh approximately 1.5 lb (0.7 kg) and are about five

Table 8.3. Outdoor Cages and Runs

Size of cage	Number/Size of opossums
Aquarium or Box (18" tall)	Litter with eyes closed
34" × 20" × 20" or 3' × 3' × 3' (86 cm × 51 cm × 51 cm)	(5–7) 4" opossums
46" × 20" × 20" (117 cm × 51 cm × 51 cm)	(5–7) 6" opossums
4' × 4' × 8' (1.2 × 1.2 × 2.4 meters)	(5–7) 6–8" opossums
4' × 4' × 8'	1 juvenile
Runs with Bedding Boxes	
7' × 4' × 8' (2.1 m × 1.2 m × 2.4 m)	(10–12) 7–9" opossums
12' × 4' × 8' (3.6 m × 1.2 m × 2.4 m)	(10–12) 7–9" opossums
Housing for Injured Adult	
2' × 2' × 2' (0.6 m × 0.6 m × 0.6 m)	
Outside Adult	
4' × 4' × 8' (1.2 m × 1.2 m × 2.4 m)	

months old and 10–12 in (25.4–30.5 cm) in body length from tip of nose to base of tail. Feed a light meal before releasing or forgo the meal and provide backup food such as 10–20 lb of dry dog or cat chow, which is scattered in an area that is somewhat protected from the elements. Release after sunset. Make sure that the weather is favorable on the release day and several days thereafter. The release site should have a year-round supply of fresh water, dense brush, and abundant natural foods.

Whenever batches of opossums are released, they should be interested in exploring the release area or run away. If any animal returns to the carrier and wants to stay there, tries to get into or on the carrier and is not interested in leaving it, or stays near the rehabilitator, it is too immature to release at that time. To do so guarantees injury or early death. If at all possible, take it back and give it more time to mature.

The moment of release ends your role as an orphan caregiver for this individual animal or litter. Your reward is knowing that you made a difference in the lives of animals that would have otherwise undoubtedly have perished without your care and nurturing.

ACKNOWLEDGMENTS

I am especially grateful to Debbie Marcum for sharing all her copyrighted opossum papers, her support, and her advice and for reviewing the original manual and training film.

To my veterinarian advisors, Scott Weldy, D.V.M. and rehabilitator, and John Kuttel, D.V.M., my thanks for sharing their time and knowledge so willingly.

Last, a special thanks to Jackie Garcia who introduced me to the world of the opossum and taught me much of what I know.

RESOURCES AND SOURCES OF PRODUCTS MENTIONED

Kendall Company, Mansfield, MA 02048; 1-800-962-9888

Opossum Orphan Care Video by Paula Taylor, RN; 1-714-536-8080

PetAg Inc., 261 Keyes Ave., Hampshire, IL 60140; 1-800-323-0877, 1-800-323-6878; www.petag.com

Purina: www.Purina.com; 1-800-778-7462

Ross Products Division, Abbott Laboratories, Columbus, OH 43215-1724; 1-800-986-8510; www.abbott.com, www.ross.com

REFERENCES

Graboski, R. 1995. Simple things that make a difference: Making water-based incubators. *Journal of Wildlife Rehabilitation* 18(2):16–17.

Marcum, Debbie. 1990. *Hand-rearing non-domestic mammals.* Suisun, CA: International Wildlife Rehabilitation Council.

White, Jan. 1993. *Basic wildlife rehabilitation lab.* 4th ed. Suisun, CA: International Wildlife Rehabilitation Council.

9
Sugar Gliders

Michele Barnes

NATURAL HISTORY

The sugar glider (*Petaurus breviceps*) has an average birth weight of 0.2 g (Fig. 9.1). Sugar gliders begin breeding in late winter (August in Australia). Females have a 29-day estrous cycle and produce one (19% of births) or, more commonly, two offspring (81% of births) after a 15–17-day gestation period (Booth 1993).

The young remain in the pouch for approximately 70 days and are then left in the group nest for an additional 30 days. Production of a second litter is common in the one breeding season.

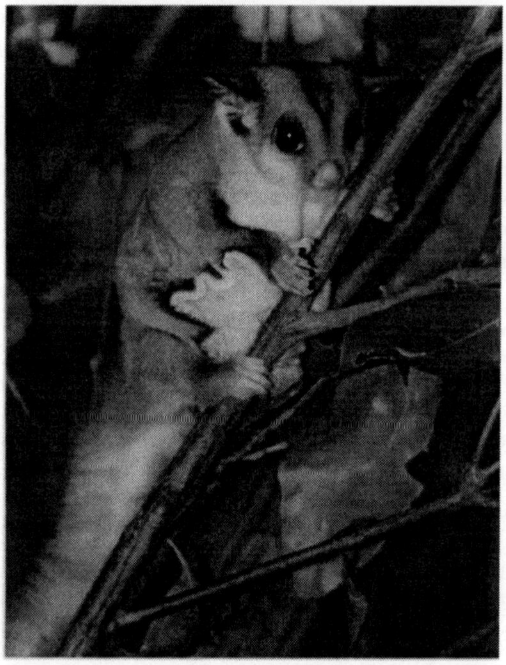

Longevity in the wild is usually 4 to 5 years, individuals may survive up to 9 years in the wild or 12 years in captivity (Booth 1998).

RECORD KEEPING

Detailed, accurate records should be maintained, as they can be a great source for future reference. Table 9.1 shows a possible format. Initial records should include things such as age, weight, body measurements, sex, distinguishing marks, parentage (if known), formula given (and at what strength), what you are housing them in (pouches, heat source, cages, etc.). Daily records should include items such as time fed, quantity given, any change in formula or introduction of solids, frequency of urine and fecal matter, consistency of feces, and behavioral notes.

EQUIPMENT

Always be prepared. Have all your hand-raising equipment on hand prior to receiving an animal whenever possible. The following items will be needed:

Artificial pouches and bedding—made from natural fibers with no loose hanging threads
Maximum/minimum thermometer—to maintain and monitor temperature
Small cage—for early stages
Large cage—for later stages when young emerge from the pouch and after weaning
Feeding aids—glider teat, syringe, measuring spoon
Electrolyte/glucose replacer—Lectade (Duvox)
Small feeding bottles—relevant for quantity of food
Bottle brush—for cleaning feeding bottles
Milton or boiling water—for sterilization of feeding equipment

Figure 9.1. Sugar glider in a tree.

Table 9.1. Format for Hand-Raising Records

Hand-raising Records	
Common Name:	Scientific Name:
House Name:	Sex:
Age:	Measurements:
Parents:	Reason:
Formula Given:	Carer:

Date	Time Fed	Amt Fed	Total	Weight	Comments

Food—milk formula; solid foods, supplements; natural foods such as blossoms, insects, various types of tree branches

Heat source (heat pad, hot water bottle)—to provide warmth

Food bowl for solids—shallow bowl that hooks to side of cage

Water bowl—shallow bowl that hooks to side of cage

Soft baby brush—for grooming

Baby wipes (Chux)/tissues—for toileting, cleaning

NapiSan (Reckitt Benckiser)—for sanitizing/cleaning pouches and bedding

CRITERIA FOR INTERVENTION

It may be necessary to intervene and hand raise young if they are failing to thrive while suckling, are sick or injured, their mother has rejected them, or they have been orphaned. Hand raising any animal requires a lot of time, effort, and patience and should not be entered into half-heartedly.

INITIAL CARE AND STABILIZATION

The initial care will be dependent on whether the young has been removed by you or rejected by its mother. The latter will require you to physically check the animal for any bleeding, breathing difficulties, broken bones, hyperthermia, hypothermia, parasites, shock, or wounds. Although basic first aid can be applied, veterinary assistance should be sought right away.

Success rates with hand rearing approach 0% for furless young, but experienced individuals may wish to try. Once the young are furred success rates approach 100% (Booth 1998).

It is important to remember when dealing with sick, injured, or orphaned animals, to try to create a stress-free environment. The young should be placed in an artificial pouch, sock, or something similar, placed on a heat source, and left somewhere quiet. Sick or injured adults should be kept at 79°F (26°C), furred young at 82°F (28°C), and furless young at 89.6°F (32°C). Artificial warmth may be provided by way of electric heat pad or hot water bottle. The heat source should preferably be placed on the outside of the cage or have towels wrapped around it to prevent the animal from coming into direct contact with it.

Air temperature should be monitored closely as overheating may be fatal and underheating could also cause problems. An internal/external thermometer is a good way to monitor the temperature without disturbing and stressing the animal. Something to keep in mind is that young animals are not toys or playthings and require lots of rest and uninterrupted sleep in order to grow.

FORMULAS, SUPPLEMENTS, AND DAILY CALORIC REQUIREMENTS

There are many low-lactose milk formulas on the market that are suitable for hand raising young gliders (e.g., Wombaroo, Biolac, Digestelac [Sharp],

Perfect Pets, and Divetelac [Sharp]). It is important that once a formula has been chosen, you stick to it, as changing may cause unnecessary problems such as diarrhea.

Remember that these formulas are a food and young will need to have access to fresh water at all times.

WHAT TO FEED INITIALLY

It is essential to establish the young animals' age before beginning to hand raise. This may be determined by a combination of head and leg measurements, weight, and milestones (Table 9.2).

Prior to offering formula it may be necessary to give high-energy fluids like Lectade (Duvox) or Pedialyte (Ross), an electrolyte/glucose replacer (if the animal has diarrhea), or Glucodin (Boots) for a period of up to 24–48 hours. High-energy fluids help stabilize the animal, combat dehydration, maintain body temperature, and rest the stomach before different foods, such as artificial milk formulas, are introduced (White 1997). Milk formula can be made up slightly diluted at first and gradually increased to full strength over a 48-hour period to reduce the possibility of causing unnecessary diarrhea. Note: Oral fluids or formula should be offered only to a warm animal.

NURSING TECHNIQUES

There are many options for nursing young gliders including, lapping from the end of a syringe, using a bottle and teat (Perfect Pets), or lapping directly from a measuring spoon as seen in Figure 9.2. Personally, I have found the latter to be the easiest method for animal and carer alike. Young may be encouraged to lap by getting them to lap/lick at a small piece of banana. Then smear banana on the end of a measuring spoon full of milk and they will often start drinking the milk while licking at the banana (Fig. 9.2). If you choose to try using a bottle and teat, be sure the size of the teat is appropriate for the age of the young. Do not try and pry their mouth open, but gently direct the teat into the side of their mouth. Also when using a teat ensure that the hole in the end is not too large.

On several occasions difficult feeders have been enticed to lap, by first offering them a grape to lap the juices from. Once they are licking the grape, it can be hollowed out for the milk to sit in.

Young gliders still in the pouch usually need to be stimulated to urinate and defecate after each feed. Using a slightly moistened cotton ball or soft tissue to tickle, not rub, around the vent area can encourage stimulation. If you are having trouble feeding your young, try toileting them during feeding. Young gliders usually give you an indication of when they are about to urinate. The best way to describe it is that they hiss. This I have found to be most helpful while enjoying a cuddle, or when they are exploring on your new couch.

FREQUENCY OF FEEDING

Feeding is age dependant, the younger the glider the more often they are fed. An unfurred glider is fed every one to two hours, just-furred gliders every four hours, gradually being reduced to once or twice

Table 9.2. Growth and Development of Young Sugar Gliders *Petaurus breviceps breviceps* from South East Queensland

Age (day)	Weight (g)	Feed (ml/day)	Milestones
1	0.2		Mouth and forelimbs most developed feature
20	0.8		Ears free from head, papillae of mystacial vibrissae visible
35	2.0	1.0	Mystacial vibrissae (whiskers) erupt, ears pigmented
40	3.0	1.5	Start to pigment on shoulders, eye slits present
60	12	3	Detaching from teat, fur emerging, dorsal stripe developing
70	20	4	Eyes open, fully furred, left in nest
80	35	6	Fur lengthens
90	44	7	
100	54	8	Emerging from nest, start eating solids
130	78		Weaned

Source: Booth (1993).

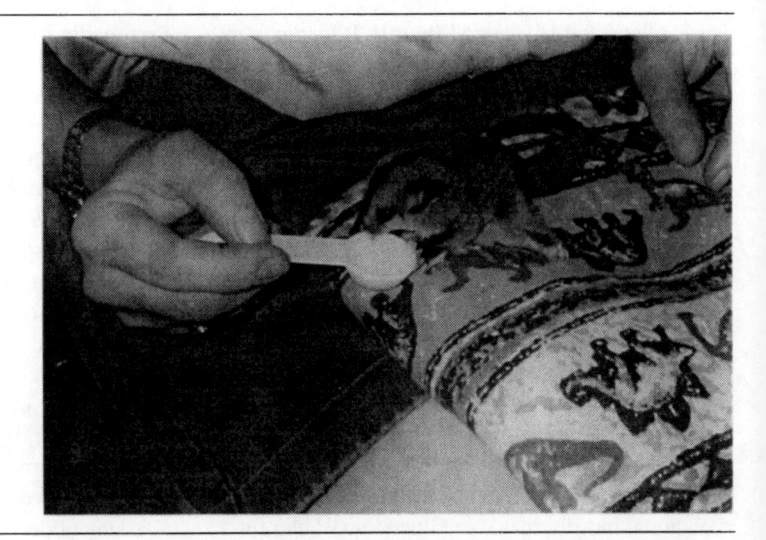

Figure 9.2. Juvenile male lapping from end of a measuring spoon.

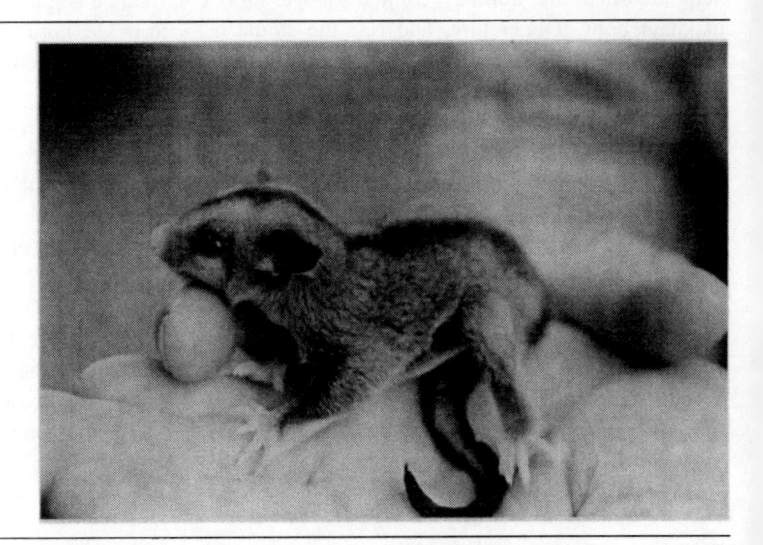

Figure 9.3. Juvenile male sugar glider.

daily prior to weaning. It is important to maintain consistency when feeding young animals.

AMOUNTS TO FEED

The amount of formula offered varies depending on the age of your glider, as seen in Table 9.2. The temperature of formula is very important and should always be checked on your wrist prior to offering it to your young. Some animals will not drink if the milk is just a little too cold or may burn their mouths if it's a little too hot. It is important not to overfeed young, as this can cause diarrhea. Once made up, formula should never be kept for longer than a 24-hour period. If formula is left out of the fridge for any extended period, it should be discarded and fresh formula made up. Strict hygiene, such as personal hygiene, sterilization of all bottles, teats, and spoons after each use, should be maintained.

EXPECTED WEIGHT GAIN

During the first two weeks, while your young settle in, it is a good idea to weigh them daily. This may be decreased to once every couple of days, then once a week, and so on until as an adult they are being weighed monthly. As scales may vary, it is suggested that you use the same one each time.

Initially, in the first 48 hours, there may be little or no weight gain and sometimes there may even be a loss. Once your glider has adjusted to his/her new diet and sleeping arrangements, you should see a gain in weight every second day if not daily (Table 9.2).

Once your glider has started eating solids, the increase in weight will become more substantial. Be cautious of overfeeding as obesity can be a problem. An adult male should weigh 115–160 g while females should weigh 95–135 g.

HOUSING

Housing requirements vary depending on the age of your glider. No matter what the age, it is very important to maintain strict hygiene standards with their cage, furnishings, bedding, food, and water bowls.

Pouch Young

Sixty-day-old young require a small pouch liner, which is placed inside a thick pouch. Old fleecy lined sweatshirts make great pouch liners when cut up and sewn into a pouch, 18 cm × 18 cm, and knitted woolen pouches work well for the outer pouch, 22 cm × 22 cm. A small cage, 42 cm × 32 cm × 36 cm, with small-gauge wire is ideal for young not yet emerged or just emerging from the pouch. The cage should be, escape proof, free from any sharp protrusions, and located in a suitable position away from domestic pets and noise.

Set the cage on top of a heat pad and monitor the temperature to attain the desired warmth, furred young at 82°F (28°C) and furless young at 89.6°F (32°C). Increase or decrease bedding around the pouch to help achieve this.

As the glider starts to emerge from the pouch ensure that you have a small water container available at all times and that there are small branches in the cage for chewing and climbing on.

Weaning/Adult

For a single glider, place the pouch inside a bird's nest box (wooden) inside a cage that is approximately 100 cm × 100 cm × 100 cm (39 in × 39 in × 39 in), with 1 cm × 1 cm gauge wire. The cage should preferably have a large door to add and remove furnishings as required.

For more than one glider, more nesting boxes and pouches should be made available to allow them to sleep separately if fighting should occur. The size of the cage also needs to be evaluated when adding more gliders. Personally, I have housed two gliders in a cage that was 150 cm long × 150 cm high and 100 cm deep (59 in × 59 in × 39 in). The two animals housed together were a compatible pair. The more gliders, the larger the cage should be.

Ensure there are plenty of climbing branches of different thickness and toys to keep them occupied. Toys that are used for birds, such as ladders, bells, balls, even stuffed animals, or something as simple as a piece of PVC pipe or small cardboard box will keep them busy. However, it is important to remember that any toy used should be free from sharp protrusions. Should you encounter problems with your animals chewing or ingesting parts of a toy or PVC piping, this toy should be removed. Branches that are loosely fitted to the cage will allow movement and will give the glider a challenge when climbing. Placement of perches is also important, fewer branches around the sides of the cage will encourage your glider to jump rather than run to the other side of the cage.

Nontoxic browse should be available at all times for the glider to chew on and also for lining nest boxes. Cages should be free from bits of wire and sharp protrusions that could cause harm to your glider. When placing food and water bowls inside the cage, be sure to put them away from any perches to prevent fouling from feces and urine.

Cage sizes for mature adults are a guide only, as bigger is always better.

IMMUNE STATUS AND SPECIAL NEEDS

There is no specific information available on the immune function in gliders; however, they appear to be immunologically fairly robust.

TIME TO WEANING

Weaning occurs at 100–110 days, and forced dispersal may occur when animals are between seven and ten months of age.

TIPS FOR WEANING FROM FORMULA TO SOLID FOOD

The food we provide for our captive animals should ideally mimic that of their natural diet (Table 9.3).

A nutritionally balanced diet, such as the one used at Australian Wildlife Experience, Dreamworld in Australia (see Table 9.4), will help to prevent problems such as obesity, viral and bacterial infections, nutritional deficiency diseases, and reduced breeding success. Resist the temptation to feed sweet foods, soluble carbohydrates, such as

Table 9.3. Definition and Composition of Dietary Components of Wild Sugar Gliders

Component	Definition	Composition
Gum	Exuded on trunks and branches by some species of acacia to bind sites of damage, particularly those made by boring insects	Complex associations of polysaccharides (cellulose, starch, and sugars), low in protein (1.3–3.1%)
Arthropods	Moths, scarab beetles, caterpillars, weevils, and small spiders	Vary in composition but contain in the region of 50–75% protein and 5–20% fat on a dry wet basis
Sap	Liquid obtained by biting through the bark of some eucalypts into the phloem	1.4% or less protein, predominantly carbohydrate of which 70–85% is sucrose
Manna	Sugary exudate produced at sites of insect damage on the leaves and branches of certain eucalypts and angophoras	Composition of sugars slightly changed from phloem sap by the action of insects' salivary enzymes
Honeydew	Sap-sucking insects ingest large quantities of sap to obtain sufficient protein and then excrete surplus carbohydrates as honeydew	About 79% mono and oligosaccharides and 9% polysaccharides
Nectar	Produced in usable quantities by larger eucalypt flowers (>5 mm diameter)	Mainly simple sugars

Source: Booth (1993).

nectar and mixtures containing honey or sugars and very sweet fruit, such as different melons. Also avoid processed carbohydrates such as breads.

To help your glider with the transition from formula to solids, you can begin by leaving a variety of their intended diet out overnight for them to sample if they choose. The size of the pieces should be small and may even need to be grated or mashed up. Spending time with your young of an evening is a great time to encourage them to sample small pieces, or juices from your fingers. Most gliders will begin the transition to solids if solids are available to them. Food bowls should be shallow and several bowls should be available if the cage is home to more than one glider.

COMMON MEDICAL PROBLEMS

Some common medical problems include

- Cloacal prolapse, which can be stimulated with excessive rubbing while toileting young.
- Obesity, which occurs regularly with captive animals and should be monitored closely. Body condition of gliders can be gauged by the thickness of their gliding membrane; it should be thin and stretchy not thick with fat.
- Teeth root abscesses, general tooth and gum disease, periodontal disease, tartar accumulation are all common, and can be caused by incorrect diet.
- Wounds, eye problems, and corneal ulcers from incompatible gliders fighting can be common.
- Nutritional osteodystrophy or hind limb paresis/paralysis is a commonly reported disease of pet sugar gliders, but has never been reported in zoo collections (Booth 1998).

Some drugs that have been used without ill effect are:

- Diazepam, 0.5–1.0 mg/kg, for sedation
- Isoflurane administered with oxygen via vaporizer, for anesthetic
- Drontal Worming Suspension for Puppies and Small Dogs; Bayer, Australia LTD, which contains febantel, 15 mg/ml; Pyrantel Embonate, 14.4 mg/ml at a dose rate of 0.1 ml/100 g; Ivomec(ivermectin), concentration 0.8 mg/ml at a dose rate of 0.2 mg/kg; Benzelmin oxfendazole, concentration 200 mg/ml at a dose rate of 10–20 mg/kg, all for worming
- Clavulox, amoxicillin, for antibiotic

Table 9.4. Daily Diet for Captive Sugar Gliders Provided at Australian Wildlife Experience, Dreamworld

Daily Diet	
5 g	Sweet corn kernels
1	Dog chow / Eukanuba
6 g	Vegetables (sweet potato, carrot, apple, but no melons or sweet fruits)
2	Mealworms
2 g	Sprouted seed
1 tsp	Nectar (see recipe below)

Supplements	
5	Pollen grains (Once per week)
2	Grey stripe sunflower seed (Once per week)
1	Almond (Once per week)
3	Sultanas/raisin (3–4 times per week)
1 g	Eco-pet (Once per week)
Insects (moths, etc.) (3–4 times per week)	

Nectar Mix	
1.25	Shelled egg
41.5 g	High-protein baby cereal (Farex)
167 ml	Cold water
335 ml	Honey
0.5 g	Calcivet
0.5 g	Soluvet
500 ml	Hot water

Table 9.5. Selected Physiological Data for Sugar Glider

Parameter	Reference Range
Heart Rate	200–300/min*
Respiratory Rate	16–40/min*
Body Temperature	36.3°C
Body temperature in torpor	≥ 15°C
Thermoneutral zone	27–31°C
Basal Metabolic Rate	2.54 w $kg^{0.75}$

*Under isoflurane anaesthesia

Some drugs cause problems. Tiletamine/zolazepam has been associated with mortality of three apparently healthy squirrel gliders when used at a dose of 10 mg/kg intramuscularly (Booth 1993). It is therefore not recommended for use in sugar gliders, although this drug combination is a very useful anesthetic agent in possum species (Booth 1993).

Any antibiotic used may upset gut flora, which may cause diarrhea. All drugs used on your animal should be given with veterinary advice only and correct dose rates administered.

Selected physiological data for sugar gliders can be found in Table 9.5.

CAPTIVE VERSUS WILD

An animal's life in captivity should always mimic that of its wild cousins. Sugar gliders are very social, active animals in the wild and there's nothing better than seeing them jumping and gliding from tree to tree in their natural environment. These animals are very easily imprinted when hand rearing, as they require much time and attention.

If your glider is being hand raised to be released, it needs to be established with a colony of gliders that are also to be released, prior to releasing. Another important factor is familiarization of local food sources and the presentation of large browse branches to encourage foraging for insects, gum, and sap.

SOCIALIZATION OR REINTRODUCTION TECHNIQUES

A dominant male glider will continually scent mark all the members of his colony with the scent gland found on his head. Juvenile sugar gliders of either sex enjoy having this gland rubbed.

Wild gliders live in family groups or colonies, so it is important for your gliders' well-being to have a minimum of two animals housed together, especially if you are unable to spend ample time with them. Depending on the size of the cage and compatibility of the animals, you may be able to house up to seven individuals together. Introduction of any new animal to the colony should be done very carefully. There are several methods of introducing new animals to a cage; they can be referred to as a soft or hard release. A soft method would be to place the new animal inside a smaller holding cage within the larger cage for several weeks, then release the new animal into the enclosure. A hard release would be to dust all animals and bedding with Fidos Free Itch powder or talcum powder and put them all together. A second method of hard release would be to cross scent all the animals that are to be housed together. This can be achieved by rubbing their scent glands together and also by covering them in each other's urine. All methods will require you to check each animal daily for injuries, as fighting is almost certain to occur.

SOURCES FOR PRODUCTS MENTIONED

Biolac, PO Box 93, Bonnyrigg NSW, Australia 2177; Ph: +61-2-9823-9874

Boots Co., Australia Pty Ltd., 101 Waterloo Road, North Ryde NSW, Australia 2113; Ph: 1-800-226-766; FAX: +61-2-9870-6100

Duvox Pty Ltd., Brotherford NSW, Australia

Eco Pet (Lamb with Vegetables): This is a type of processed dog food in Australia and contains crude protein 15% min, crude fat 12.5% min, crude fiber, 3% min, and salt 0.8%. From Pet Health Food Product, 17 Amberley Crescent, Dandenong Victoria 3175, Australia. Ph: +61-3-9792-1505; 1-800-659-940

Farex/High Protein Baby Cereal. From Heinz Watties Australasia, Locked Bags 57, Malvern Vic., Australia 3144; Ph: +61-3-9864-5757; FAX: +61-3-9864-5524

Nipples and formulas in the United States: Perfect Pets, Inc., 23180 Sherwood Road, Belleville, MI 48111-9306; 1-734-461-1362; FAX 1-734-461-2858; E-mail GSCHROCK1@aol.com; PetAg Inc., 261 Keyes Ave., Hampshire, IL 60140; 1-800-323-0877, 1-800-323-6878; www.petag.com

Reckitt Benckiser, 44 Wharf Road, West Ryde NSW 2114, Australia

Ross Products Division, Abbott Laboratories, Columbus, OH 43215-1724; 1-800-986-8510; www.abbott.com, www.ross.com

Sharp Brothers Lab, 12 Hope Street, Ermington NSW, Australia 2115. Ph: +61-2-9858-5622; FAX: +61-2-9858-5957

Wombaroo Food Products, PO Box 151, Glen Osmond, SA Australia 5064; Ph: +61-8-8277-7788; FAX: +61-8-8277-7045

REFERENCES

Booth, Rosemary. 1993. General husbandry and medicine of sugar gliders. In *Current veterinary therapy XIII*, edited by Robert Kirk. Philadelphia, PA: Saunders.
———. 1998. General husbandry of sugar gliders, handout, Wildlife seminar—marsupials, 28 March, at Department of Animal Sciences, Ithaca Campus, Brisbane Institute of TAFE, Fulcher Road, Red Hill, Queensland, Australia.
White, Sharon. 1997. First aid emergency care. In *Caring for Australian wildlife*, edited by Ken Eastwood. Terrey Hills, NSW 2084, Australia: Australian Geographic Pty Ltd.

ADDITIONAL READING MATERIAL

Booth, R. General husbandry and medicine of sugar gliders. In *Current veterinary therapy XIII*, edited by Robert Kirk. Philadelphia, PA: Saunders.
MacPherson, Caroline. 1997. *Sugar gliders, a complete pet owner's manual*. Hauppauge, NY: Barron.

10
Macropods

Rosemary Booth

NATURAL HISTORY

There are over 50 Australian species and 15 New Guinea species of kangaroos, wallabies, and rat-kangaroos grouped in the superfamily Macropodoidea (Flannery 1995; Maynes 1989). The main species kept in zoos are red-necked wallaby (*Macropus rufogriseus*), red kangaroo (*Megaleia rufa*), eastern grey kangaroo (*Macropus giganteus*), western grey kangaroo (*Macropus fuliginosus*), parma wallaby (*Macropus parma*), and tammar wallaby (*Macropus eugenii*). Currently, the total numbers of these species held in zoos contributing to ISIS (International Species Information System) are 1039, 849, 324, 265, 165, and 121, respectively (subspecies grouped). Table 10.1 lists some natural history data for these species.

The feature that most clearly distinguishes marsupials from most other mammals is the immaturity of their young at birth (Tyndale-Biscoe and Janssens 1988). This places a greater emphasis on lactation in marsupial reproduction. Some species of kangaroo can simultaneously suckle two young of different ages from adjacent teats, secreting milk of two different concentrations (Tyndale-Biscoe and Janssens 1988).

The best studied macropodid is *M. eugenii* and its development is indicative of the general pattern. It is born after a 28-day gestation weighing 300–400 mg (0.01% of maternal weight). The joey remains permanently attached to one teat for one hundred days by which time it weighs approximately 100 g. At about day 140, the eyes open, the ears reflect from the head, and the underfur is visible. By day 160, the joey is able to stand, the pelage is thickening, and it produces a concentrated urine indicative of complete nephrogenesis. By day 180, thyroid function is fully developed and the joey is now homeothermic. The joey may be seen with its head out of pouch nibbling grass at this time but the first pouch emergence occurs around day 190. Weaning can be considered to commence from this time as herbage forms an increasing proportion of the diet, however peak milk intake occurs at day 240. The joey permanently exits the pouch at about day 250 and ceases to suckle between days 300 and 350 (Tyndale-Biscoe and Janssens 1988).

Macropods have been hand reared successfully in Australia for many decades, with most orphans resulting from road trauma or shooting. The greatest wealth of experience has developed with volunteer wildlife carers who primarily hand rear animals for release back to the wild.

The challenges in hand rearing macropods are to simulate the functions of the pouch (which provides both psychological security and a temperature controlled environment until the joey is homeothermic) and to offer a satisfactory milk replacer, which can mimic the changing needs of the developing marsupial during pouch life.

RECORD KEEPING

During hand raising it is important to keep a daily record of milk intake, fecal and urine production, fecal consistency, hydration, and behavioral notes including attitude and appetite. Body weight should be measured daily initially, but once stabilized, weekly is sufficient. It is also desirable to measure head length, tail length, and foot length monthly and plot all measurements on a graph to emphasize trends. Any unexpected plateaus in weight gain or linear growth are indications for a full clinical examination by a veterinarian.

EQUIPMENT

Commercially made latex teats are available for macropods (Smith; Wombaroo). The hole in the teat is best made with sharp scissors and should be big

Table 10.1. Selected Natural History Information for Macropods Commonly Kept in Captivity in Zoos

Species	Macropus rufogriseus	Megaleia rufa	Macropus giganteus	Macropus fuliginosus	Macropus parma	Macropus eugenii
Adult female weight	14 kg	27.3 kg	27.6 kg	27.6 kg	3.5 kg	5.0 kg
Neonatal weight	450 mg	817 mg	740 mg	828 mg	510 mg	370 mg
First off teat		70 d			120 d	105 d
Permanent pouch exit	270 d	235 d	319 d	310 d	212 d	250 d
Weaning	360 d	360 d	540 d	540 d	300 d	270 d
Sexual maturity	11–21 m (F) 13 m (M)	14–20 m (F) 24–36 m (M)	18 m (F) 48 m (M)	14 m (F) 31 m (M)	9–12 m (F) 13 m (M)	8 m (F) 24 m (M)
Birth season (Australia)	Jan-Aug	All year	Oct-Mar	Oct-Mar	All year	Jan-Jun
Estrous cycle	31.9	34.8±0.6	45.6±9.8	34.9±4.4	41.8±7	30.6
Gestation	29.4	33.2±0.2	36.4±1.6	30.6±2.6	34.5±0.1	29.3
Postpartum estrus	Yes	Yes	No	No	No	Yes
Embryonic diapause	Yes	Yes	Yes	No	Yes	Yes

Source: Data from Tyndale-Biscoe and Renfree (1987).

enough that when inverted, milk drips very slowly from the teat. Latex teats need to be replaced regularly as they become sticky or the hole becomes too large. The teats fit onto a range of plastic or glass bottles. Hygiene is extremely important. All feeding equipment should be kept free of milk residue by washing in detergent and scrubbing with a bottle brush. They must then be thoroughly rinsed before being sterilized.

Equipment required to hand rear macropods includes:

Artificial pouch (e.g., sheepskin bag)
Cotton pouch liners (e.g., pillow case)
Heat source (e.g., electric heat pad with thermostat)
Thermometer
Glass/plastic bottles, 50–200 ml
Macropod teats
Tissues/cotton wool for toileting
Moisturizing lotion (e.g., aqueous cream)
Electronic scales for weighing
Calipers and tape measure
Antibacterial solution/boiling water for sterilizing bottles and teats
Antibacterial washing powder to hygienically launder pouch liners

CRITERIA FOR INTERVENTION

Furless or lightly furred joeys are under constant close maternal care within the pouch. If a joey of this age is found away from its mother, then intervention is required. It is a survival technique of macropods to jettison pouch young when being chased by predators, and this occurs in captivity with moderate frequency in response to a range of stressful stimuli such as manual capture by keepers, or chasing by other animals. The pouch young is "thrown" by simultaneous relaxation of the pouch sphincter muscle and contraction of the longitudinal subcutaneous muscles of the pouch that in effect makes the pouch disappear. Very small pouch young, which are still permanently attached to the nipple, are not a great burden to a fleeing mother, and furred young, which can come and go from the pouch, can often be safely reunited with their mother after a chase. The at-risk group is the unfurred, intermittently attached, pouch-dependent young. Unweaned orphans will also require hand raising. Fostering of valuable species to lactating females of a different species but of similar (1) maternal size, (2) length of pouch life, and (3) stage of lactation is possible. All three criteria must be met and the young of the recipient mother must be removed to achieve successful cross-fostering. This has been used as a tool in endangered species programs to "double clutch" valuable macropod species but the technique is still relatively experimental (Merchant and Sharman 1966; Schultz 1999).

ASSESSMENT OF THE POUCH YOUNG

On presentation, the joey should receive a full clinical examination including temperature, pulse, and respiration (TPR). A normal uncompromised joey should resist handling, seek a pouch, and vocalize. Marsupials have a lower metabolic rate than eutherian (placental) mammals and this is reflected in the slow resting heart rate and low body temperature. Normal rectal temperature is 96–99°F (35.5–37.0°C) (Speare 1988). Ensure the thermometer is placed in the rectum, not just the cloaca, to obtain an accurate indication of core body temperature. The resting heart rate for adult *M. rufa* is 40 bpm measured by telemetry (Fanning and Dawson 1989). Smaller species and young animals have a higher resting heart rate (range 70–200 bpm). Normal respiratory rate is in the range of 20–40 bpm. Normal macropodid young should have prominent and readily palpable paired cervical thymi. Prolonged elevation of cortisol for any reason may cause premature thymic involution and effect ability to respond to infections.

INITIAL CARE AND STABILIZATION

Orphaned or mismothered young are usually presented hypothermic, so warming in a pouch with a heating unit set at 90–93°F (32–34°C) is the first requirement. A digital thermometer with a probe can be used to monitor the air temperature surrounding the joey to avoid overheating. Young marsupials will be distressed if they are not enclosed in a substitute pouch. Subcutaneous or intravenous fluid therapy with solutions containing glucose is indicated if there has been prolonged hypothermia and milk deprivation. The lateral tail veins or recurrent tarsal veins are suitable sites for intravenous infusions. The joey should be weighed and measured during the initial examination so that its age can be estimated and its feeding requirements can be calculated while it is warming up.

FORMULAS

Throughout lactation, the composition of marsupial milk changes, generally with increasing levels of fat and protein and decreasing levels of carbohydrate in late lactation. Compared with eutherians, suckling macropods have a low tolerance for lactose that is not due to low levels of intestinal lactase activity, but the result of intracellular localization of lactase activity (Messer, Crisp, and Czolij 1989). This means that lactose cannot be digested into monosaccharides until after it has been transported into enterocytes, apparently by relatively slow pinocytosis. Eutherians digest lactose with an enzyme located extracellularly on the microvillous membrane (Messer et al. 1989). For this reason, low-lactose milks are preferable for macropods.

Most work on macropod lactation has been carried out on *M. eugenii*. In this species total protein increases significantly during lactation and consists predominantly of whey proteins. The relative concentration of amino acids is quite constant with some exceptions such as the increase in sulphur-rich amino acids during hair follicle development. In early lactation the lipid concentration is low (2% of whole milk). There is a dramatic increase in lipids to around 25% that coincides with the decline in carbohydrates and the emergence of the young from the pouch (Merchant 1989). At this time there is a increase in energy requirement in the young for independent thermoregulation and locomotion. Triglycerides account for more than 90% of milk lipids throughout lactation. The predominant fatty acids in the triglyceride fraction are palmitic and oleic acid. This pattern has been confirmed in *M. r. banksianus* and *M. rufa* (Merchant et al. 1989).

It has been suggested that changes in milk carbohydrate concentration are related to the establishment of conditions in the gut suitable for the microorganism populations necessary for the digestion of herbage (Janssens and Messer 1988). In *M. eugenii* the carbohydrate concentration varies from 3% on day 7 peaking at 13% at day 180 then declining rapidly to 1% until the end of lactation (Merchant 1989). For most of lactation the predominant carbohydrates are the higher oligosaccharides with a pattern of increasing size followed by a decrease in size to monosaccharides by the end of lactation. Galactose and glucose predominate as the major saccharide units.

The energy content of *M. eugenii* milk increases as lactation proceeds from 250 kJ/100 g at day 7, to 500 kJ/100 g at day 180 with a rapid increase to a peak of 1150 kJ/100 g by days 250 to 280 (Green, Merchant, and Newgrain 1988). This increase in energy content is directly due to the increased lipid in late lactation.

Copper and iron concentrations are substantially higher in marsupial milks than eutherian milks, particularly in early lactation when the neonatal liver has a limited storage capacity. The copper concentration is initially around 5 mg/l decreasing to 0.1–1.0 mg/l; and the iron concentration is initially around 20–23 mg/l decreasing to 5–7 mg/l after pouch emergence for *M. eugenii* and *M. r. banksianus* (Merchant 1989). By comparison, in eutherians copper concentration in milk is in the order of 0.1–0.6 mg/l and iron, 0.3–0.5 mg/l. Supplementation is not generally required for hand reared joeys, but should be considered if attempting to hand rear very young orphans.

Wombaroo and Biolac (Smith; Perfect Pets Inc.; see Resources below) are commercially available marsupial milks with different concentrations of the major components to match the needs of joeys in different stages of development. The development of Wombaroo macropod milk replacers appears to have been associated with better growth rates and better coat condition although there is a lack of objective, controlled experimental evidence to allow recommendation of one product over another. Divetelac (Sharpe), a product with a long history of success with macropods, has recently changed formulation, so the new product cannot be assumed to be as suitable. Passionate debate has occurred on which is the best milk to use, but it is possible to raise joeys on almost any low-lactose formula provided close attention is paid to achieving an adequate growth rate and to overall management.

WHAT TO FEED INITIALLY

Orphaned macropods are very susceptible to dietary diarrhea as they adjust from mother's milk to an artificial formula. It is good practice to dilute formula with an oral rehydration electrolyte solution on the first two to three days in captivity to allow adjustment to the new formula. Half strength on day 1, two-thirds on day 2, three-quarter strength on day 3, and full-strength milk on day 4 is an example of a suitable regime. If it takes longer than this to adjust to full strength milk there is the risk of insufficient energy being supplied to the joey.

A moderately strict routine of feeding should be established for each stage of development. Milk should be fed at a temperature close to body temperature (30–36°C, 86–97°F). This is generally achieved by immersion in a warm-water bath. If the joey is a slow feeder, rewarming during the feed may be required. Temperature of milk affects acceptance, so if a joey is a difficult feeder, double-check the milk temperature with a thermometer. Table 10.2 summarizes the requirements of *Macropus rufogriseus banksianus* as a model for other macropod species.

NURSING TECHNIQUES

Joeys feed best in the pouch, curled in a half circle on the lap of their carer, who has one hand covering the eyes and guiding the joey to stay on the teat (see Fig. 10.1). This prevents disturbing visual stimuli from distracting the joey. A plastic bottle is an advantage when teaching a joey to suckle because drops of milk can be carefully squeezed from the end of the teat. Patience is essential. Aspiration is common. Don't attempt to feed new joeys until they have been warmed up or they will be unable to suckle properly and will be more likely to aspirate milk. Some joeys pass milk from their nostrils intermittently during feeding, which is disconcerting to the carer but is rarely associated with aspiration. This can be minimized by reducing the size of the hole in the teat to slow feeding, and perhaps by increasing the frequency of feeding to avoid frantic sucking.

The macropod mother stimulates the joey to void urine and feces by licking its cloaca (Fig. 10.2a). The hand-reared joey needs to be toileted after every feed by gently stroking the cloaca with a moistened tissue or cotton wool while it is within the pouch (Fig. 10.2b).

TUBE FEEDING

Tube feeding is rarely required, but if it is, nasogastric tubing is simpler than the orogastric route. Lubricate the tube and direct it inferiorly through the nasal cavity.

FREQUENCY OF FEEDING

The number of feeds per day depends on the age and state of health of the animal. Small furless or just-furred joeys require small frequent feeds every two to three hours including throughout the night. Older furred joeys require feeding every three to four hours. The amount and frequency of feeding gradually decreases once the joey starts to leave the pouch and begins eating solids. Table 10.2 indicates the frequency of feeds required for the various stages of joey development.

AMOUNTS TO FEED

In general joeys should be fed approximately 10–20% of their body weight daily. Wombaroo provides charts of total daily intake derived from weight $^{0.75}$ and length for various species. Divide the total daily intake evenly by the number of feeds per

Table 10.2. Developmental Milestones and Requirements for Hand-Reared Macropodids Based on the Red-necked Wallaby *Macropus rufogriseus banksianus*

Age (months)	Weight (approx)	Features	Milk feeds	Warmth	Special requirements
4	200 g	Furless, eyes closed, ears down but free, yellow custard feces.	7–8 bottles/ 24 hrs	32°C	Pouch bound. Apply lotion to skin twice daily.
5	450 g	Furless, eyes open, ears erect, thicker yellow feces.	6 bottles/ 24 hrs	32°C	Pouch bound. Apply lotion to skin daily.
6	800 g	Very fine covering of fur. Concentrated urine. Toothpaste consistency feces.	5 bottles/ 24 hrs	30°C	Pouch bound. Apply lotion to tail and feet daily. Offer dry grass and soil within pouch.
7	1200 g	Short sleek fur, homeothermic, soft olive green pellets.	4 bottles/ 24 hrs	28°C	Starting to emerge from pouch. Very incoordinated. Offer access to grass outside with constant access to pouch and under supervision.
8	1700 g	Fur becoming fluffy. Soft dark green pellets.	3 bottles/ 24 hrs	20–25°C	Gaining confidence out of pouch. Access to well-fenced grassy enclosure during the day. Group orphans together.
9	2300 g	Dense fur. Firm dark pellets.	2–1 bottles/ 24 hrs	Ambient	Very confident out of pouch. Access to well-fenced, predator-proof, grassy enclosure day and night.
10	3000 g	Coordinated and increasingly flighty.	Weaned	Ambient	Pouch may be removed. Provide natural shelter. Reduce human contact.
11–12	4–5 kg	Independent			No human contact if for release.

Source: Modified from Sharon White, unpublished.

day recommended in Table 10.2 for the stage of development.

EXPECTED WEIGHT GAIN

If body weight changes are plotted on a graph beside expected growth for that species, then any slowing of growth will be immediately evident and action can be taken to discover the problem before it is too late. Relative growth rates are constant for most of pouch life up until pouch vacation when growth rates slow. Expected weight gain of *M. giganteus* and *M. rufogriseus banksianus* young are shown in Figure 10.3.

HOUSING

The young macropod requires an accessible pouch at all times until permanent pouch exit, access to grazing and/or browsing, and drinking water in a container that can't be knocked over (Fig. 10.4). At night they should be placed in a predator-proof enclosure with a roof, and opaque but flexible fencing. When macropods take flight they rush head long into fences often with fatal consequences. Loosely strained chain-link fence covered with dark shade cloth is ideal. Posts supporting fences should be on the outside so animals can't crash into them as they "fence run." Small macropods require tussocks

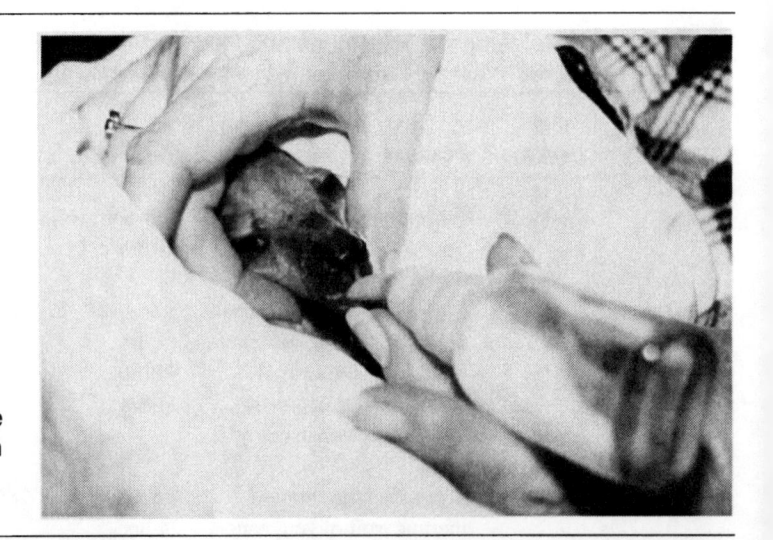

Figure 10.1. Feeding a five-month-old, furless joey from a 50-ml glass bottle and latex macropod teat. Joeys should be fed within the pouch to maintain temperature until they are homeothermic.

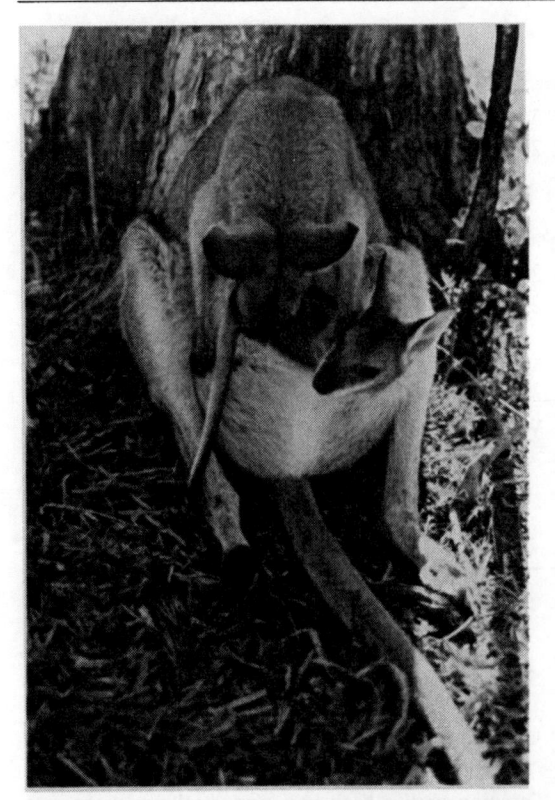

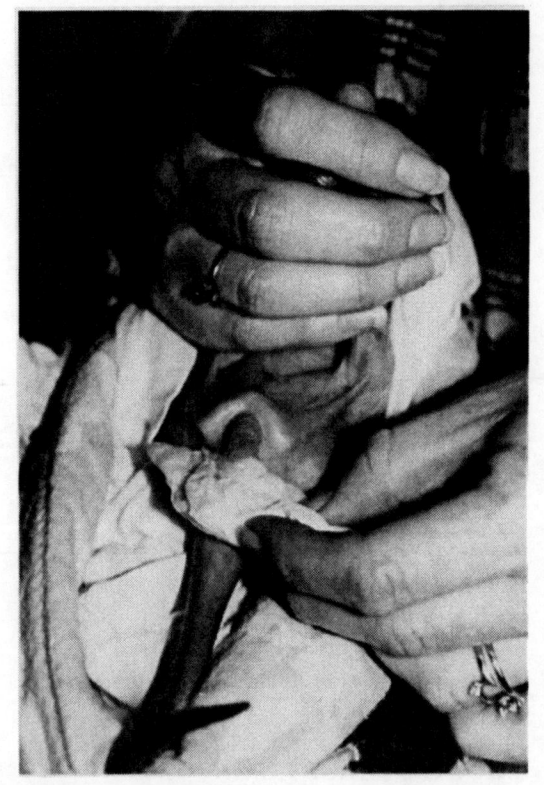

Figure 10.2. (a) The mother stimulates the joey to void urine and feces by licking its cloaca. (b) The hand-reared joey needs to be toileted after every feed by gently stroking the cloaca with a moistened tissue or cotton wool while it is within the pouch.

or low shrubs to provide cover and a sense of security. Judicious planting in a corridor parallel to the fence assists capture. Shade trees or artificial shelters are also necessary.

PASSIVE AND ACTIVE IMMUNITY

Maternal immunoglobulins and milk macrophages play a critical role in the protection of pouch young

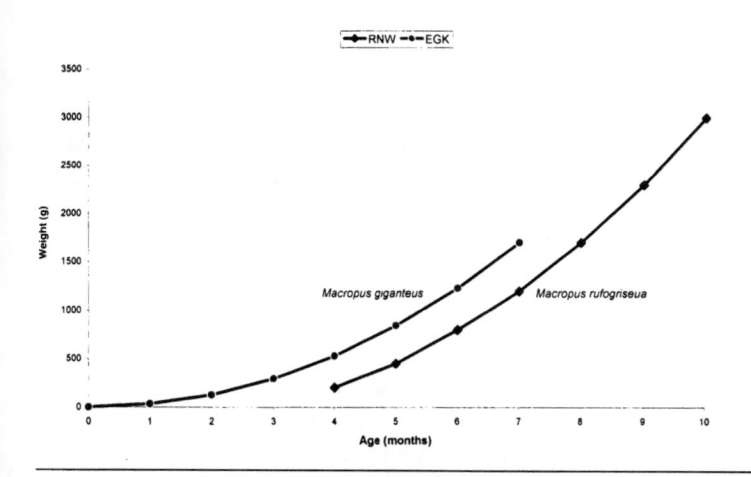

Figure 10.3. Expected body weight increase with age for eastern grey kangaroo (*Macropus giganteus*) and red-necked wallaby (*Macropus rufogriseus*). (Based on Wombaroo information booklet and and Sharon White, unpublished.)

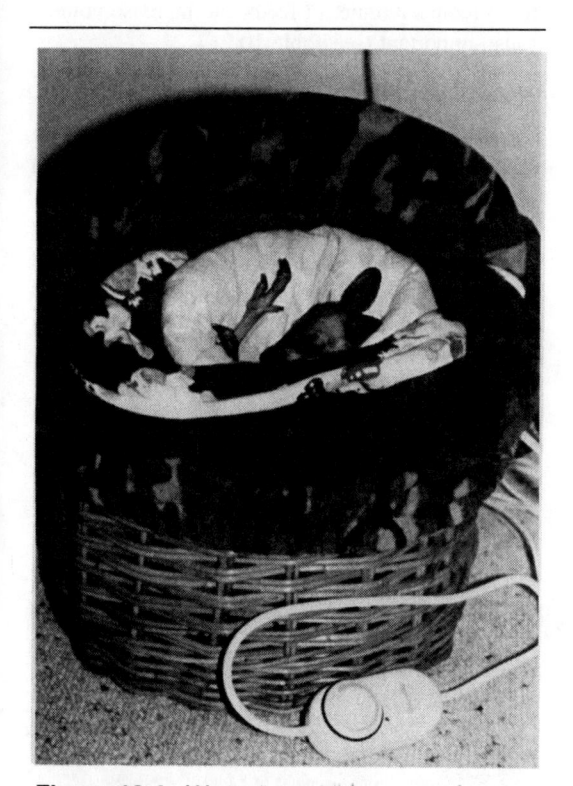

Figure 10.4. Warm "pouch" for young joeys.

against infection (Merchant 1989). A colostrumlike secretion has been identified at birth in marsupials (Deane and Cooper 1988). In the Quokka (*Setonix brachyurus*), maternal immunoglobulins in the milk are absorbed from the gut until first pouch exit at 170 days. In this species, this passively acquired antibody has a half-life of eight to nine days and has virtually disappeared from the blood four to six weeks after cessation of suckling (Yadav 1971).

Active immunity starts to develop from approximately day 10 when Hassall's corpuscles can first be identified in cervical thymus of *S. brachyurus*, and antibody response to antigen can be detected. In common wallaroo (*Macropus robustus*), pouch young serum has been found to have an IgG level of 0.2 mg/ml at day 14, which rose only slightly by day 95. A sudden rise in IgG was detected, initiated between day 95 and 110, which coincides with the first release of the teat, which presumably makes the ingestion of harmful bacteria more likely (Deane and Cooper 1988). The orphaned young raised on artificial milk is at greater risk from infectious disease, and high standards of hygiene are essential.

POUCH EMERGENCE

It appears that thermal intolerance between mother and young is the main stimulus for the joey to vacate the pouch (Janssens and Rogers 1989). As the joey matures it gradually gains thermoregulatory independence. Most macropods finally leave the pouch at the time when they are approximately 20% of the maternal weight (Rose 1989). The age at pouch emergence for six species of macropods is shown in Table 10.1. During hand raising it is important not to prematurely subject a joey to separation from its pouch.

TIME TO WEANING FROM FORMULA TO SOLID FOOD

There is variation in the time taken from first ingestion of grass when the head first emerges from the pouch, to complete weaning depending on the species (Fig. 10.5). Table 10.1 provides an indication of the age to expect weaning for various species. Table 10.2 provides a guide to when to reduce bottle feeds.

TIPS FOR WEANING

Macropod joeys should be offered solid foods from the time they are finely furred and sit with their head out of the pouch. Fresh grass with roots and dirt attached, chopped apple and carrot, lucerne pellets, soft hay, and browse (edible leaves such as melaleuca and eucalyptus) are all suitable. Kangaroos and wallabies are foregut fermenters and inoculation of the gut with appropriate bacteria presumably occurs from exposure to the feces of adult animals of the same species. Hand-raised joeys should be given access to fresh adult fecal pellets that have been confirmed free of parasite oocysts.

COMMON MEDICAL PROBLEMS

Diarrhea

Diarrhea is the most common problem encountered with orphaned joeys. To successfully manage the joey with diarrhea, a systematic approach must be adopted and a prompt response is required. Initially diet, temperature stress, and psychological distress are the most common causes of diarrhea. As the symptoms persist, and the gut flora is altered, specific and opportunistic pathogens begin to play a bigger role. Chronic mismanaged diarrhea leads to irritable bowel syndrome with consequences of malabsorption and failure to thrive.

Noninfectious Causes

Diet

Changes in diet cause changes in gut motility. As the joey adjusts from its mother's milk to any artificial formula, there is often a transitional period of diarrhea or, less often, constipation. Milk should be iso-osmotic with plasma to avoid osmotic diarrhea. Lush green grass can also cause diarrhea during weaning.

Overfeeding

Feeding too much or too frequently can exacerbate any problems that the gut may be having adjusting to the milk, so careful calculation of total daily intake and estimation of number of feeds required per day is important. Correct identification of timing to reduce number of feeds and increase volume is also important (see Table 10.2).

Temperature Stress

Temperature fluctuations or inadequate heating are effective ways to produce a profuse watery diarrhea in a joey. "Stress lines" may also appear in the toenails and growth rate will be poor due to energy lost trying to maintain body temperature. Inconsistent growth from any source will produce this toenail abnormality. A small uncoordinated joey trapped in a pouch is also susceptible to hyperthermia, so regular double-checking of the temperature within the pouch is essential. Older joeys can get themselves out of the pouch if it gets too hot.

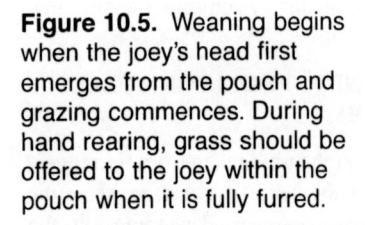

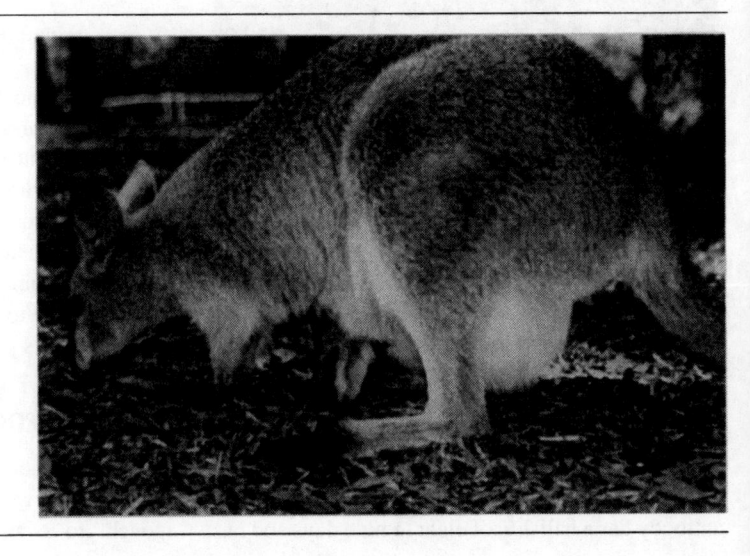

Figure 10.5. Weaning begins when the joey's head first emerges from the pouch and grazing commences. During hand rearing, grass should be offered to the joey within the pouch when it is fully furred.

Bad Management

Bad management includes everything from lack of routine, variety of carers, noisy environment, poor attention to hygiene, poor toileting technique, poor pouch design, premature separation from pouch, separation from carer when out of the pouch, difficulty getting back into pouch when alone, to poor feeding technique. Anxiety from any source can cause significant diarrhea. Be sensitive to the joey's need for a quiet peaceful environment. Be serene and nurturing rather than businesslike and brusque. Do not use the joey as a playmate for children or domestic pets.

Irritable Bowel Syndrome

An irritable bowel is the outcome of chronic, unresolved diarrhea. The decreased transit time of digesta through the gut does not allow adequate digestion, so malnutrition results and death may ensue from starvation, dehydration, or intercurrent disease. Changes to the gut mucosa due to chronic inflammation may make treatment unsuccessful. Prompt diagnosis and treatment of diarrhea in the early stages are required to prevent it.

Infectious Causes

Bacteria

Bacteria are often blamed but rarely guilty in the early stages of diarrhea. In cases unresponsive to symptomatic treatment, fecal culture is advisable to determine which organisms are involved to instigate appropriate antibiotic therapy.

A study of joey fecal flora from 31 clinically healthy joeys and 31 joeys with clinical diarrhea found the following pathogens associated with the following types of diarrhea: (1) hemolytic *E. coli* was strongly associated with acute liquid diarrhea in newly captured joeys; (2) *Salmonella* spp. were associated with chronic pasty diarrhea and long-term captivity; and (3)*Klebsiella* spp. were associated with long-term captivity and acute and chronic liquid diarrhea (Cargill and Frith 1991). Little antibiotic resistance was detected in most isolates in this study, however 36% of isolates (including 100% of *Klebsiella*) were resistant to ampicillin/amoxicillin; 18% of isolates were resistant to streptomycin; and 10% were resistant to sulfa/sulfa-trimethoprim. Nonhemolytic *E. coli* and *Streptococcus* spp. were common isolates from joeys with normal feces and can be considered normal fecal flora (Cargill and Frith 1991).

First-line antibiotic therapy is best with the broad-spectrum sulfa/sulfa-trimethoprim drugs unless fecal culture indicates otherwise. The dose rate used is as for other species: 5 mg/kg of the trimethoprim component P/O OID for five to seven days.

Yeasts

When numbers of bacteria in the gut have been reduced by antibiotic use, yeasts such as *Candida* and *Torulopsis* are able to take advantage of the lack of competition. Under these circumstances, yeasts can become serious pathogens. In addition to diarrhea, they may cause white cheesy lesions in the mouth leading to dysphagia and sickly sweet breath. Generalized dermatitis may also occur in unfurred joeys. *Candida* spp. are associated with chronic pasty diarrhea and long-term captivity. *Torulopsis* spp. are associated with acute pasty diarrhea and recent capture (Cargill and Frith 1991). Any joeys receiving antibiotic therapy should simultaneously receive a course of nystatin to control yeasts at a dose of 5000–10,000 U/kg PO TID for 7–14 days.

Coccidiosis

Coccidiosis is a major disease of macropods and is caused by protozoans in the genus *Eimeria*. Animals stressed by transportation or weaning seem most susceptible particularly *M. giganteus* and *Macropus parryi* (Pretty-faced wallaby). Hand-reared individuals seem most susceptible, so milk-transferred maternal immunity may play a role in protection. In *M. giganteus* it seems the major pathogen is *E. wilcanniensis* (formerly *kogoni*)(Beveridge 1993). Simultaneous infection with several species is usual and it is frequently impossible to tell which is the major pathogen (Beveridge 1993). Coccidian parasites are typically host specific. Transmission is via ingestion of oocysts shed in the feces contaminating grazing areas. Warm, wet weather enhances oocyst survival.

Coccidiosis may present as sudden death with no evidence of diarrhea. In less-acute cases, clinical signs include depression with dull eyes, hunched posture, dull coat, anorexia, and diarrhea leading to dehydration and hypoproteinemia. Death may occur despite intensive treatment. Diagnosis is based on history, clinical signs, species, and the presence of oocysts in the feces. Absence of oocysts in the feces does not preclude diagnosis as intermittent shedding occurs. Postmortem diagnosis should be suspected if there is hemorrhagic enteritis with multiple pale foci 0.5–3 mm diameter in the small intestine.

Coccidiocidal drugs such as toltrazuril (Baycox) at a dose of 20 mg/kg P/O or diiodohydroxyquinolone (Zoaquin) at 20 mg/kg P/O for three days are more successful for treatment than coccidiostats such as amprolium, ethopoboate, or diclazuril. Intravenous fluid therapy with a balanced electrolyte solution is usually required if clinical disease is present.

Pelleted food incorporating coccidiostats has been widely used for captive colonies of macropods. This potentially induces drug resistance in the protozoan and may gradually reduce the fitness of the host to deal with a "normal" parasite. Optimizing stocking rates and maintaining a normal social structure helps to reduce stress and minimize fecal contamination of pasture to provide a drug-free preventative program. Daily removal of fecal pellets from enclosures particularly around feeding stations is an essential component of good macropodid husbandry. Rotational grazing is also a useful way to minimize parasite load on pasture.

Plasma transfusions have been used experimentally in an attempt to provide passive immunity to hand-raised *M. giganteus* specifically to prevent clinical coccidiosis. This involves anesthetizing joeys of 3–3.5 kg and transfusing them with 10 ml/kg plasma collected from an adult animal of the same species. At least 25 joeys have received this treatment without adverse effect and it appears to either prevent or alleviate the severity of coccidiosis (Blyde, phone conversation with author).

Helminthosis

Helminths are rarely responsible for diarrhea during hand rearing, but should be considered in the list of differential diagnoses. The principle pathogen in juvenile macropods is the blood-sucking nematode of the small intestine *Globiocephaloides trifidospicularis,* which causes anemia, hypoproteinemia, diarrhea, and mortality when burdens number from 400 to 1500 (Arundel et al. 1990). Young recently weaned macropods are most susceptible, particularly during midwinter when worm burdens peak in conjunction with nutritional and cold stress.

Ivermectin is a safe and effective treatment used at dose rates recommended by the manufacturer for sheep. Benzimidazoles can also be used with caution as toxicity has occurred.

Pneumonia

Pneumonia is the second most common problem in orphaned joeys after diarrhea (Speare 1988). Aspiration pneumonia from impatient feeding is a common cause. Some joeys routinely discharge milk through the nostrils during and after feeding even when fed slowly. This does not always lead to aspiration pneumonia, but alarming sounds can be auscultated from the chest after feeding. These sounds are often referred from the pharynx but if they persist an hour after feeding pneumonia must be suspected. Clinical signs include dyspnoea, anorexia, and depression. Coughing is rare. Radiography assists diagnosis. Gram-negative bacteria are the most common isolates. Recovery is possible if appropriate antibiotic therapy is provided early enough and if energy intake can be maintained. Therapy should be based on culture and sensitivity of a transtracheal wash. Amikacin at 10 mg/kg I/M BID for five to seven days is often effective. Once pneumonia is present, animals are more prone to further aspiration due to the incompatibility of suckling and gasping.

Cataracts

Cataracts have developed in joeys raised on a variety of diets including mother-reared captive and wild joeys. The etiology is unknown. The estimated prevalence is less than 5% in orphaned joeys (Speare 1988). Most occur when joeys are starting to graze. It appears that there is a critical period when the lens is susceptible to whatever the problem is. Very rare cases have resolved after a period of months. It had been suggested that an inability to digest dietary lactose led to galactosemia, which then caused osmotic damage to the lens. This has subsequently been refuted by Speare who measured blood galactose in four affected and five unaffected joeys and found no elevation in individuals with cataracts.

CAPTIVE VERSUS WILD

Macropods are very prone to imprinting but appropriate hand raising can avoid it. Two main problems associated with imprinting include sexual and nonsexual aggression from male hand-raised macropods toward people, and neurotic submissive head tremoring and shaking in response to people. The key to avoiding imprinting is to provide only sufficient nurturing to give a sense of security, avoid subjecting the animal to stimuli that are not relevant to the species (e.g., children, dogs, TV), detach the joey from the carer at the age that it would separate from its mother (see Table 10.1), and expose it to its own species from as close to the time of pouch emergence as possible. The joey should be raised to (1) be fit and healthy (physically and mentally), (2) maintain condition on natural foods, (3) recognize its own species, (4) be familiar with the social behavior of its species, (5) show appropriate levels of fear of humans and predator, and (6) not show evidence of being imprinted on humans.

The timing of psychological detachment from the carer is very important and is most aided by the companionship of other animals of the same species. Creching of orphans for a number of months prior to release or introduction to a captive group is the ideal way to do this. Eastern grey kangaroos, western grey kangaroos, red kangaroos, and wallaroos mature to a size big enough to be dangerous to humans. It is inappropriate to hand raise males of these species unless you take considerable care not to imprint the animals and to socialize them with their own kind from an early age (Bach and Lodewikus 1998; Bellamy 1994; Cooper and Johnston 1994; Green and Merchant 1988; Kirkpatrick 1965; McCracken 1991; Sharman, Frith, and Calaby 1964; White 1997).

ACKNOWLEDGMENTS

Wildlife carer Sharon White provided growth and development data for Table 10.2 and Figure 10.5, photographic subjects, and editorial assistance. Red-necked wallaby mothers with young were photographed at Lone Pine Koala Sanctuary.

RESOURCES AND SOURCES OF PRODUCTS MENTIONED

Perfect Pets Inc., 23180 Sherwood Road, Belleville MI 48111-9306, USA; Phone 1-734-461-1362; FAX 1-734-461-2858; E-mail GSCHROCK1@aol.com

Sharpe Laboratories Pty Ltd., 12 Hope St., Ermington NSW, Australia 2115

Smith (Geoff and Christine), PO Box 93, Bonnyrigg NSW, Australia 2177

Wombaroo Food Products, PO Box 151, Glen Osmond SA, Australia 5064

REFERENCES AND SUGGESTED READING

Arundel, J. H., K. J. Dempster, K. E. Harrigan, and R. Black. 1990. Epidemiological observations on the helminth parasites of *Macropus giganteus* Shaw in Victoria. *Australian Wildlife Research* 17:39–51.

Bach, C., and C. Lodewikus. 1998. Birth date determination in Australasian marsupials. Sydney: Australasian Regional Association of Zoological Parks and Aquaria.

Bellamy, T. 1994. Hand rearing native animals, Dubbo, Post Graduate Committee in Veterinary Science.

Beveridge, I. 1993. Marsupial parasitic diseases. In *Zoo and wild animal medicine current therapy 3*, edited by M. E. Fowler. Philadelphia, PA: Saunders.

Cargill, C., and F. Frith. 1991. Joey diarrhea project—Preliminary report. *Vetlab Newsletter*, Department of Agriculture, South Australia(36):10–13.

Cooper, D., and P. Johnston. 1994. Welfare of kangaroos and wallabies in captivity. Continuing Education Program, 1994 Study guide. Sydney: Macquarie University School of Biological Sciences.

Deane, E. M., and D. W. Cooper. 1988. Immunological development of pouch young marsupials. In *The developing marsupial models for biomedical research*, edited by C. H. Tyndale-Biscoe and P. A. Janssens. Berlin: Springer-Verlag.

Fanning, F. D., and T. J. Dawson. 1989. The use of heart rate telemetry in the measurement of energy expenditure in free-ranging red kangaroos. In *Kangaroos, wallabies and rat-kangaroos*, edited by G. Grigg, P. Jarman, and I. Hume. Chipping Norton, NSW: Surrey Beatty & Sons Pty Ltd.

Flannery, T. 1995. *Mammals of New Guinea*. Chatswood NSW: Reed Books.

Green, B., and J. Merchant. 1988. The composition of marsupial milk. In *The developing marsupial*, edited by C. H. Tyndale-Biscoe and P. A. Janssens. Berlin-Heidelberg: Springer-Verlag.

Green, B., J. Merchant, and K. Newgrain. 1988. Milk consumption and energetics of growth in pouch young of the tammar wallaby, *Macropus eugenii*. *Australian Journal of Zoology* 36(2):217–28.

Janssens, P. A., and A. M. T. Rogers. 1989. Metabolic changes during pouch vacation and weaning in macropodoids. In *Kangaroos, wallabies and rat-kangaroos*, edited by G. Grigg, P. Jarman, I. Hume. Chipping Norton, NSW: Surrey Beatty & Sons Pty Ltd.

Janssens, P. A., and M. Messer. 1988. Changes in nutritional metabolism during weaning. In C. H. Tyndale-Biscoe and P. A. Janssens. *The developing marsupial models for biomedical research*. Berlin: Springer-Verlag.

Kirkpatrick, T. H. 1965. Studies of macropodidae in Queensland 2. Age estimation in the grey kangaroo, the red kangaroo, the eastern wallaroo and the red-necked wallaby, with notes on dental abnormalities.

Queensland Journal of Agricultural and Animal Sciences 22:301–10.

Maynes, G. M. 1989. Zoogeography of the macropodoidea. In *Kangaroos, wallabies and rat-kangaroos*, edited by G. Grigg, P. Jarman, and I. Hume. Chipping Norton, NSW: Surrey Beatty & Sons Pty Ltd.

McCracken, H. 1991. *Husbandry and veterinary care of orphaned marsupials*. Melbourne, Australia: Melbourne Zoo.

Merchant, J. 1989. Lactation in macropodoid marsupials. In *Kangaroos, wallabies and rat-kangaroos*, edited by G. Grigg, P. Jarman, and I. Hume. Chipping Norton, NSW: Surrey Beatty & Sons Pty Ltd.

Merchant, J., and G. B. Sharman. 1966. Observations on attachment of marsupial pouch young to the teats and on the rearing of pouch young by foster-mothers of the same or different species. *Australian Journal of Zoology* 14:593–609.

Merchant, J., B. Green, M. Messer, and K. Newgrain. 1989. Milk composition in the red-necked wallaby, *Macropus rufogriseus banksianus* (Marsupialia). *Comparative Biochemistry and Physiology a Comparative Physiology* 93(2):483–88.

Messer, M., E. Crisp, and R. Czolij. 1989. Lactose digestion in suckling macropods. In *Kangaroos, wallabies and rat-kangaroos*, edited by G. Grigg, P. Jarman, and I. Hume. Chipping Norton, NSW: Surrey Beatty & Sons Pty Ltd.

Rose, R. W. 1989. Comparative growth in the macropodoidea with particular reference to *Bettongia gaimardi*. In *Kangaroos, wallabies and rat-kangaroos*, edited by G. Grigg, P. Jarman, and I. Hume. Chipping Norton, NSW: Surrey Beatty & Sons Pty Ltd.

Schultz, D. J. 1999. Cross fostering of brush-tailed rock-wallaby *Petrogale penicillata penicillata* young into surrogate tammar *Macropus eugenii* and yellow-footed rock-wallaby *Petrogale xanthopus xanthopus*. Jervis Bay. *Proceedings of the Wildlife Disease Association*. Sydney, Australia.

Sharman, G. B., and H. J. Frith, and J. H. Calaby. 1964. Growth of the pouch young, tooth eruption, and age determination in the red kangaroo, *Megaleia rufa*. *CSIRO Wildlife Research* 9:20–49.

Speare, R. 1988. *Clinical assessment, diseases and management of the orphaned macropod joey*. Sydney: Post Graduate Committee in Veterinary Science, University of Sydney, Australia.

Tyndale-Biscoe, C. H., and P. A. Janssens. 1988. *The developing marsupial models for biomedical research*. Berlin: Springer-Verlag.

White, S. 1997. *Caring for Australian wildlife*, edited by I. Connellan. Terrey Hills, NSW: Australian Geographic Pty Ltd.

Yadav, M. 1971. The transmission of antibodies across the gut of pouch young marsupials. *Immunology* 21:839–51.

11
Hedgehogs

Ian Robinson

NATURAL HISTORY

Hedgehogs are nocturnal insectivorous mammals characterized by a coat of hard spines (Fig. 11.1). Hedgehogs belong to the order Lipotyphla, family Erinaceidae. This family is split into two subfamilies, the hairy hedgehogs, or moon rats (Galericinae), and spiny hedgehogs (Erinaceinae). The order Lipotyphla also contains the family Tenrecidae, which includes the hedgehog-tenrecs. Hedgehog-tenrecs are small spiny insectivores, similar to but smaller than hedgehogs. They are naturally found on the islands of Madagascar and the nearby Comores, but have also been introduced to Mauritius and Reunion.

Moon rats (Galericinae) have no spines, but are furry with ratlike tails. They come from the forests of Southeast Asia and are increasingly threatened by deforestation.

Spiny hedgehogs (subfamily Erinaceinae)

Four genera and 14 species of spiny hedgehog are recognized. They are spread widely throughout Europe, Asia, and Africa, but are absent from Southeast Asia, Australasia (European hedgehog introduced into New Zealand), and North or South America (Table 11.1).

Hedgehogs are not strongly represented in zoological collections although they are increasingly present in "nocturnal houses." However, in western Europe the wild western European hedgehog (*E. europaeus*) is held in great affection and is perhaps the most rescued and rehabilitated species in the world. The numbers of individuals rescued and released back into the wild each year by dedicated rehabilitators numbers thousands, and the information in this chapter comes from the work of these rehabilitators.

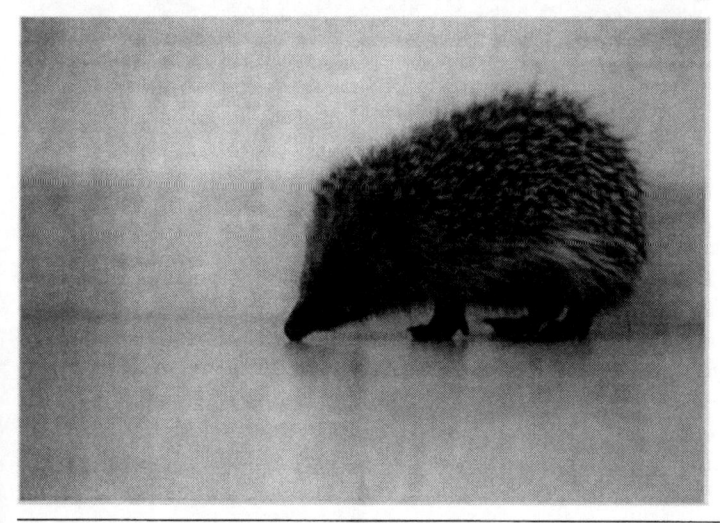

Figure 11.1. Juvenile hedgehog.

Table 11.1. Scientific and Common Names of Hedgehogs and Their Distribution

Scientific name	Common name	Distribution
Erinaceus europaeus	Western European hedgehog	Western Europe
Erinaceus concolour	Eastern European hedgehog	Eastern Europe and Asia
Erinaceus amurensis	Chinese hedgehog	China
Atelerix algirus	Algerian hedgehog	North Africa
Atelerix albiventris	Central African (white bellied) hedgehog	Central Africa
Atelerix frontalis	Southern African hedgehog	Southern Africa
Atelerix sclateri	Somalian hedgehog	Somalia
Paraechinus aethiopicus	Ethiopian hedgehog	North Africa
Paraechinus hypomelas	Brant's or long spined hedgehog	Middle East
Paraechinus micropus	Indian hedgehog	Desert areas of Pakistan and India
Hemiechinus auritus	Long eared hedgehog	North Africa to Mongolia
Hemiechinus collaris	Hardwicke's or collared hedgehog	Pakistan, North West India
Hemiechinus duuricus	Daurian hedgehog	Mongolia, Manchuria
Hemiechinus hughi	Hugh's hedgehog	Central China

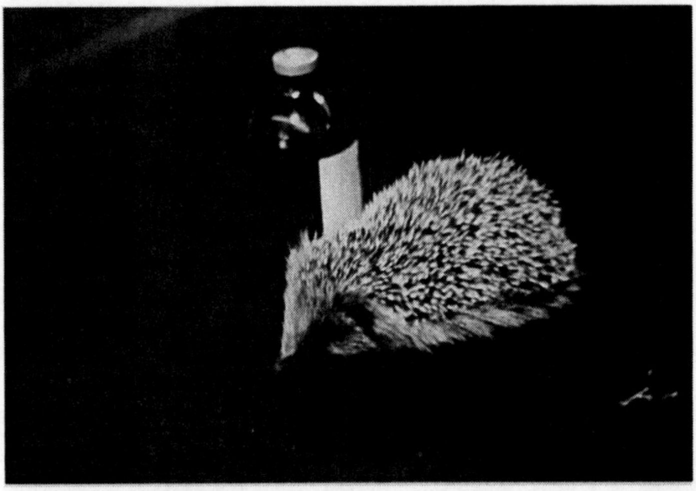

Figure 11.2. Juvenile hedgehog on table.

Adult Appearance

The dorsal surface of the body is covered in spines with no hair. Hair is present over the face and in a skirt around the edge of the spiny coat. The spines can be erected by strong "erector pili" muscles. Also, strong subcutaneous muscle layers allow the hog to roll into a ball. These muscles are the panniculus, which spreads over the back of the hedgehog like a coat, and the circular orbicularis muscle, which acts like a purse string to close the ball and protect the vulnerable head, legs, and belly (Fig. 11.2).

To unroll a hedgehog for examination, place it on a flat table. Gently tickle the middle of the back with a couple of fingers. Persistence will usually result in the hedgehog gradually unrolling. Then move the other hand under the rear of the animal and gently grasp the back legs. Now lift the back legs into the air, being careful to leave the front legs on the table. The hedgehog will be reluctant to take its front legs off the table and will stay stretched out in a "wheelbarrow" position. However, any excess stimulation will result in instant rerolling. Other techniques that are useful include placing the hedgehog on a glass or clear plastic plate, and waiting until it unrolls. The underside can then be examined through the plate.

When disturbed, hedgehogs will snort, and often will make little upward jumping movements with their spines erect to deter would-be aggressors. This behavior is normal, although the snorting is often mistaken for respiratory distress.

Another unusual hedgehog habit is "self anointing." It seems to be triggered by unusual scents. The hedgehog will start to produce copious saliva and to anoint its spines. Sometimes hogs will contort into strange positions to reach inaccessible parts of their bodies. The reason for this behavior is unknown. It has been suggested that in the wild hedgehogs chew toad skin, containing poisons, and anoint themselves with the poison to make their spines a more effective defense. This is highly speculative, although the behavior has been observed in the wild.

Both these behaviors can be observed from quite a young age, so be prepared to encounter them.

Natural Behavior

Adults are solitary, but share overlapping home ranges, each of which may extend over several acres. Each hedgehog builds several nests in its home range and will visit the nearest nest at the end of a night's foraging, spending the daylight hours concealed. It is abnormal to find a hedgehog out of its nest and active during the hours of daylight. The home range is not defended or marked, although aggressive behavior may occur during the mating season.

Radiotracking studies indicate that both adult and juvenile hedgehogs released after a period in captivity rapidly adopt natural behavior patterns, although some dispersal from the site of release may take place.

Table 11.2 outlines growth of the hedgehog from newborn to four months.

A female produces two litters per year. Juveniles must weigh approximately 500 g to survive their first hibernation. Hibernation occurs at temperatures below 36°F (8°C), although hogs will emerge during spells of warm winter weather. In the autumn as food supplies become scarce, small juveniles (150–300 g) from second litters can be found out during the day, often weak and emaciated. These hedgehogs can be successfully reared through the winter and will remain active and feeding, if maintained in an artificially heated (frost-free) environment.

RECORD KEEPING

It is useful to keep track of the following:

Body weight—best kept as a rolling mean or graphically. It is difficult to weigh a wriggly hedgehog accurately, and weight can fluctuate daily, especially when hoglets start to wean themselves. However, an underlying upward trend is essential.

Volume or food taken each feed; comments on feeding behavior.

Toileting—passing urine and feces; comments on color and consistency.

Evidence of self-feeding.

Any other comments.

EQUIPMENT

These items are needed for hand rearing:

1. Syringes or feeding bottles for orphan kittens (Catac; PetAg). Teats used for orphan kittens are adequate for all but the tiniest hoglets.

Table 11.2. Biological Data

Age	Normal weight	Appearance
Newborn	12–20 grams	White spines covered by a swollen cutis producing a smooth surface. Ears and eyes closed. Umbilical remnant visible.
2–3 days		Brown spines start to grow.
7 days	50 grams	Hair starts to grow.
12–14 days		Eyes start to open.
21–23 days	100 grams	Deciduous teeth start to erupt.
3–5 weeks	100–200 grams	Youngsters leave nest and go on foraging expeditions with mother.
4–6 weeks		Families split up and juveniles become independent.
7–9 weeks	250–300 grams	Permanent teeth begin to erupt.
4 months		Last deciduous teeth lost.

Smaller teats can be made by dipping a blunted hypodermic needle into model maker's latex, allowing it to dry and then repeating the process to build up layers until the teat is the required thickness.
2. Scales, preferably electronic digital type, measuring 1-g intervals.

CRITERIA FOR INTERVENTION

Intervention is most often called for in the following cases: (1) nest disturbed, infants (hoglets) abandoned by mother; and (2) autumn juveniles, too small to hibernate and out during the day.

INITIAL CARE

Hoglets may be hypothermic when first found abandoned. Place in an incubator at 86°F (30°C) and ensure they are thoroughly warm before feeding. Feed at two- to four-hour intervals depending on weight. Very tiny hogs may require feeds every two hours. Once they are 60 g or more, feeds every four hours are adequate, and over 80 g can go through the night without a feed. The first feed should be oral rehydration fluid (such as Pedialyte [Ross]). Consecutive feeds should then be one-fourth, one-half, and three-fourths Esbilac with Pedialyte until full-strength milk is finally used. This not only treats any dehydration, but also allows the gastrointestinal tract to adjust to the new diet.

WHAT TO FEED

Feed hoglets a milk substitute such as liquid Esbilac (PetAg) or similar puppy or kitten milk replacer. We find ready-made liquids more reliable than powdered milk as they eliminate mixing errors and lumps, which can cause gastrointestinal upsets. To avoid wastage, open a can and pour the excess into plastic ice-cube trays and place them in the freezer. Each feed, a fresh frozen cube may be defrosted. Goat's colostrum is a popular natural alternative to proprietary brands, but must be from milkings during the first 48 hours after kidding.

DAILY ROUTINE

Before the first feed in the morning, weigh each hoglet. In the wild, hoglets average 4–5 g weight gain per day from birth to independence at 250 g plus. Hand-reared hedgehogs should gain weight from 1.5 g/day under 60 g to 6–7 g per day when fully weaned.

Feed each individual with teat and syringe or bottle as preferred. Hoglets naturally press their front feet into their mother's mammary glands to stimulate milk letdown. Therefore, allowing the hoglet to simulate this natural behavior can aid suckling. Do not dangle them in the air, but hold them on a surface with a good grip and allow them to push forward against the resistance of your hand. Hogs of 60–80 g should take 5 ml per feed. Between 80 g and 100 g, 7–10 ml per feed is common and the frequency of feeding may be reduced. Also at this weight, hoglets will start to lap milk from a bowl, further reducing the need for hand feeding.

After feeding, the hoglet must be "toileted," or encouraged to pass urine and feces by stimulating the perineum. This may be done with a damp cotton bud. An adequate quantity of both must be produced. If the perineum starts to look sore after repeated stimulation, petroleum jelly or a soothing emollient ointment can be used—homeopathic remedies such as calendula are popular for this purpose. Color and consistency of feces can be a useful indicator of health. Normal feces when on an all-milk diet are pale greenish brown and the consistency of toothpaste.

HYGIENE

All equipment should be washed and sanitized after use. Between feeds, washing in detergent and keeping immersed in sterilizing fluid (with sterilizing tablets—Unichem) suitable for human babies is adequate. Syringes should be disposed of and renewed frequently, preferably daily. Teats and bottles should be autoclaved or steam sterilized daily if possible. If a number of litters are being reared, they should be isolated from each other and separate equipment should be kept for each litter. All surfaces, scales, and other items should be sanitized between handling each litter. Disposable gloves should be worn and changed between each litter. Practice good barrier nursing technique to prevent the possible spread of infections between litters.

HOUSING

Incubator or vivarium with heat source and thermostat are ideal. Hoglets should start off maintained at 86°F (30°C). While under 100 g, they are best kept together in an artificial nest. We use plastic margarine tubs lined with soft tissue paper. Once over 100 g, hoglets start to become more active. They are best provided with a temperature gradient that allows them a nesting area in the hot spot, and a slightly cooler area where they can be active and where food is provided. When their body weight is between 150 g and 200 g, the temperature may gradually be reduced to room temperature before moving to the next stage.

TIPS FOR WEANING

Hoglets are first offered milk in a bowl to lap. Then when lapping is established they are offered tinned invalid diet (Hill's AD Prescription Diet) mixed with an insect mix intended for birds (Bogena Universal or KayTee Exact Softbill diet). At first they seem to mainly walk in this then lick it off themselves. Sometimes offering a little of the mix on the end of a finger will start them eating. As quantity eaten increases, hand feeding can be reduced. Daily weight gain should be maintained and if at any time weights start to go down, then reverse the process and increase by one milk feed. Once weaned and weighing 200 g or more, young hedgehogs are moved out of the incubators and "hardened off." We use plastic water tubs for this purpose. They are a suitable size, hedgehogs can't escape because they have high smooth walls, and they are easy to clean and sanitize between litters. Here they are bedded on shavings and have room to forage for themselves and make nests in the shavings—nest-making behavior is essential to survival in the wild. They are fed twice daily and cleaned out and weighed twice weekly. If it is cold, a ceramic radiant heat lamp is placed over one end of the tub.

During this time they are gradually changed from weaning diet to adult diet (see Table 11.3). Hedgehogs are kept inside in tubs until they reach 350 g. During the summer they are then moved outside to natural enclosures prior to release. In the autumn and winter they are kept inside at room temperature until they reach 500 g. They are then released during mild spells or in the spring.

COMMON MEDICAL PROBLEMS

Hedgehogs have been described as walking biohazards and are susceptible to a multitude of diseases, several of which are zoonotic (passed to humans). Good hygienic practice is therefore essential at all times when handling hedgehogs.

GI Tract Infections

Salmonellosis. British hedgehogs commonly carry *Salmonella enteriditis* phage type 11. Fortunately this is of low infectivity to humans but still has zoonotic potential. Other Salmonellae are not uncommon.

Table 11.3. Adult Hedgehog Diet

Mix together:

1 tin puppy food
1 tin cat food
1 Pancrex V capsule (mixed pancreatic enzyme supplement)[1]
1 teaspoon SA37 (multivitamin mineral supplement)[2]

Feed small quantity according to size of individual animal.
Feed in double bowls as they do not spill the water as easily.
Feed BID (twice daily) at 8 a.m. and 8 p.m. unless otherwise directed.

[1]Pharmacia & Upjohn Ltd., West Sussex, England.
[2]Intervet UK Ltd., Cambridge, England.

Coccidiosis. Both *Eimeria* spp. and *Isospora* spp. occur in hedgehogs and can cause disease in unweaned hoglets.

Internal Parasites

Most parasites require a secondary host, a slug, snail, or insect, to complete their life cycle. Therefore, hedgehogs must have access to natural food to become infected. In the wild, late-born hogs too small to hibernate are often heavily infected with a range of parasites, due to accumulation of infection in the food chain over the summer.

Gut Worms

Nematodes. Capillaria spp. are very common and can cause disease. Intestinal fluke *Brachelaemus erinacae* also commonly cause clinical signs. Tapeworms (cestodes) and thorny headed worms (acanthocephala) are also common, but often with no apparent ill-effect.

Lung Worm

Capillaria aerophila and *Crenosoma striatum* can occur in nearly 100% of autumn juveniles and are a cause of significant disease and mortality.

Skin Diseases and External Parasites

Ringworm. Trichophyton mentagrophytes ver. erinacei occurs commonly in western European hedgehogs and can cause disease. Also, approximately 20% of individuals are symptomless carriers. This disease is probably the most important zoonosis of hedgehogs, and is certainly the most commonly contracted zoonosis of rehabilitators in the U.K.

Mites. Caparinia tripilis are common and can be synergistic with ringworm infection. Both sarcoptic and demodectic mange also occurs.

Fly-strike (Myiasis). Injured or debilitated hedgehogs are commonly targeted by blowflies, which lay clusters of eggs on the skin between the spines and around all body orifices. When they hatch, the maggots can invade the mouth, anus, ears, and genitalia, and also burrow beneath the skin, especially around skin wounds. Great care must be taken of hedgehogs during the summer when blowflies are present to check for and remove any eggs or maggots.

SOURCES FOR PRODUCTS MENTIONED

Bogena NL, Postbus 120, 5320 AC Hedel, Netherlands; www.bogena.com

Catac Products Ltd., Catac House, 1 Newnham St., Bedford MK40 3JR England; www.catac.co.uk

Hills Pet Nutrition, USA; 1-800-445-5777; www.sciencediet.com

KayTee Exact Softbill diet, www.kaytee.com

PetAg Inc., 261 Keyes Ave., Hampshire, IL 60140; 1-800-323-0877, 1-800-323-6878; www.petag.com

Ross Products Division, Abbott Laboratories, Columbus, OH 43215-1724; 1-800-986-8510; www.abbott.com, www.ross.com

Unichem, Surrey, England

REFERENCES AND FURTHER READING

Reeve, Nigel. 1994. *Hedgehogs*. London: T.&A.D. Poyser Ltd.

Robinson, I., and A. Routh. 1999. Veterinary care of the hedgehog in practice. *Journal of Veterinary Post Graduate Clinical Study* 21(3):128–37.

12
Sloths

Judy Avey-Arroyo

NATURAL HISTORY

Two of the five species of sloths found in the Neotropics are found in Costa Rica where Aviarios del Caribe Sloth Rescue and Rehabilitation Center is located. All species of sloths have three toes (i.e., three digits on the rear legs), therefore it might be preferable to forgo the old terminology of two-toed and three-toed sloths and instead call them two- and three-fingered sloths (Fig. 12.1).

The average birth weight of a two-fingered sloth (*Choloepus hoffmanni*) is 350–550 grams, and for a three-fingered sloth (*Bradypus variegatus*) is 300–450 grams. Births occur year-round for both species found along the Caribbean lowlands of Costa Rica (two-fingered to 3300 meters and three-fingered to 2400 meters), which are moist-to-rainy year-round. Little is known about seasonality of births throughout the rest of the country. Births may be seasonal due to the distinct dry and wet seasons of the Guanacaste/Pacific regions, the extended dry season limiting new bud/leaf growth during part of the year for nursing mothers and weaning young.

RECORD KEEPING

Keep a daily log of food intake (milk and solids), fecal and urine production, fecal consistency, body weight, and behavioral notes including attitude and appetite. Both species have erratic fecal output times. For infants up to one month of age, urination is quite regular, every 3 to 5 days; fecal output can range from every 3 to 4 days up to 12 days. Fecal output should then become regular, every 3 to 8 days, depending on the individual. In both species defecation almost always occurs with urination; however, it is not unusual for urination to occur without defecation. Body weight should be logged daily for general record keeping but actual body weight gain (or loss) will be found by weighing immediately after defecation and urination, giving an accurate reading for weight gain or loss. This schedule of weighing should be continued for at least the first year, then monthly weight checks should be sufficient, always just after defecation and urination.

FORMULAS

Both species of sloths from newborn until they reach about 12 weeks of age are a challenge to hand raise, the three-fingered being the more difficult. There have been no milk composition studies carried out on either species, at least none have been published, so there are no hard and fast nutritional rules to follow.

When infant sloths arrive at the center, because there is no history, both species of any age are rehydrated by giving them 5 ml of Pedialyte (Ross) per

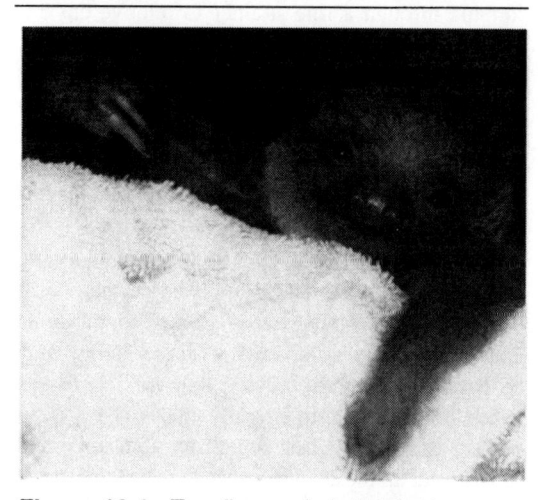

Figure 12.1. Two-fingered sloth infant.

500 g body weight every 20 to 30 minutes during the day. Use an eyedropper or a pet nurser to deliver the fluids. Continue giving the fluids until the infant has urinated at least twice. This process may take two to three days, depending on the hydration status of the infant. Once the infant is sufficiently rehydrated and is urinating, the oral fluids may be discontinued. The infant sloth will then urinate normally after that.

Two-fingered Sloths

Five two-fingered sloths have been successfully hand reared at the Aviarios Center. On arrival, two were newborns and three were between three and four weeks of age. Two were raised on fresh goat milk (goat was milked each morning), and three on powdered whole goat milk (Meyenberg Powdered Goat Milk, Jackson-Mitchell). A new version, Meyenberg "Instant," is now available. At Aviarios, the former formula is preferred due to successful results, and to date there have been no opportunities to test the instant version from newborn to weaning. However, at the time of writing, an infant two-fingered sloth that arrived at the center at approximately four days after birth is being hand reared on the Meyenberg "Instant" formula and at 61 days old is doing very well.

The powdered milk must be prepared for that day's use (if you are feeding through the night, prepare enough formula for each 24-hour period), discarding any left over. Mix one level tablespoon Meyenberg powder with one tablespoon boiling water, forming a paste with no lumps. Add warm water to equal 2 fluid ounces (60 ml). Pass the formula through a fine strainer to remove any remaining lumps that might clog the nipple hole. This formula should be reduced by half with sterile water (one-half of the mixed formula and one-half water) for the first two days feedings after the infant's arrival (no matter the age), gradually reducing the amount of extra water to reach the full-strength formula, over a four-day period.

Heat fresh goat milk just to the boiling point, refrigerate, and throw away leftovers at the end of the day's (or 24 hours) needs. Store-bought whole goat milk and fresh goat milk, after sterilizing, may be frozen in ice-cube trays. Remove the frozen cubes, transfer them to a tightly closed heavy plastic bag (Ziploc Freezer Bag from Johnson), and squeeze out all the air. The cubes may be kept for up to six weeks in the freezer.

Measure the amount of milk needed for one feeding into the Pet Nurser and warm it in a hot-water bath. It should be just above warm, not hot. Always test it on your wrist. Microwave heating is not advised, as it can cause a breakdown in the milk resulting in digestive upsets. When the infant sloth is approximately five weeks old, or 500 g, 1 tsp (5 ml) of Esbilac powder (PetAg) may be added to the 2 oz (60 ml) of goat milk formula, and by seven weeks of age, 2 tsp (10 ml) are mixed into the formula. The feces will show tiny white flecks, which is normal for baby sloths fed Esbilac.

A two-fingered sloth that weighs more that 1000 g or is five months old on arrival at a rescue center should not be given the goat milk formula, instead offering hard-cooked egg and dark meat from chicken as a source of protein, along with vitamin/mineral drops such as ACTIVON Junior or Poly-Vi-Sol (Stein; Bristol-Meyers). A three-fingered sloth over 850 g or four months of age should be given only leaves with vitamin/mineral drops. Worth repeating again: upon arrival to a rescue center both species should be given a rehydration formula such as Pedialyte (Ross) as a matter of course until the sloth has urinated at least twice. Dehydration may be diagnosed by the appearance of the eyes and mucous membranes, and additionally in two-fingered sloths by the appearance of the palms of the hands and feet. They should appear smooth, shiny, and slightly plump. The skin of both species is very tight on the body and cannot be lifted up in the usual manner to test for the dehydration.

Cow's milk appears to be the common denominator in infant sloth mortality. Infant sloths of both species who were fed cow's milk in any form before arriving at Aviarios Rescue Center presented with unstoppable diarrhea and died. Their digestive systems appeared to be irreparably damaged.

Other formulas (Nestle's canned Evaporated Milk + water; Esbilac; KMR; whole cow's milk) have been tried at various zoos, with two-fingered orphans, with varying degrees of success (Merritt 1986). Several of these formulas have been tried at Aviarios Rescue Center, but without success, making both fresh and powdered goat milk the formula of choice for us.

Three-fingered Sloths

The center has not successfully hand reared a three-fingered sloth from neonate to three months of age on arrival, therefore, the urgency of conducting

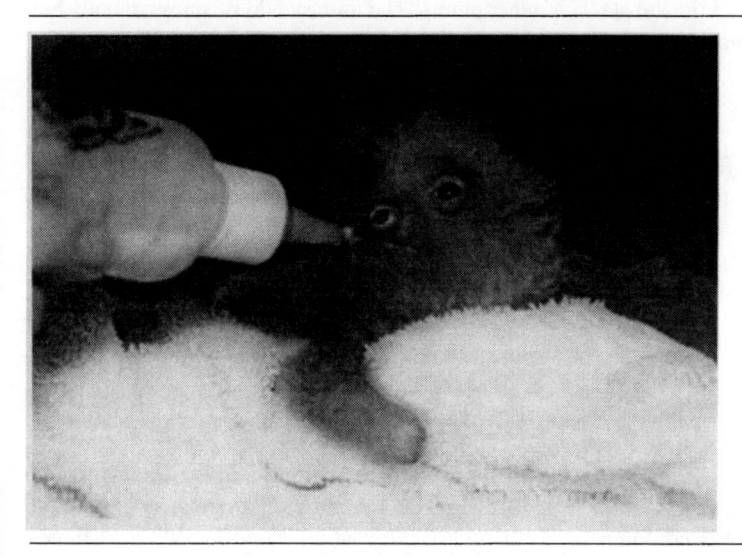

Figure 12.2. Bottle-feeding a sloth.

mother's milk composition studies remains. We continue to work with different formulas when these infant sloths are brought to the center.

NURSING TECHNIQUES

Both species of sloths will readily nurse from a Four Paws 2-oz Pet Nurser (Poly). Using a hot needle, make a small hole in the new nipple that, when the bottle is squeezed, releases a fine stream of milk. Before first use, boil the nipples in water with three drops of dish soap for four minutes to remove the burned rubber taste. Boil again in clear water to remove all traces of soap. (The infant could refuse an untreated nipple and thereafter refuse to nurse from the Pet Nurser nipple.) Bottles, nipples, and eyedroppers must always be boiled before each use.

If the infant is under 500 g, its mouth is probably too small to accommodate the Pet Nurser nipple, and you will have to use a glass eye/ear dropper with a straight tip (Optic). Permanent teeth erupt before birth. Only the two-fingered sloths have canines and neither species has incisors, so care must be taken to keep the tip of the eyedropper in the center of the mouth where there are no teeth, and not allow the sloth to move the glass eyedropper to the side of the mouth to bite. Insert the tip of the dropper no more than 1/4 in (0.6 cm) and squeeze the bulb drop by drop, encouraging the infant to suckle. Avoid having to refill the dropper several times during a feeding session, as interrupting nursing could result in the infant losing interest. To accomplish this, fill the tube with formula, invert and squeeze the air out of the tube, reinsert the dropper into the formula and take up more formula; repeat the process until all the air has been expelled from the eyedropper and the bulb and glass tube are filled with formula. The infant may then be fed smoothly and you won't have to stop and refill the tube. Remove the tip from the mouth to allow air to enter the eyedropper as the sloth drinks the milk, but only briefly. A feeding may take up to a half hour to complete, so you must be patient. A healthy infant will suckle with brief pauses until it reaches satiation.

An infant of 600 g should easily suckle from the Pet Nurser nipple. During feedings, hold the infant stomach-side down at no more than a 30-degree angle, preventing accidental inhalation of formula, which could result in inhalation pneumonia and death. The angle should be approximately that which the infant experiences when mother-raised. Babies lie on their mothers' stomachs while suckling and eating their first solid foods. They do not gain the ability to take in food, eat, and swallow while hanging upside down until at least six months of age. After about four months of age, as the infant progresses in age and size, you may deviate from this position and angle of approach.

FREQUENCY OF FEEDING

Newborn sloths of both species require round-the-clock feedings every two hours for at least the first

30 days, allowing the body temperature time to stabilize and to ensure that the suckling response is strong and dependably present. The feedings between midnight and 6 A.M. may be discontinued as the infant gains strength and size. If in doubt, continue with at least one nighttime feeding, however no more than eight weeks are necessary. At about one month of age both species will vocalize when they are hungry, the three-fingered with a shrill, whistlelike call, and the two-fingered with a bleating, more humanlike "maa, maa" sound.

AMOUNTS TO FEED

Newborns of both species to four weeks should take 5–10 ml of formula per feeding every two to three hours. Four to eight weeks, 8–15 ml every four hours, increasing as the infant demands. Weight gain is the best indicator to increase milk consumption. Milk should be continued to at least five to six months of age for the two-fingered sloth and to four months for the three-fingered sloth if milk was offered and accepted before the fourth month, during which time the amount has been increased to 80 ml over a 12-hour period. Two drops of liquid vitamin/mineral solution for each 20 ml of formula should be given by glass eyedropper from newborn to approximately 800 g weight or 12–13 weeks of age. As growth rate and weight gain level off, increase to three drops. All infant two-and three-fingered sloths should be offered water by eyedropper or Pet Nurser two to three times per day. A good indicator of excellent health in the two-fingered young sloth is the appearance of the palms of the hands and feet. They should be smooth, shiny, and rather plump. The nose should be shiny, smooth, but not wet. Two-fingered sloths sweat through the nose; tiny drops appear when the animal is excited or too hot. Bright eyes and a dry smooth nose are good indicators of a healthy three-fingered baby sloth. Both species should appear alert and at about two to three weeks of age should show a keen interest in their surroundings, by sniffing and pulling objects to the mouth, batting at an extended finger, pulling it to its mouth to bite. The infant two-fingered sloth licks everything it comes in contact with; a very good reason to wash the hands well before handling babies.

EXPECTED WEIGHT GAIN

At birth, a two-fingered sloth should weigh 350–550 g; by 4 months, approximately 1000 g; at 6 months 1300 g; at 12 months, 2400 g. A three-fingered sloth weighs approximately 300–450 g at birth and at 6 months, approximately 1200 g (Fig. 12.3).

Body weight should be logged daily for general record keeping, but actual weight gain or loss will be shown by weighing immediately after urination and defecation. A weight gain of approximately 20 g or more in a two-fingered sloth should be expected each week for the first 2 months, 30 g or more per week in the third and fourth months, with a weight of approximately 2400 g by 12 months of age. Weight gains haven't been recorded for the three-fingered sloth from birth through three months. However, a gain of 30 g or more should be expected per week. Because sloths defecate and urinate at great intervals, it is rather difficult to moni-

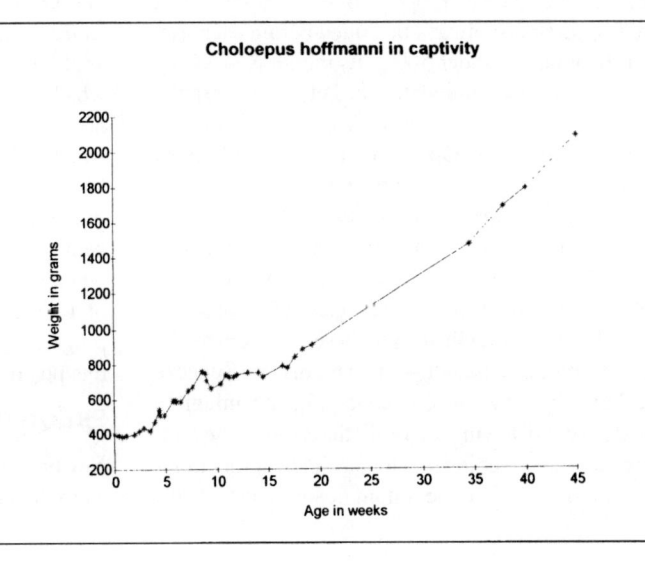

Figure 12.3. Expected weight gain from birth to 45 weeks for a male *Choloepus hoffmanni* in captivity.

tor daily progress. If an infant doesn't gain weight, or actually loses weight after defecation and urination and seems otherwise healthy, increase the frequency of feedings, that is, every three hours and through the night if under three months, or more solid foods more frequently if over three months.

HOUSING AND SPECIAL COMFORT NEEDS

Both species of sloths are heterothermic; body temperature fluctuates with the ambient temperature, dropping by as much as 5°C during the night or times of heavy rain. Mothers and babies both have sparser belly hair allowing the heat from the mother's body to transfer to the infant. For these reasons it is very important to maintain a constant temperature for the infant until at least three months of age. This may be accomplished with an isolette (incubator) used for human babies. Ideally the isolette will have a built-in humidity source. For a newborn to a three-month-old, whose need for warmth is most critical, should an isolette not be available, use an electric heating pad (Sunbeam P.N.) with at least 6 in (15 cm) of terry-cloth towels folded on top of the heating pad, which is set on the lowest setting. The heating pad must be placed flat in the bottom of a cardboard box, with the box measuring at least 20 in (51 cm) high, and the bottom being the same size as the heating pad (13 in × 16 in or 33 cm × 40 cm). The temperature in the box must always be monitored. An indoor/outdoor thermometer may be taped to the inside wall of the box and should register between 70 and 80°F (25–27°C).

A rolled terry-cloth towel or stuffed animal (remove all plastic pieces; i.e., eyes, noses) should be provided as a surrogate mother for the baby to lie on and cling to. Babies should always be picked up or handled on the surrogate mother as their adaptation to cling to their mother is so strong that they easily panic if not allowed to cling. When the sloth reaches four months of age the box may be replaced with a plastic-coated wire cage (30 in × 16 in × 20 in) or (75 cm × 40 cm × 51 cm) with a washable solid plastic floor. The heating pad can be eliminated but ample towels should be provided under which the sloths will burrow for warmth as much as for security. Terry-cloth towels must always be checked for holes and/or frayed edges with strings because, as the babies move and turn about, their heads or legs may become entangled causing strangulation or cut-off circulation.

When the sloth is about five to six months of age, a tree branch of appropriate diameter for the nails may be securely attached to the cage for climbing. The bones and muscles aren't sufficiently developed for the sloth to hang upside down independently until then.

At around four to five months of age, the young of both species may be introduced to a "toilet tree." This may be a small living tree outdoors of approximately 3–4 in (7.5–10 cm) in diameter, or, if a living tree is unavailable, any similar substitute. Place the young sloth on the ground at the base of the tree with its arms and legs wrapped around the tree trunk (this might require two people, one person handling the front legs and one handling the back legs). This may be done every day and will encourage the sloth's natural instinct to defecate at the base of a tree. The three-fingered sloth uses its tail (3–4 in long as an adult) to move leaf debris and soil away in order to deposit feces in the resulting depression. The two-fingered sloth wiggles its behind on the ground to accomplish the same result. Toilet training is beneficial to sloths in captivity as well as those scheduled for release to the wild.

IMMUNE STATUS AND SPECIAL NEEDS

Great care must be taken in handling orphaned newborn infants of both species as they are not protected by the immunoglobulins from the mother's colostrum. It is a given that those babies separated from their mothers cannot be returned to their mothers in the wild because of the difficulty in identifying the actual mother and returning the baby to her in the canopy. Many rescued sloths of both species, in the tropical countries in which they are found, are removed from homes in which they have been kept as pets. They are susceptible to sarcoptic mange due to stress caused by improper diet and/or handling. In a zoo situation, there are most likely extenuating circumstances by which a baby is orphaned or separated from its mother that preclude returning it to its mother.

Infants of either species orphaned after three months of age, with care taken in their diet, handling, and housing, are generally hardy, and thrive.

Baby sloths of both species spend the first four to five months of life clinging to their mothers' bellies, therefore it is recommended that an infant be held and cuddled against the caregiver's chest as often as possible and for as long as possible at every opportunity throughout its development. Holding the infant on its surrogate mother, encourage it to move onto the caregiver's chest where it will cling while being supported with one hand, then cover it with a small hand towel or infant receiving blanket. It

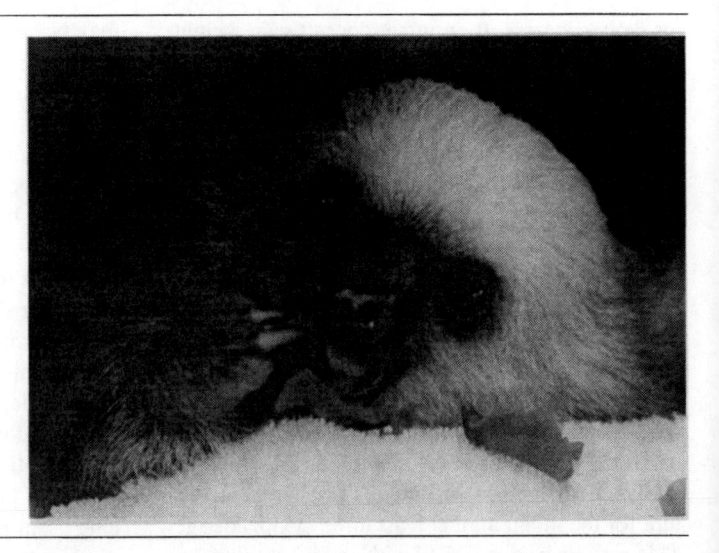

Figure 12.4. Introducing solid foods to a sloth infant.

seems to willingly leave the surrogate mother for the caregiver. Reverse the process to return it from the chest to the surrogate mother and into its nest box. This handling seems to be a very important factor in the infant's will to live. A few moments cuddling after the nighttime feedings seems to be critical for the infant's well-being.

Baby sloths don't appear to mind being handled by different persons if handling is begun early on. It is a very good idea to accustom the two-fingered sloth who is to remain in captivity to being handled by various persons. This will help lay a foundation of trust to enable caretakers to handle the same sloth as an adult without causing undue stress, as a two-fingered sloth can deliver terrific injuries with its teeth and nails if it feels threatened. An infant three-fingered sloth requires cuddling and contact with human handlers until it reaches approximately 10–12 months of age—the age of social weaning from the mother. Three-fingered sloths are always docile and may be handled throughout their life without harming their handlers. The juvenile may then be introduced into a cage (9 ft × 9 ft × 6 ft or 3 m × 3 m × 2 m) with a cement floor with drainage for ease of cleaning, using 1 1/2-in cyclone fencing wire, along with its sleep box until ready for release. If a two-fingered sloth is to remain in captivity, it is recommended that regular handling be continued throughout its life.

The young of both species begin to play, batting at an extended finger, sniffing, licking, and testing with the teeth, at around two weeks. They must be encouraged to explore and to develop an interest in their surroundings.

Exposure to the early morning sun for at least a half hour for infants up to five months old is very important for thermoregulation. When toilet training is begun, at least an hour outdoors in the early morning or late afternoon is recommended.

TIME TO WEANING

Two-fingered sloths are generally eating on their own at 6 to 7 months, however they have been observed in the wild suckling at 10 1/4 months (hand-reared two-fingered sloths should be weaned from milk by 8 months). Social weaning by the mother could occur any time between one year and a year and a half.

A three-fingered sloth is usually weaned from mother's milk at around four months. From two to three weeks, it is eating leaves, first from around the mother's mouth, until at about three months it is pulling leaves to its mouth from branches as its mother feeds herself. The baby ventures away from its mother for short excursions at four months, and climbs well. It has not been documented at what age the three-fingered sloth is socially weaned from the mother, but commonly thought to be approximately 8–10 months.

TIPS FOR WEANING FROM FORMULA TO SOLID FOOD

For two-fingered sloth babies begin weaning from formula to solids by offering each new food item before the scheduled milk formula feeding (Fig. 12.4). If an infant refuses after several attempts, the preferred food item (e.g., carrots, green beans) may be pureed and added to the formula in the bottle. To allow the heavier consistency to pass through the nipple, enlarge the hole using the same method as you would a new nipple (see Nursing Techniques above).

Solid Foods—Two-fingered Sloths

Beginning at five weeks of age, or around 600 g body weight, introduce solid foods to the diet. Begin with steamed green beans. They should be quite soft for ease in biting off pieces and chewing. Begin by feeding one to two beans once a day, allow about 8–10 days to pass to ensure that the infant is handling the solid food well. Continue adding other steamed foods such as carrots, chayote (green summer pear squash), yellow (winter) squash, or sweet potatoes (yams). At about 1000 g (three months of age, approximately), as the infant has developed a taste for these food items, begin adding fruits, such as bananas, mangos (both green and slightly ripened), grapes (the seeds must always be removed), apples, and other sweet fruits. Protein in the form of muscle (thigh and leg) meat from chicken (cubed and boiled in water for one minute) and hard-cooked egg can also be added at this time. Beginning at about four months, add to the diet a high-protein bread cubed and softened in goat milk, and at about five and a half months add an excellent quality puppy food, such as Eukanuba, IAMS, or Science Diet, completely softened in goat's milk during the first two months, then switching to water. After the sloth is eating the dog food well, discontinue the protein bread. Always wait two bowel movements after each introduced food item to determine if there are digestive problems. There should be no problems, and any new food could cause soft stool, but if very loose stool or diarrhea occurs, discontinue food item and try again in two weeks to allow more time for the digestive system to mature. The feces of an infant sloth with a milk diet will be light tan to caramel colored, elongated to about 1 cm with a rather rough textured surface. They may form a single compacted pellet until the digestive system stabilizes with a new diet. As solids are added, the pellets become darker brown, almost black in color, rounder, smoother, and separated, and they should be firm.

To facilitate the sloth feeding itself with its hands, the vegetables and fruits may be cut into long, narrow pieces, following the form of the green beans.

If the sloth does not take readily to these new foods, you will have to be creative in your approach. Young sloths sample new foods, thus developing a taste for them, by licking around the mother's mouth as she eats. By placing a new food item between your pressed lips (avoiding contact with your saliva) and offering it to the sloth face to face, the baby should be attracted and reassured that it is safe to eat. Sloths will rarely, if ever, overeat, so follow the baby's lead as far as capacity. If a release into the wild is to be attempted, the introduction of leaves and fruits, which wild sloths in the release area are seen to eat, should begin at around three months of age. At five to six months of age, the ratio of food should be approximately 80% specific tree leaves, vegetables, and fruits, and 20% protein. As discussed above, this protein source will gradually change at four to five months of age, from mostly milk to muscle meat of chicken, high-protein bread, and softened puppy food. By eight months, the sloth should be weaned from milk. Baby sloths will always display specific likes and dislikes in food, as well as intermittent or irregular acceptance of proffered foods.

Telemetry-monitored release of a two-fingered sloth has never been attempted, or reports have not been published of any attempts. Keep in mind that if a hand-reared two-fingered sloth is to be released, the diet should reflect the types of food that it will look for and find in the release area. Solid foods should be made up mostly, then, of the various types of leaves and wild fruits that wild sloths in the release area are observed to be eating. The domestic vegetable and fruits and protein sources should still be given, but in lesser quantity in ratio to the wild sources and diminishing in quantity as the sloth reaches release age. Fresh leaves must be harvested every day and refrigerated until used. The remaining leaves should be thrown out at the end of the day. Neither species drinks water in the wild, obtaining all the required moisture from their food. Therefore, it is very important that their food be absolutely fresh.

Solid Foods—Three-fingered Sloths

The three-fingered sloth infant should begin showing an interest in eating leaves at around three weeks of age, sampling them from the mother's mouth as she eats. Three-fingered sloths have never been successfully kept outside of the tropics, because their need for a minimum of 60% humidity precludes most zoo situations, and their need for copious amounts of specific rain forest leaves limits the supply that can be grown in zoo facilities. No satisfactory substitutes have been found for tropical leaves.

The optimum chance for success in hand rearing a three-fingered sloth is keeping it in its natural environment, and feeding it freshly harvested leaves, such as cecropia (Cecropiaceae: *Cecropia obtusifolia, Cecropia insignis*; Spanish name: Guarumo), sangrillo (Fabacae: *Pterocarpus officinalis*; Spanish names: Sangrillo and Sangregao), strangler fig (Moraceae: *Ficus crassiuscula*; Spanish name: Matapalo), or others that local three-fingered sloths feed on. They are especially fond of the fruit of the cecropia, which resembles long bean pods, and is seasonal from area to area. Feed only one new leaf type at a time to observe the reaction, such as changes in the stool. The feces of an infant three-fingered sloth are tiny, round, and black, about the size of BBs, becoming larger as the sloth grows (feces of adult sloths are shiny black, round, and pea-size). The pellets can number from 100 to 200 for each evacuation, which occurs every two to eight days.

COMMON MEDICAL PROBLEMS

Both species of sloths are very difficult to hand rear before they reach three months of age. Infants of both species orphaned or separated from their mothers after the age of three months are generally quite easy to care for and are generally quite hardy.

Gastrointestinal problems arising from improper diet and/or inadequate milk formulas fed to infants before their arrival to rescue centers are the usual reason for infant mortality.

Anemia has been found in two-fingered sloths but not studied in the three-fingered sloth.

Unknown (unstudied) species of tapeworm have been found in all ages and both species of sloths. Ascarids have been found in fecal examinations in the two-fingered sloth.

Sloths climb power poles in villages and along roadsides and frequently experience severe burns from contact with high voltage wires. They are often hit by cars as they cross roads and highways.

Mange (*Sarcoptes* spp.) occurs with some frequency, particularly in the three-fingered, and clinical signs include pustular dermatitis characterized by large, hardened scabs, but with no alopecia.

There has been an instance of a two-month-old two-toed sloth arriving at the center with canine distemper and infecting a second infant, both of which succumbed. There are no investigations to date of a possible vaccine against canine distemper for sloths in captivity.

Captive adult animals usually cannot wear down their nails as they grow, and these will curl into the palms of the hands and feet, making it necessary to trim the extra length.

A guillotine-type dog nail trimmer works well on both species. Begin trimming in increments of 3 cm (1/8 in) until the remaining portion of nail on the hand is about 9 cm (3 1/2 in); the nails on the feet approximately 6 cm (2 3/8 in). The bone of the last phalange of the fingers and toes extends to nearly the tip of an adult nail that is naturally maintained in the wild, therefore great care must be taken with trimming the nails. Nail trimming is generally well tolerated by an adult three-fingered sloth if it has been conditioned from an early age. However, an adult two-fingered sloth must be subdued, either chemically or physically with a net or squeeze cage, even if it appears docile in most situations. The sloth will normally attempt to bite with its very sharp teeth and may grab a caregiver's hand and bite with astonishing speed and severe consequences.

RELEASE

Captive Versus Wild

There has been only one documented release, with radio telemetry, of a hand-reared three-fingered sloth (none for the two-fingered) and that release successfully occurred at Aviarios del Caribe Sloth Rescue Center in Costa Rica. Very little is understood about the ways in which the mothers of either sloth species teach their young to be independent, increasing the difficulty of a successful release of a hand-reared sloth of either species back into the wild. Other rehabilitated sloths of both species at Aviarios Rescue Center are awaiting radio telemetry monitored release.

Introduction of Hand-Reared Young Back to the Exhibit

Two- and three-fingered sloths of both sexes are usually quite tolerant of one another in an exhibit if it is large enough to support a sleep box for each individual to choose as its own; they will sometimes choose to sleep together. A hand-reared juvenile ready to move back to the exhibit should be introduced with its own sleep box with which it is familiar, along with a towel placed on the floor of the sleep box, as it burrows under, or covers itself with the towel. The towel may be eliminated if the sleep box is too high for easy access of weekly towel changes.

ACKNOWLEDGMENTS

I thank Laurie Gage for asking me to put into usable form my experiences and knowledge of hand rearing young sloths gathered over the years. Thanks also to Linda Yauk for her encouragement, belief, and little purple editing pencil. Thanks to the many people who over the years have brought injured and orphaned sloths to Aviarios, entrusting their care to us, and to those who have supported the rescue center with donations and their joy of learning about these fascinating creatures. A special thanks from my soul for the many beautiful sloths who have come to Aviarios for help and have given so much in return. They are my teachers. And a special mention to Mowgli, Bella, Jasper, and Tuffy, the adorable infant sloths who appear in the illustrations. The sloths would especially like to thank Cali and Chago, the humans who go into the steaming, teeming jungle every day, and harvest fresh leaves. The Costa Rican Ministry of Natural Resources has been wonderfully supportive with permits and licensing for the establishment of the rescue center, and in helping us initiate education programs for the conservation of Costa Rica's wildlife. I am grateful to the scientists and biologists who have studied sloths and written reports on their findings. We deeply thank the many volunteers, without whose help our work would have been nearly impossible. They gave so much and took away with them a great respect for the rainforest and the fascinating sloths who inhabit it. My husband, Luis Arroyo, deserves sainthood for supporting me, the sloths, and the rescue center through the years, financially and spiritually, allowing me the opportunity to learn more about and further develop the care and hand rearing of sloths. Without his love and care we would still be crawling instead of making long strides. Thanks Sloth Papa!

One last very special thank you to Buttercup, the three-fingered sloth, who started it all when she arrived at our door as a three-month-old orphan in September 1991!

SOURCES OF PRODUCTS MENTIONED

Bristol-Meyers Squibb Ecuador of Mead Johnson & Company, Evansville, IL, USA

Eukanuba: www.eukanuba.com

IAMS: www.iams.com

Jackson-Mitchell, Inc., PO Box 934, Turlock, CA 95381, USA

Johnson (S.C.) & Son, Inc., Racine, WI 53403-2236, USA

Optic Shop, Pro-Optics, Inc., 317 Woodwork Lane, Palatine, IL 60067, USA

PetAg Inc., 261 Keyes Ave., Hampshire, IL 60140; 1-800-323-0877, 1-800-323-6878; www.petag.com

Poly Nurser, Hauppauge, NY 11788

Ross Products Division, Abbott Laboratories, Columbus, OH 43215-1724; 1-800-986-8510; www.abbott.com, www.ross.com

Science Diet: www.sciencediet.com

Stein Laboratory, S.A., Apto. Postal No. 930-1007, Centro Colon, San Jose, Costa Rica, 1-800-STEINSA (1-800-783-4672)

Sunbeam P.N., 46251-505-971 Z-2047; 1-800-56-SUNBEAM

RESOURCES

Information contained in this chapter has essentially been obtained through personal experience over 11 years working with sloths at Aviarios del Caribe Sloth Rescue and Rehabilitation Center in Costa Rica, from bits and pieces of information collected over the years from zoos that exhibit two-fingered sloths, and from various studies on both species reported in wildlife journals. For further information e-mail Judy Arroyo at aviarios@costarica.net; website: www.OGphoto.com/aviarios.

REFERENCES

Beebe, W. 1926. The three-toed sloth. *Zoologica* 7(1).
Merrit, D., Jr. 1985. The two-toed Hoffmann's sloth, *Choloepus Hoffmanni* Peters. In *The evolution and ecology of armadillos, sloths, and vermilinguas*, edited by G. G. Montgomery. Washington, DC: Smithsonian Institution.
———. 1986. *Hand-rearing Edentates, Lincoln Park Zoological Gardens*. Washington, DC: Smithsonian Institution Press.
Montgomery, G. G., and M. E. Sunquist. Habitat selection and use by two-toed and three-toed sloths. In *The ecology of arboreal folivores*, edited by G. G. Montgomery. Washington, DC: Smithsonian Institution Press.
Vogel, I., B. de Thoisy, and J-C. Vie. 1998. Comparison of injectable anesthetic combinations in free-ranging two-toed sloths in French Guiana. *Journal of Wildlife Diseases* 34:555–66.

13
Ground and Tree Squirrels

Dawn Smith

NATURAL HISTORY

There are over 20 species of ground squirrels, including burrowing species and a few others that utilize tree nests and aboveground food caches, in addition to their ground burrows. The tree squirrels, three species of which are common to the United States, are all arboreal, and utilize tree nests exclusively (Table 13.1).

RECORD KEEPING

Keep a daily log of food intake, fecal and urine production, fecal consistency, hydration, body weight, and behavioral notes including attitude and appetite. Weight loss, dehydration, or diarrhea can quickly become life threatening if not caught in the early stages. A change in behavior may be indicative of impending illness or a move to the next phase of development, both of which require prompt attention.

EQUIPMENT

For feeding 1, 3, 6, and 12 cc Luer-tip syringes should be available. Measuring cups, measuring spoons, and a food blender or processor are needed for making formula. A bottle warmer or other warm-water source will be necessary to heat the formula. Heating formula in a microwave is not recommended as it tends to alter protein composition, which may affect nutritional value.

Neonates with eyes closed may be housed in a variety of simple boxes or cages. Heat, in the form of a heating pad or incubator, should be provided. Incubators are preferred because they allow ideal humidity to be maintained, in addition to providing heat. If heating pads are used, they should be placed under half of the cage or box housing the animals. By leaving half the enclosure unheated, healthy babies can move closer or further from the heat source as they begin to thermoregulate on their own. Once eye slits are defined (approximately two weeks of age), it is best to move the babies to the next type of enclosure (wire multilevel cage with branches for tree squirrels, terrarium with dirt or shavings for ground squirrels). By doing so, the animals will be exposed to as natural an environment as possible as their eyes open and they begin to explore.

CRITERIA FOR INTERVENTION

Wild squirrels that are warm and well hydrated may be left for several hours under observation to determine whether the parents will return. Many females build a second emergency nest, so even if the original nest is destroyed, the babies should be left in a safe place near their original nest. If the neonates are cold, they should be taken in and first provided with a warm, dark, quiet place to recover. If, after a short period of warming, the neonate(s) are active,

Table 13.1. Natural History of Squirrel Pups

Species	Birth weight	Litter Size	Weaning age
Ground squirrel	7–8 grams	1–7	6 weeks
Tree squirrel	15 grams	2–6	10 weeks

Table 13.2. Age Determination of Squirrels

Weeks	Aging characteristics
0–1	Body is pink and hairless/eyes and ears sealed
1–2	Hair begins to grow, skin color darkens, eyelids obvious
2–3	Fur coloration takes on adult pattern, lower incisors erupt
3–4	Eye slits begin to open at corners
4–5	Eyes open
5–6	Upper incisors erupt, ears open
6–7	Weaning occurs in ground squirrels
10	Weaning occurs in tree squirrels

an attempt may be made to put them in the area of the original nest. Do not allow them to become chilled a second time. Provide a small box with low sides that the mother may easily enter and exit. Lining it with an old towel or piece of fleece will keep the babies warm while giving the parents time to retrieve them, if they have not deserted the area. Inserting a hot water bottle or other heat source underneath the towel will help keep the babies warm on cold days, while waiting for a possible reunion.

Captive-born squirrels may require hand rearing if the mother is not caring for them. Lack of weight gain and/or vigor is an indicator of the need for intervention.

ASSESSMENT OF THE NEONATE

Before initiating the hand-rearing process, the squirrel should have a complete physical examination. Age, weight, temperature, pulse, respiration, and hydration should be assessed. The animal should be manually flea-combed to remove as many external parasites as possible. In areas at high risk for plague, a pyrethrin-based powder suitable for use on kittens may be used to kill any fleas not removed by combing. Attention must be paid to the overall health of the individual as flea powders may be toxic to compromised neonates. Wild-born squirrels should also be checked for injuries from falls or predators. See Table 13.2 for developmental information that will aid in assessing the age of newborn squirrels.

INITIAL CARE

When admitting wild-born neonates, body temperature should be evaluated immediately, as hypothermia is their most common problem. Hypothermic infants will be nonresponsive and cool to the touch. These animals must be thoroughly warmed before attempting to feed. Warmed subcutaneous fluids may be administered immediately. Warm oral electrolyte solution may be given as soon as the normal core body temperature has been reestablished. Hydration status should be determined next, as neonates that have not eaten dehydrate rapidly. Once a neonate is well hydrated and has a normal core body temperature (100–102°F or 37.8–38.9°C), dilute formula may be introduced.

FORMULAS AND CALORIC REQUIREMENTS

For a thorough review of the composition of squirrel milk with a comparison to various formulas, see Marcum (1997). Many recipes have been used successfully to raise baby squirrels, and most include or consist of commercially mixed powders. New to the market is Formula 32/40 (Fox Valley). This product does not yet have a substantial track record, but so far appears to be promising. MultiMilk, Zoologic 30/55, or Esbilac (all available from PetAg) have been used either as stand-alone formulas when mixed with water, or in various combinations. (See Table 13.3 for a comparison of formulas and an analysis of squirrel milk.) Daily caloric requirements for these animals range between 0.4 and 0.8 kcal per gram body weight per day, with the highest requirements occurring in the earliest developmental stages. These formulas are designed as completely balanced nutrition for unweaned squirrels. As such, they should not be supplemented. As weaning age approaches, a variety of natural foods should be made available.

WHAT TO FEED INITIALLY

It is best to initiate feedings with a straight electrolyte solution to ensure the gastrointestinal tract is functioning well. A strong, well-hydrated baby may only need one electrolyte feeding before beginning to be gradually converted to the milk replacement formula. Once the neonate is hydrated, feed one-fourth formula and three-fourths electrolytes. Increase to half formula and half electrolytes, then three-fourths formula and one-fourth electrolytes, and finally, full-strength formula. If, at any point in this process, the baby is not tolerating the feeding (i.e., vomits, has diarrhea, gas, or bloating), the ratio should return to the last well-tolerated level. Severely dehydrated babies may require a very slow

Table 13.3. Squirrel Formulas

Formula	Solids (%)	Protein (%)	Carbs (%)	Kcals/cc
Fox Valley 32/40 (2:3)	25.0	8.0	3.8	1.70
Esbilac/MultiMilk[1] (1:1/2:2)	21.7	7.3	2.3	1.33
Esbilac/MultiMilk[1] (1:1:2)	26.7	8.8	2.1	1.65
Esbilac/Cream (1:1/3:1.5)	23.4	6.3	3.1	1.55
Squirrel Milk[2]	25–39	7.4–9.2	3.0–3.7	1.57–2.67

Notes: Numbers in parentheses are ratios of the ingredients listed with the last number being the amount of water to add.
[1]MultiMilk is equivalent to Zoologic 30/55.
[2]Data on squirrel milk composition from Marcum (1997).

introduction to full-strength formula. Electrolytes alone may be given the first day, then the percentage of formula may be increased over the next 72 hours to full-strength formula on day four. Neonates that are also severely emaciated may require a small amount of formula (one-fourth of the feeding or less) early on to prevent hypoglycemia.

NURSING TECHNIQUES

Squirrels should be fed in the sternal position. They are very strong sucklers if healthy. The newborn (pinkie or hairless baby) will need to be started on a 1-cc syringe for ease of determining and controlling intake. Depressed infants may be stimulated to drink by angling the syringe upward to tickle the roof of the mouth, or by moving the syringe in and out of the mouth. The size of the syringe should be regularly increased to match the infant's intake. Bottle-feeding often presents problems since the squirrels will adapt to one particular type of nipple and will quickly chew through it as their teeth mature. In addition, gas and bloating are more common with this feeding method, as the infant tends to swallow large amounts of air. Syringe feeding offers the advantage of better control of quantity as the baby learns to nurse. A combination of the two methods has been used in some facilities, where a nipple is fitted over the end of the syringe (Fig. 13.1). However, this may limit the size of the syringe that may be used. Squirrels must be stimulated to urinate and defecate at every feeding until it is determined that they are able to do so on their own, usually at about four to five weeks.

FREQUENCY OF FEEDING

On admission, neonates should be fed electrolyte solution every hour until normal hydration is achieved. Then feedings should be reduced to every two hours. At approximately two weeks of age, the squirrel may be fed every four hours with one late-night feeding (six times/day). At four weeks, the night feeding may be eliminated and the number of feedings reduced by one feed every two days, but only as long as weight gain is consistent. If the squirrel gains weight for two days in a row, it may be cut back on syringe feedings.

When working with small numbers of animals, it is best to closely monitor individuals by weight, as animals develop at differing rates. The California Wildlife Center has documented the cases of three female tree squirrels, all approximately five to six weeks of age on admission, that thrived on one syringe feeding per day by seven weeks of age. One infant started eating solid foods (determined by the fact it was dragging food into the nest with crumbs everywhere) by six weeks of age. It takes many babies longer to wean; six to seven weeks for ground squirrels and ten weeks for tree squirrels, but it is important to attempt to get them to independence as quickly as possible. Any animal that loses weight, or fails to gain on a reduced number of feedings, should be brought back to the level at which it was doing well until it is gaining weight steadily again.

AMOUNTS TO FEED

The amount to feed is based on a combination of overall health, stomach capacity, and individual tol-

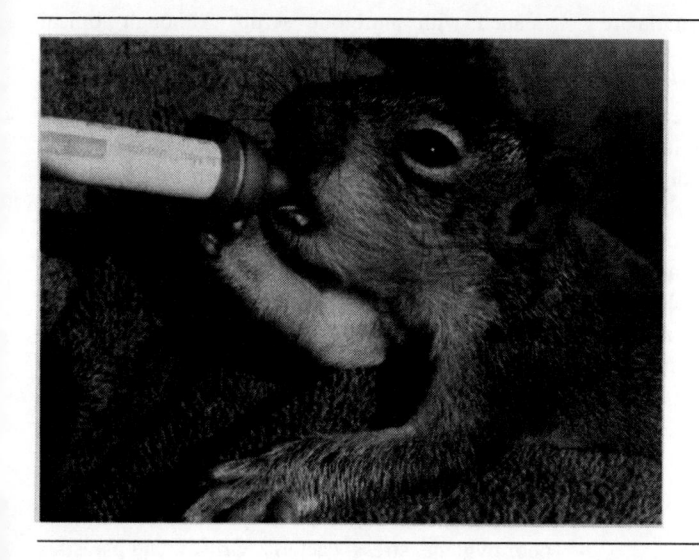

Figure 13.1. Feeding a ground squirrel (photo by Jackie Wollner, California Wildlife Center).

erances. A good rule of thumb is to start at 5% of body weight (i.e., 0.5 cc per 10 g body weight). As the baby progresses, gradual increases in the amount fed can be attempted as long as there are no indications of digestive upset. When the young reach weights over 100 grams, feeding 7% of body weight per feed (or 7 cc/100 g) is well tolerated by most squirrels, but significantly exceeding this amount may result in diarrhea.

HOUSING

Housing of neonates may initially be as simple as a cardboard box, but if an incubator or brooder box is available, that is preferable, especially for "pinkies" or hairless babies. The temperature should be 85–90°F (29.4–32.2°C) and the humidity should be 70–80%. Once the infants' eyes are open, they will need escape-proof and chew-proof housing such as fine mesh (less than 5 cm) wire cages or small airline pet carriers. See Casey and Casey (1998) for a simple design for a starter cage. Old towels or pieces of polyester fleece may be used as bedding. Loose threads should be removed from any bedding fabric. Terry cloth should not be used as some animals may catch their toenails in the loose weave.

Ground squirrels should be transferred into a terrarium filled with wood shavings or clean, soft soil once they are active and weaned. Cedar shavings should not be used as they may cause a skin reaction. If using wood shavings or if the cage is not deep enough to provide two or more feet of soil, a tunnel system of cardboard tubing from paper towels or PVC piping must be provided. Ground squirrels will need a large terrarium in which to develop burrowing skills. Sections of hard plastic piping such as PVC provide hiding places. Monitor carefully if using PVC piping as the squirrels may chew and ingest the plastic.

Tall cages will be needed for tree squirrels to practice their climbing skills. A hiding place such as a hollow tree trunk or a wooden nest box placed in a tree is recommended for tree squirrels that are going to be released, so that they can acclimate to outdoor temperatures with shelter available.

TIME TO WEANING AND TIPS FOR WEANING ONTO SOLID FOOD

Ground squirrels generally wean earlier than tree squirrels, at around six weeks of age. They are much more likely to reject feedings or evade the feeder as they discover solid food. Once their eyes have opened, the babies will begin to explore their environment, often beginning to handle and/or chew items found in their cage. Items of interest will be taken from the surface of the soil or shavings and cached in their tunnels. If these items have been present from the beginning, there will be the added benefit of their recognizing the smell of normal foods.

Tree squirrels will need to be given fewer syringe feedings and need to be provided with a variety of natural foods to push them into the weaning process. They are much more likely than ground squirrels to habituate to the syringe. Small shallow bowls with solid food items soaking in formula are more likely to draw their attention. Fresh fruit is another item they are likely to taste early in the weaning process. Caution should be taken with quantities of fruit provided as they will often overindulge, leading to diarrhea and other digestive upsets. Monitoring weight frequently during the weaning process will allow the caregiver to determine how well the animal is self-feeding. The addition of Purina or Kaytee brand rodent lab block on the bottom of the cage will give the babies a nutritionally well-balanced food item to chew on, and lessen the chance of the squirrels chewing on the cage itself.

COMMON MEDICAL PROBLEMS

Parasites

Fleas and ticks are commonly found on wild-born squirrels. For the health and safety of staff, it is important to remove these parasites. However, the use of chemicals on neonates should always be approached with caution. Manual removal is best. A fine toothed comb is necessary for flea removal and pair of tweezers will be needed for pulling the ticks. Fleas and ticks can be dropped into a bowl of alcohol or acetone to kill them.

Fleas also transmit squirrel pox (Fibromatosis). If lesions are present, they should be cleaned daily. Treatment with ivermectin is recommended.

Lice and sarcoptic mange may also be seen in wild-born squirrels. Animals with either of these parasites should be isolated. A carbamate-based flea powder should be used to treat for lice, once the neonate is determined to be stable. Ivermectin is given for sarcoptic mange but, again, the infant should be stabilized before treatment is initiated. Fly eggs and maggots are often found in the ears, mouth, eye slits, and other areas of very young squirrels, and must be removed promptly.

Common injuries include head and spinal trauma secondary to falls, being hit by cars, or being attacked by dogs or cats. Many urban squirrels unfortunately land on concrete when they fall from their nests, and are admitted to rehabilitation centers with bloody noses. These babies often benefit from a short course of steroids, such as dexamethasone, to combat associated head trauma. Veterinary assistance should be sought in these cases, when possible, as treatment will vary dependent on the severity and location of the lesions. Cat and dog bites are common in wild-born squirrels. Small, superficial wounds can be cleaned with antibiotic scrub. Although topical antibiotics would theoretically be of value, these animals will generally lick their wounds, quickly removing anything applied externally. Oral antibiotics should be used sparingly, especially in neonates due to secondary GI effects and concerns for developing antibiotic resistance in the environment. If the wounds are penetrating or if abscesses are present, veterinary assistance should be sought.

While being hand reared, gastrointestinal (GI) problems often occur. Diarrhea and bloating are most common but caregivers should be alert to the possibility of constipation or aspiration of formula as well. When treating the symptoms, it is also important to attempt to determine the source of the problem. Overfeeding is the number-one culprit in GI upsets, but incorrect temperature of formula, poor hygiene, stress, bacteria, viruses, and parasites may also be a primary or secondary factor. Symptomatic treatment for diarrhea and bloating can include discontinuing feeding for at least one feed, feeding dilute formula or electrolyte solution and giving subcutaneous fluids to prevent dehydration. Course and duration of treatment will vary dependent on the age and overall condition of the animal and the severity of the symptoms.

RELEASE: CAPTIVE VERSUS WILD

Neonates being raised for captive display should be handled regularly as they transition from nursing to self-feeding. It is important to spend time with the animals during this phase so that human beings become a normal and welcome part of their environment. Because they are highly social, separating them from the other squirrels for periods of time, while providing opportunities to interact with caregivers, will enhance this process. Hand feeding of solid foods will also encourage them to approach handlers.

Squirrels intended for release to the wild should have minimal contact with their caregivers. They should always be housed with conspecifics, and talking should be kept to a minimum in their presence. Human-habituated squirrels may be significant hazards to public health and safety. Tree squirrels being prepared for release should be housed in a large cage with natural plant cover and some trees or large branches for climbing. An old, hollow log will provide a natural nesting site. If none is available, a nest box may be used. For squirrels that will remain in captivity, the nest box is preferred as it can be cleaned and disinfected and provides easy access to the animal.

SOURCES FOR PRODUCTS MENTIONED

Fox Valley Animal Nutrition, Inc., PO Box 146, Lake Zurich, IL 60047; 1-800-679-4666

PetAg Inc., 261 Keyes Ave., Hampshire, IL 60140; 1-800-323-0877, 1-800-323-6878; www.petag.com

REFERENCES AND FURTHER READING

Casey, A. M., and S. J. Casey. 1998. Simple things that make a difference: Design and plans for a juvenile squirrel cage. *Journal of Wildlife Rehabilitation* 21(2):30–31.

Fosco, L. 1997. *Rehabilitation of North American tree squirrels.* In-house training manual. San Rafael, CA: WildCare.

Hanes, P. C. 1997. *Ground squirrel rehabilitation.* Suisun, CA: International Wildlife Rehabilitation Council.

Hanes, P. C., and Jennifer Simmons. 1990. Rehabilitation of tree squirrels. Suisun, CA: International Wildlife Rehabilitation Council.

Marcum, D. 1997. Rehabilitation of North American wild mammals: Feeding and nutrition. Suisun, CA: International Wildlife Rehabilitation Council.

Whittaker, J. O. 1995. National Audubon Society field guide to North American mammals. New York: Alfred A. Knopf.

14
Insectivorous Bats

Susan M. Barnard

NATURAL HISTORY

There are 47 species of bats in the United States. Although nectar-feeding bats visit and pollinate some of our desert plants, they are not native to this country. Only insectivorous species will be encountered for hand rearing.

The average birth weight depends on the species and ranges from one-half to six grams. Births are seasonal. Throughout most of the United States they occur May through July.

Important: The bat under care MUST be identified to species as requirements differ from species to species.

RECORD KEEPING

Maintain a log on the milk replacer type(s) being used. Record food intake, daily weight, and fecal consistency. Note when fur begins to appear.

EQUIPMENT

The following items should be on hand:

1-cc syringes (for feeding and hydrating)
25-ga × 5/8 in (1.6 cm) hypodermic needles (for subcutaneous injections)
Lactated Ringer's solution without glucose
Mother's Helper or Zoologic 33/40 puppy milk replacers (PetAg) Modified 3 1/2 French, open-ended tom cat catheter to narrow the feeding tip when using
Syringes to feed pups (most species). Narrowly pointed eyedroppers are also suitable.
Clean artist brush or eye make-up foam applicator to deliver milk to Molossid pups
Glass (not plastic) petri dishes: 100 × 20 mm for mealworms when weaning, and 60 × 15 mm for water
Avitron multivitamins
Avimin multiminerals
Fortified mealworms (see Diet for Mealworms below)
Blender
Styrofoam container (approximately 12 in D × 19 in L × 14 in H [30.5 cm D × 48.3 cm L × 35.6 cm H]) until pup is weaned (see Barnard 1995, for further details)
Appropriate-sized twig when housing pups in the genus *Lasiurus*
Heating pad(s)
Paper towels
Mealworm bags, pillow cases, or other nonfrayed cotton items
Masking, or other adhesive-type tapes
Scale weighing in grams (accurate to at least 0.10 g)
Durocraft fine-mist humidifier

CRITERIA FOR INTERVENTION

Bats are reservoirs for rabies. Only vaccinated individuals should handle bats. Bat babies require hand rearing when they are found on the ground by the public. They may be found if they have fallen from a roost (e.g., eaves of a house, tree), or when they fall off of their mothers during flight. In captivity, bats become orphaned when their mothers abandon them because of overcrowding or other stresses. They are often found on cage flooring by the bat worker.

Orphaned bats may range in age from newly born to a week or more old. Anyone preparing to hand raise an infant bat MUST be able to identify the species and estimate the pup's age. This is a difficult task for inexperienced bat carers: Depending on the species, they can be born with or without fur. Eyes may or may not be open, and some newborn species are so large at birth that they equal the weight of some adult species.

All bats presented for hand raising must be hydrated and weighed before any other action is taken. If one is uncertain as to where to begin, call a bat rehabilitator in the area. For more information, visit http://lads.com/basicallybats/rehablist.html.

INITIAL CARE

Bats have been hand fed with varying degrees of success, using paint brushes, eye make-up sponges, eyedroppers, and syringes. Modified urethral and feeding catheters of appropriate size can be attached to syringes to deliver milk accurately, especially to very small pups (e.g., *Pipistrellus* spp.).

Maintaining adequate hydration is probably the most important factor in rearing pups. Experience has shown that some species dehydrate when offered oral electrolytes in combination with milk (Barnard 1991, 1995). Such solutions should not be used when feeding bats a milk diet, nor should they be used as a substitute for water when mixing milk formulas. Fluid replacement for clinically dehydrated, unweaned pups should be accomplished by subcutaneous injection.

FORMULAS, SUPPLEMENTS, AND INFANT GROWTH

Bat milk varies in composition, not only among species (Jenness and Studier, 1976), but also during the course of lactation (Kunz, Phone conversation with author). Unfortunately, formulas currently available for hand raising infant animals do not approximate the nutrient composition of natural bat milks, and therefore choices selected for rearing bats have been determined through trial and error.

The nutrients in milk replacers vary enough to affect growth rates. In order to evaluate a pup's growth, weigh it each morning before its first meal. If an individual infant fails to gain weight on the prescribed formula, it may become necessary to increase the fat content. This should be done conservatively because oversupplementing with fat causes diarrhea. Add heavy whipping cream in 0.50-ml increments to approximately 25 ml of prepared milk replacer to achieve a steady weight gain. Feed approximately 0.05 ml per gram of body weight.

WHAT TO FEED INITIALLY

A pup should not be fed until it has been hydrated and warmed to a body temperature of approximately 95°F (35°C) (or human body temperature). This can be accomplished by holding it gently in the palm of the hand.

Neonates are born with milk teeth, which allow them to cling to their mothers' teats. These teeth are useless for eating insects, so food should consist of a prepared milk diet. Mix powdered Mother's Helper (Lambert) or Zoologic 33/40 (PetAg) as directed on the label. Do not add supplements such as syrups or vitamins because they may cause diarrhea, and lead to serious dehydration. Avoid the use of milk replacers such Esbilac, Unilact, and KMR (all PetAg products). Butterfat has been added to these milk replacers causing the death of numerous pups of a variety of species.

To maintain hydration, offer oral fluids to pups one-half to one hour after each feeding. Deliver 0.05 cc fluid per gram of body weight of the following solution: one drop Avitron, two drops Avimin (Lambert) in 25 ml tap or distilled water.

NURSING TECHNIQUES

Before feeding pups, warm the formula in a hot-water bath. Check the temperature by placing a drop or two on the inside of the wrist; it should feel warm, not hot. Feed a pup on its belly or side, with its head lower than its feet, to prevent it from aspirating fluids into its lungs (see Fig. 14.1).

FREQUENCY OF FEEDING AND AMOUNTS TO FEED

Insectivorous pups require frequent feedings, approximately every two to three hours. If they refuse food at two-hour feeding intervals, or if formula is still visible in their stomachs (this is easily seen through the skin of the abdomen), feed approximately every three hours, or adjust the feeding schedule as necessary. For pups weighing over 4 g, feedings should begin around 6 A.M. and can be discontinued at 11 P.M. to midnight. Pups weighing 4 g or less require at least one feeding during the night. Feed approximately 0.05 ml per gram of body weight.

EXPECTED WEIGHT GAIN

The single most important way in which one can determine if a baby bat is growing properly is to weigh it daily. Most pups lose weight or remain stable until they learn how to take formula from the substitute teat. Depending on the species, weight gains will vary. For example, an eastern pipistrelle bat, *Pipistrellus subflavus*, should gain approximately 0.5 g per week for the first six to eight weeks. At maturity, this bat's weight fluctuates between 5 g and 9 g. The medium-sized big brown

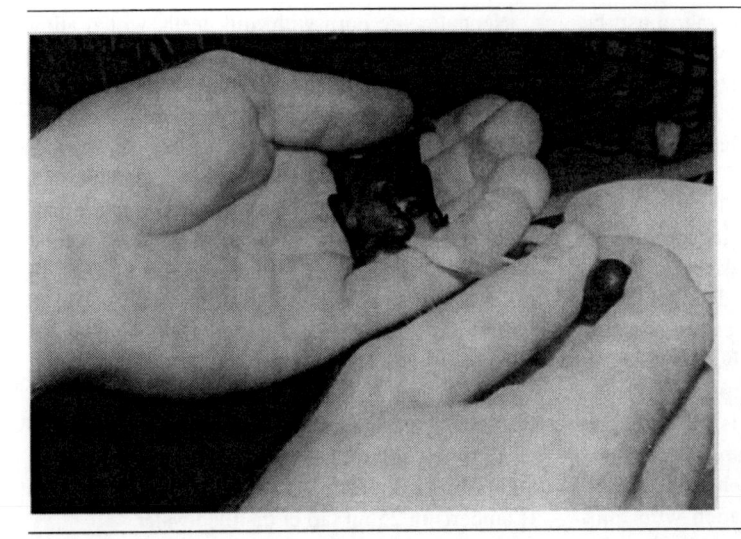

Figure 14.1. When feeding a baby bat, tilt it slightly downward to prevent it from aspirating formula into its lungs. (Photo courtesy of Forest Park Nature Center, Peoria Heights, IL.)

bat, *Eptesicus fuscus*, is typically 18 g to 23 g at maturity. Its infant growth rate should be approximately 1.5 g per week for the first eight weeks. The hoary bat, *Lasiurus cinereus*, is a relatively large bat, and its adult weight may reach 30–35 g. For the first eight weeks, the pups should gain approximately 3 g per week.

SPECIAL NEEDS

Infant bats will lap milk readily, a drop at a time, from the palm of the hand or directly from one of the objects discussed above. Avoid the use of nursing bottles, as these can cause fatal colic (Barnard 1988–1990). Before feeding a pup, wash hands thoroughly to prevent contaminating any formula that pups may lick from the palm of the hand.

It is not known why some species fail to thrive on milk replacer. For example, *Lasiurus borealis* and *Pipistrellus subflavus* bloat and/or dehydrate when fed exclusively milk formula. This problem is sometimes overcome by offering these pups milk replacer once a day and a blended mealworm diet for the remaining meals, or by alternating the two food sources.

After each feeding, wet a cotton swab with lukewarm water and massage the pup's anus to stimulate defecation. Note, however, that they may not defecate after every meal. Normal stools are firm and black; although, it is usual for pups to have cream-colored stools for a day or two until they adjust to the milk replacer.

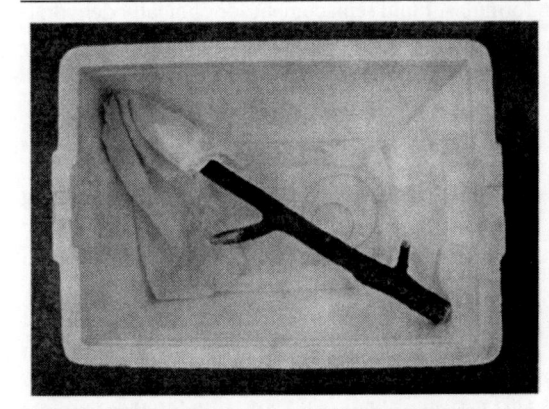

Figure 14.2. Pups of a tree-roosting bat species require a branch on which to roost (or a mesh-lined container top) to allow them to hang naturally. (From Barnard 1995)

Special attention must be paid to the roosting habit of lasiurine bats: these infants will soil themselves if they are not allowed to hang from a thin rough branch (see Fig. 14.2), or mesh on a cage top.

HOUSING: CAGING AND ENVIRONMENT

Place a pup in a Styrofoam container measuring approximately 12 in D × 19 in L × 14 in H (30.5 cm D × 48.3 cm L × 35.6 cm H) until it is weaned (see Barnard 1995, for further details). Air can be provided by punching one row of holes with a pencil around the middle of the container. *Be sure to punch the holes from the inside to the outside of the container.* Always tape the top of the container to prevent a pup from escaping. Whether baby bats are hand raised at home or in a windowless office, they should be exposed to the same photoperiod as the person doing the hand raising. Maintain container temperatures between 80°F (26.7°C) and 84°F (28.9°C), and relative humidities of 55–80%. *Warning: Many facilities place pups in incubators to maintain warmth and humidity. When housed in these devices, small species often die of dehydration.*

Monitor heating pads closely because they can malfunction, resulting in fatal burns. Pups of small bat species can be kept warm by placing the nursery container with the pup in a larger one with the heating pad wedged between the walls of the two containers, as shown in Figure 14.3. The insulating properties of the two containers also protect the pup against rapid temperature changes when the heating pad must be unplugged for short periods. If the two-container system is not used, then a heating pad can be placed between the nursery container housing the bat and any wall. Do not place a heating pad directly inside a small Styrofoam container because even at the lowest setting, the pad may generate enough heat to produce hyperthermia in the pup. When providing warmth with a heating pad, never place it under the cage bottom. Bats generally seek out the highest point in a cage, and forcing them to the bottom for warmth may be stressful. Also, heating pads on cage bottoms cause bats to lie horizontally, rather than in the normal upside down position which, over an extended period of time, may result in swollen joints.

Place nursery containers with pups in a room small enough that humidity can be regulated with a fine-mist humidifier (e.g., Durocraft). Be sure to follow the manufacturer's instructions on the care of the humidifier.

For proper growth, pups require room to exercise. Juveniles of crevice-dwelling species (e.g., big brown bats) should be placed in hard-sided caging with wood walls (see Figs. 14.4a, b, c).

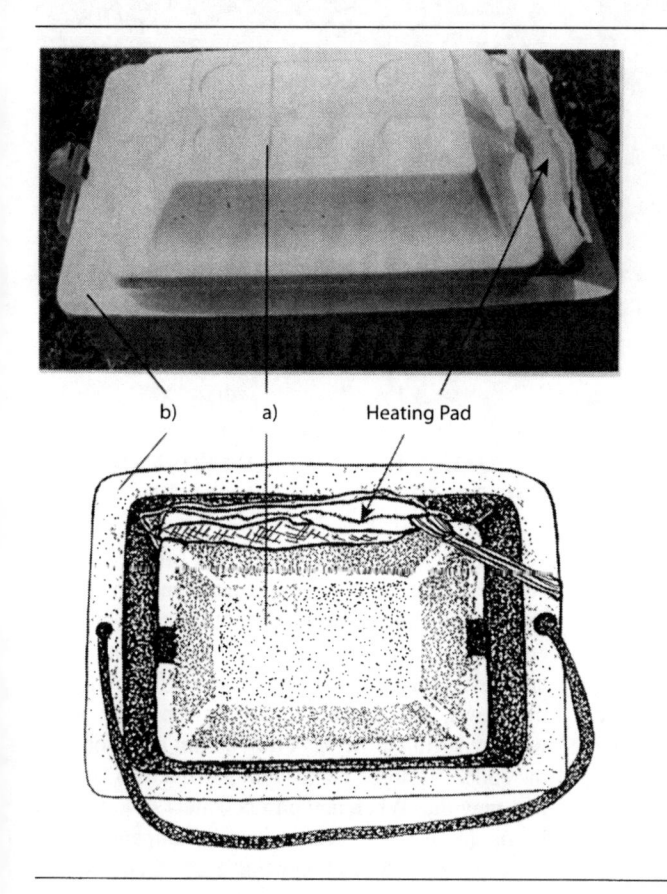

Figure 14.3. To prevent overheating a pup with a heating pad, place the small container with pup (a) inside a larger container (b). Wedge the heating pad between the two containers as shown by the arrows. (From Barnard 1992)

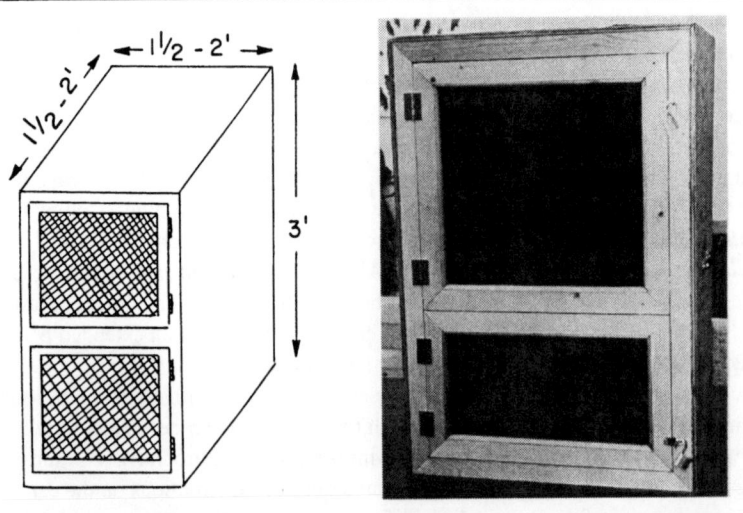

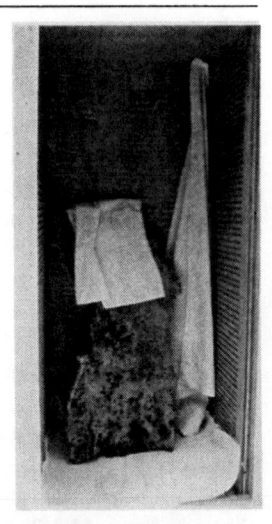

Figure 14.4. Juveniles of crevice-dwelling bat species should be housed in wooden cages. (a) Cage dimensions; (b) constructed cage; (c) cage interior. (From Barnard 1995)

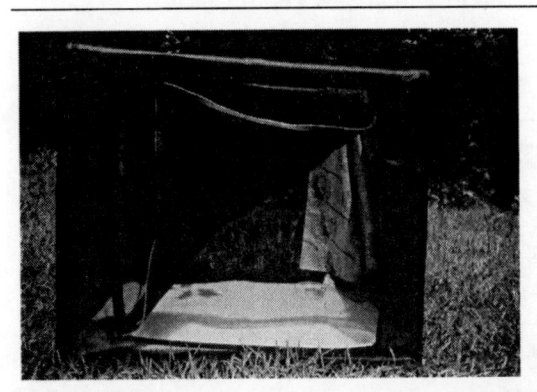

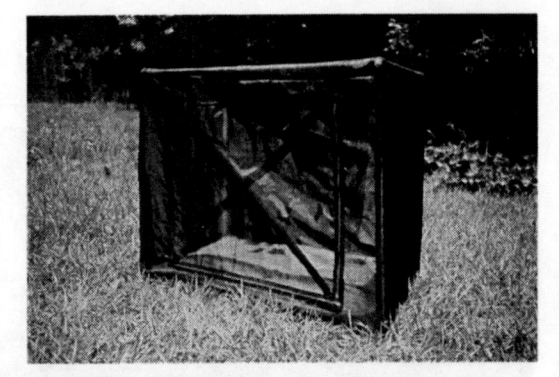

Figure 14.5. Juveniles of tree-dwelling bat species should be housed in soft-sided caging. (a) Door unzipped and pinned open; (b) door zipped closed.

Place lasiurines (e.g., red bats) in an appropriately sized (65 gal) soft-sided cage (see Fig. 14.5). The cages (called reptariums) may be purchased online at http://www.thatpetplace.com.

TIME TO WEANING

Most insectivorous pups are ready to be weaned at about three to four weeks of age. This is also the age when they are ready to fly. They do not have to be taught; it is instinctive. Milk teeth have been replaced by permanent teeth, and the infant is ready to receive chitin (the substance forming insect exoskeletons) in its diet. Chitin is important to the bat for the continued formation of firm stools.

TIPS FOR WEANING FROM FORMULA TO SOLID FOOD

To wean bats onto mealworms, cut off the insect's head and squeeze its viscera into the pup's mouth as one would squeeze a tube of toothpaste. Whenever bats are willing, allow them to chew on the chitinous exoskeletons of the mealworms to strengthen their jaws. This process, however, can leave mealworm viscera on the bat's fur. Within a day or two, the soiled fur loses its insulating properties and the pup may die. When any pup becomes soiled, clean its fur immediately with a warm, dampened swab stick, gauze pad, or cloth handkerchief. Allow it to dry naturally near a the heating pad. Never dry a bat with a hair dryer.

To teach a juvenile to associate food with a dish, feed it over one containing fortified mealworms, and always feed it from the end of a blunt forceps, not the fingers. After the bat has eaten its ration, offer it a few drops of fresh water. When a bat feeds regularly on whole mealworms (about 10 to 40 or more, depending on the species) with their heads intact, it should be housed and fed as an adult in the appropriate cage type (see Figs. 14.4 and 14.5).

The blended mealworm diet and the diet for mealworms are given below:

Blended Mealworm Diet[1]
Blend together:
Mealworms[2] . . . . 3 g
Olive oil . . . . .1 drop
Vitamin/Mineral Water[3] . . . . .1.5 ml

[1] Freeze surplus and defrost as needed.
[2] Large mealworms weigh approx. 0.10 g
[3] Vitamin/Mineral Water is prepared by mixing together 1 drop Avitron multivitamins and 2 drops Avimin multiminerals in 30 ml tap or distilled water.

Diet for Mealworms
Per 10,000 mealworms:
Oat bran . . . . .1/2 cup
Wheat bran . . . . .1/2 cup
Cornmeal . . . . .1/2 cup
Powdered Vionate multivitamins . . . . . . .1/2 cup
Bone meal powder (sterilized) or calcium
    carbonate powder . . . . .1/2 cup
Leafy greens, unchopped (e.g., collards,
    spinach, cabbage, mustard greens, kale, etc.)
    . . . . .several
    leaves
Sweet potato and/or apple . . . . .1/2 each

COMMON MEDICAL PROBLEMS

Bloat

Bloat is commonly observed in hand-raised, neonate bats that ingest air during feeding. Colic may be avoided by offering formula in such a way that ingestion of air is minimized. For example, avoid using bottles with nipples when feeding insectivorous bat pups.

Occasionally, newborns are orphaned before their intestinal tract develops normal flora. Certain milk replacement formulas contain ingredients that are difficult for pups to digest (Barnard, 1991, 1992, 1995) and thus cause bloat. If the underlying cause is not diagnosed quickly, the condition is usually fatal. In these cases, it may be necessary to medicate them by alternating simethicone (Mylicon or Phazyme, available over-the-counter) and metoclopramide hydrochloride (Reglan, available by prescription) syrup five to ten days into the hand-raising period. Mix these products separately, adding one drop of product with four drops of tap or distilled water. Add two drops of the mixtures to 1 ml of formula. Alternate these medications at every meal for up to ten days. Do not mix medications together.

Dehydration

Virtually all sick, injured, or orphaned bats become dehydrated. Mortalities may be reduced substantially by rehydrating them immediately, and before further treatment. Give subcutaneous injections of lactated Ringer's solution (without glucose) at a dosage of 0.05 ml/g/day. Insert the needle on the bat's back just posterior to the shoulder blades. Depending upon the severity of the medical problem, a bat will rehydrate within one to three days. It will usually accept food after the second or third injection of lactated Ringer's solution, and food must be offered by hand to insure it receives adequate nutrition. A dehydrated bat probably has not fed voluntarily because it produces little or no saliva, making it difficult for the animal to swallow.

Diarrhea

Diarrhea in captive bats is usually associated with diet and/or stress. Dietary causes include the feeding of spoiled food. "Bat glop" (a pureed diet containing various mixtures of dairy products, commercial baby foods, commercial cultivars of produce, and other commercially available foods), fed as a substitute for live, fortified insects may also cause diarrhea. Other dietary causes of diarrhea include overfeeding, or oversupplementation with multivitamins or fat.

Stress may induce diarrhea. Stressors include shipping, cage changes, overhandling, incompatible cage mates, a noisy environment, and, depending on the species, exposure to inappropriate lighting and/or prolonged exposure to humidities below 30% or above 80%. Viruses, bacteria, and endoparasites can also cause diarrhea in bats.

Wing Injuries

Simple fractures usually heal within a month with minimal or no medical assistance. Euthanasia should be considered when pups are presented with compound fractures.

Respiratory Disorders

Respiratory problems in bats are similar to those in other mammals. Pneumonia can encompass a variety of causes including parasites, fungi, bacteria, viruses, chemical inhalation, and fluid aspiration (especially in hand-raised infants). Symptoms include nasal and oral discharge, gaping, audible, and labored breathing, depression, anorexia, and emaciation. Treatment for respiratory disease in bats is the same as it is for other mammals.

Infectious Diseases

Rabies is the most widely reported disease in bats. The AZA Bat TAG (1995) reported that there are no rabies vaccines presently recommended for bats (but see Wiggins 1995). Furthermore, they reported that any vaccine administered to a bat might interfere with tests for rabies detection (see Wiggins 1995).

Membrane Problems

Small holes in the wing membrane do not affect a bat's ability to fly and should be left alone.

Hair Loss

Unnatural hair loss can be caused by dietary deficiencies, disease, or poisoning. Inexperienced caregivers also tend to leave pups on milk replacer too long. The weaning process should begin within three weeks of birth. In species that are born without fur, weaning should begin at the onset of fur growth.

Parasites

Bats worldwide support endo- and ectoparasites similar to those found in other mammals. In captivity, mites are the most difficult to control when strict quarantine is not observed. Of particular interest is the fact that bat ectoparasites usually disappear after several weeks when caging and bedding are cleaned daily. Avoid chemical eradication.

Coccidiosis has been treated successfully with trimethoprim sulfamethoxazole suspension (concentration of 40 mg of trimethoprim and 200 mg of sulfamethoxazole per 5 cc) at a dosage of 15 mg/kg, PO BID, for eight to ten days (Barnard, 1991, 1995).

Fenbendazole is effective against intestinal nematodes in bats at a dosage of 50 mg/kg, PO SID, for three days; repeated in three weeks if necessary (Barnard 1991, 1995), or at a single dose of 75–100 mg/kg, PO; repeated in ten days (AZA Bat TAG 1995). Although ivermectin has been recommended for treating intestinal nematodes in bats (AZA Bat TAG 1995), it is my opinion that its use should be avoided.

Praziquantel is recommended for cestode infections at a dosage of 7.5–15 mg/kg, IM or PO (AZA Bat TAG 1995).

Trematodes are difficult to treat, and even a high dose of praziquantel is usually ineffective (AZA Bat TAG 1995).

Poisoning

Accidental poisoning can occur when pesticides and disinfectants are used indiscriminately. The major cause of poisoning in insectivorous species is from ingestion of pesticides sprayed in the environment. Typical symptoms of poisoning include a hunched back; drawn-up legs; excessive salivation; rapid respiration; increased, irregular, or slow respiration; tremors; incoordination; hindquarter weakness and/or stiffness; and lethargy. When poisoning is suspected, administer supportive therapy. Treatments include activated charcoal, calcium gluconate, atropine sulfate, diuretics, and fluids. Follow the manufacturer's recommended dosages. Also, controlling central nervous system stimulation with diazepam or barbiturates may be indicated.

RELEASE: CAPTIVE VERSUS WILD

Bats are highly specialized animals with complex lives. Many species learn "bat life" from their mothers (Barclay 1982; Bateman and Vaughan 1974; Bradbury 1977; Brigham and Brigham 1989; Vaughan 1976; Vaughan and Vaughan 1987). Young bats observe and mimic their mothers and/or conspecifics to learn how, what, and where to hunt, but a high percentage of them still die during their first year of life. Survival requires adequate hunting skills, identification of appropriate shelters (e.g., day and night roosts, hibernacula), knowledge of migratory routes, avoidance of predators, and appropriate social skills with conspecifics. Bats must also be in excellent condition, both physically and behaviorally, or their chances for survival are limited.

Captive-reared, insectivorous bats have been taught to catch insects in flight within the confines of a building. Such bug-catching abilities, however, may not translate into survival in the wild. Rehabilitators must hold themselves accountable when releasing hand-raised or captive-born bats by making every effort to evaluate the success or failure of their release programs. This might be achieved with the use of implanted electromagnetic transponders (Barnard 1989) in combination with identification bands and radio-tracking devices (Adkins and Wasserman 1993; Albrecht and Helversen 1994; Dicke 1994). Until affordable and workable release programs can be developed for captive-reared, insectivorous bats, they should remain in captivity. Rehabilitators who hand raise insectivorous bats, and who are not working on *bona fide* release studies, may wish to consider the following options:

1. Some bats, such as those in the genera *Eptesicus*, *Nycticeius*, and *Tadarida*, adapt well to captivity and can be sent to appropriate institutions for use in education and conservation programs. Anyone not able to care for a hand-reared bat for the duration of its natural life (up to 20 years), should make every effort to find it a permanent home at a zoological park, museum, or nature center.
2. Species that do not adapt well to captive conditions, such as *Lasiurus* and *Mormoops*, might have a better chance of living if displayed to the public in relatively large, naturalistic exhibits.
3. Another option is euthanasia, preferably before the hand-raising process begins.

Rehabilitation considerations proposed for human-raised orphaned bats also apply to those born in captivity to wild, releasable mothers. Wild, insectivorous bats who give birth in captivity may abandon their pups when released. Any wild animal suddenly taken captive, regardless of the reason, must perceive the situation as "dangerous." Lactating females, therefore, increase their chance of surviving, and reproducing again, by lightening their burden with the abandonment of their young.

SOURCES OF PRODUCTS MENTIONED

Durocraft Corporation, 490 Boston Post Road, Sudbury, MA 01776-9102

Lambert Kay, Division of Carter-Wallace, Inc., Cranbury, NJ 09512-0187

PetAg Inc., 261 Keyes Ave., Hampshire, IL 60140; 1-800-323-0877, 1-800-323-6878; www.petag.com

REFERENCES

Adkins, B., and J. Wasserman. 1993. Suitability of captive-reared bats for release: A post-release study of a captive-reared big brown bat (*Eptesicus fuscus*). *National Wildlife Rehabilitation Symposium Proceedings* (Sacramento, CA) 11:119–26.

Albrecht, K., and O. V. Helversen. 1994. Development of foraging behavior of young noctule bats, *Nyctalus noctula*, revealed by radio tracking. *Bat Res. News* 35:13.

Allen, G. M. 1939. *Bats*. Cambridge, MA: Harvard University Press.

American Zoo and Aquarium Association Chiropteran Taxon Advisory Group (AZA Bat TAG). 1995. *Fruit bat husbandry manual*. Gainesville, FL: Lubee Foundation, Inc.; Kensington, MD: AZA Bat TAG.

Barclay, R. M. R. 1982. Interindividual use of ecolocation calls: Eavesdropping by bats. *Behavioral Ecology and Sociobiology* 10:271–75.

Barnard, S. M. 1988–90. *The maintenance of insectivorous bats in captivity*, editions 1, 2, and 3. Atlanta, GA: Zoo Atlanta.

———. 1989. The use of microchip implants for identifying big brown bats (*Eptesicus fuscus*). *Animal Keepers Forum* 16:50–52.

———. 1991. *The maintenance of bats in captivity*. Atlanta, GA: Zoo Atlanta.

———. 1992. Rehabilitating bats: Caring for orphans. *Wildlife Rehabilitation Today* Spring:45–47.

———. 1995. *Bats in captivity*. Springville, CA: Wild Ones Animal Books.

Bateman, G. C., and T. A. Vaughan. 1974. Nightly activities of mormoopid bats. *Journal of Mammalogy* 55:45–65.

Bradbury, J. W. 1977. Social organization and communication. In *The biology of bats*, vol. 3, edited by W. A. Wimsatt. New York: Academic Press.

Brigham, R. M., and A. C. Brigham. 1989. Evidence for association between a mother bat and its young during and after foraging. *American Midland Naturalist* 121:205–7.

Dicke, C. 1994. A post-release study of a juvenile pallid bat. *Wildlife Rehab* 17:3–5.

Kunz, T. H. 1989. Phone conversation with author. Boston University, Boston, MA.

Vaughan, T. A. 1976. Nocturnal behavior of the African false vampire bat (*Cardioderma cor*). *Journal of Mammalogy* 57:227–48.

Vaughan, T. A., and R. P. Vaughan. 1987. Parental behavior in the African yellow-winged bat. *Journal of Mammalogy* 68:217–23.

Wiggins, G. 1995. Management of rabies in a colony of pallid bats (*Antrozous pallidus*) at the North Carolina Zoo. In *Proceedings of the American Association of Zoo Keepers National Conference*, Denver, CO.

15
Lemurs

Cathy V. Williams

NATURAL HISTORY

There are more than 50 recognized taxa of Lemuriformes (Mittermeier et al. 1994). Lemurs range in size from mouse lemurs weighing as little as 25 grams (*Microcebus* spp.) to Indri (*Indri indri*) weighing 6–8 kg. Given the diversity of dietary and environmental requirements found among different species, this chapter will focus on four diurnal species kept in captivity for which successful hand-rearing techniques have been developed; ring-tailed lemurs (*Lemur catta*), ruffed lemurs (*Varecia variegata*), true lemurs (*Eulemur* spp.), and sifakas (*Propithecus* spp.) (see Fig. 15.1).

Under natural conditions births are seasonal and in the Northern Hemisphere the majority occur between December and April. This seasonality is related to photoperiod sensitivity and out-of-season births can occur when light cycles are manipulated in captivity. Patterns of maternal care differ among lemur species. Some lemurs carry their young continuously the first few months of life while others leave their offspring in a nest or protected area. Of the species covered in this chapter, ring-tailed lemurs, true lemurs, and sifakas carry their young and ruffed lemurs use nests.

The average birth weight and number are as follows:

Ring-tailed lemurs: 65–85 g, singletons or twins
True lemur: 55–105 g, singletons or twins. Weights are subspecies dependant.
Ruffed lemurs: 80–125 g, litters of one to five
Sifakas: 90–115 g, singletons

SUPPLEMENTATION VERSUS HAND REARING

In this chapter the term "supplementation" is used to indicate nutritional support given while an infant is housed with its dam or other members of its own species. Hand rearing refers to an animal raised in a

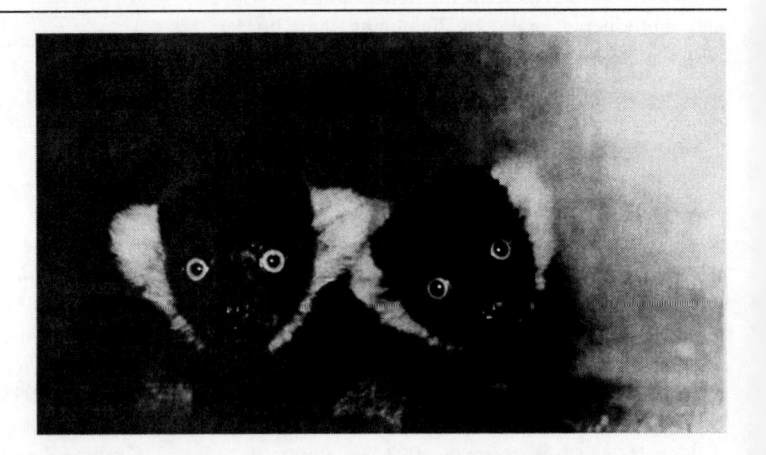

Figure 15.1. Black and white ruffed lemur twins.

nursery environment away from adults of its own species. In my opinion, hand rearing should be done only in extreme circumstances when other options have been exhausted. Hand-reared infants are more likely to exhibit abnormal social or behavioral traits and be aggressive as adults than are supplemented infants. This is less a concern in species that nest than in those that carry their young. Additionally, infants that nurse from their dams, even on a limited basis, are less likely to develop nutritional deficiencies that may occur in fully formula-reared infants. Even complete supplemental nutrition can be accomplished while infants stay with the mother or family group. At the Duke University Primate Center, successful hand supplementation of orphaned sifakas has been accomplished while infants were housed either with their father or older sibling, thereby eliminating the need to rear them in a nursery setting.

RECORD KEEPING

When supplementing or hand rearing lemurs, it is important to keep detailed records. Use a daily log to record body weight taken at a consistent time each morning, food intake, fecal production and consistency, and behavioral notes including appetite and attitude.

EQUIPMENT

Due to the small volumes of formula consumed by neonatal lemurs, feeding with syringes or eyedroppers rather than bottles and nipples is more reliable. As infants gain weight and formula volumes increase, they can be switched to a pet nurser if desired. Useful supplies include syringes (3, 6, and 12 cc) and red rubber catheters or feeding tubes (8–12 French). In addition, have on hand a mortar and pestle, gram scale, bottles for mixing and storing formula, an incubator and thermometer for young infants, hot-water bottles, disposable gloves, towels, and a surrogate such as a stuffed animal for clinging species.

CRITERIA FOR INTERVENTION

Nutritional support is necessary when infants are weak, fail to gain weight, become ill or orphaned, or in the event of maternal illness, neglect, or abuse. Low birth weight by itself is not a reason to intervene as long as the mother is attentive and the infant is vigorous and gains weight steadily. In species in which mothers carry their infants, normal newborns cling horizontally across the mother's lower abdomen or upright at a slight angle while nursing

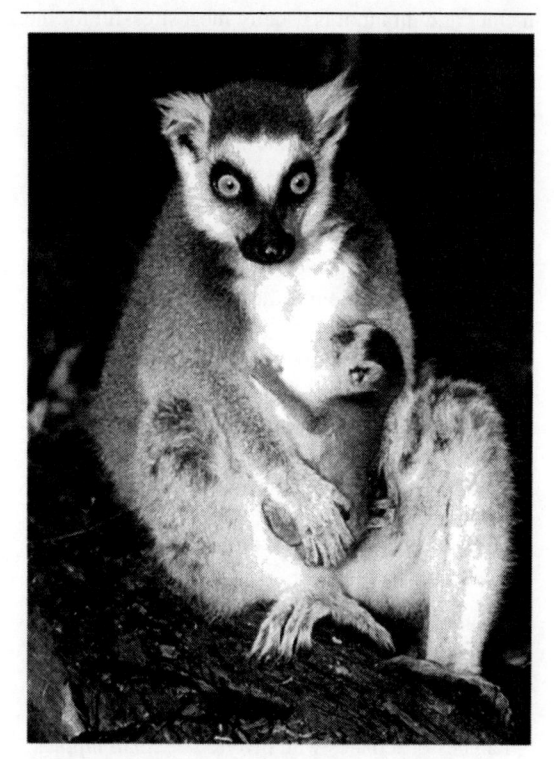

Figure 15.2. Ring-tailed lemur dam with infant in normal nursing position.

(Fig. 15.2). An infant's grip should tighten when it is startled or the mother moves. As the infant ages it gradually shifts to riding on the mother's back. In species that leave their young in a nest, mothers stay with their infants almost continuously the first few days after birth tucking them underneath her thus keeping them warm and allowing them to suckle.

CARE AND ASSESSMENT OF NEONATES

Lemur infant mortality is highest in the first 72 hours after birth. Recognizing and correcting problems early in the neonatal period can often prevent the need for long-term intervention. Careful observations of an infant's behavior and accurate daily weights are the best measure of health status. If possible, obtain a weight the day of birth, then twice weekly until the infant is one month old, then weekly until weaned. A one to two day drop in weight is acceptable but longer plateaus or decreases in weight gain are reason for concern. If a question exists as to the status of an infant, removing it from the mother for a physical exam, including a temperature and weight, is necessary. While physically removing a clinging infant can be traumatic for the mother and infant, it is usually most stressful for the handler. One person restrains the dam or distracts her with a food treat while a second removes the infant. Normal newborns vocalize loudly, eyes are open and alert, movements are vigorous, and the grip in hands and feet is strong. Droopy eyelids, infrequent or weak vocalizations, hypothermia (body temperature less than 96°F or 35.5°C), and weak grip are all signs of trouble.

A common problem in neonates is the failure to begin nursing after birth. Infants normally begin nursing within a few hours of birth and infants that do not nurse during the first 8–12 hours lose strength rapidly. They may cling in abnormal positions such as to the dam's leg, arm, or back. Once the infant's strength wanes, its head begins to drop and the grip becomes weak, until it finally falls off the mother. Infants may not be able to nurse for several reasons, including:

- Neonatal weakness due to a premature or traumatic birth
- Inability to initiate nursing because of irregular maternal anatomy as encountered with obese females or females with inverted or small nipples
- Inability to nurse often enough (Agitated females move frequently thereby preventing infants from suckling for sufficient amounts of time.)
- Maternal neglect (Maternal factors predisposing toward neglect include illness, first-time birth, or increased agitation. Dams may also reject hypothermic or weak offspring.)

Hypothermia, hypoglycemia, and dehydration are commonly encountered problems. A hypothermic but otherwise healthy neonate can be warmed, given oral electrolytes and dextrose, and returned to a maternally competent dam. If a dam neglects her offspring but is not aggressive, isolating the mother and infant(s) for several days in a small confined space, such as an airline kennel, may induce a reluctant dam to care for her young. Infants may need partial support in the form of oral or subcutaneous fluids, feeding, or warming until a dam begins showing interest in her offspring.

The longer mother and infant are separated, the greater the likelihood the mother will reject the infant when returned. Maternal rejection may occur after separations of 24 hours or less in the case of newborns. Therefore, housing the mom in close proximity to the sick infant and maximizing visual, olfactory, and physical contact improves the chance the mother will accept the infant when it is returned to her.

FORMULAS, SUPPLEMENTS, AND DAILY CALORIC REQUIREMENTS

Information on the composition of normal lemur milk is limited but available data indicate composition varies widely between species (Tilden 1997). In general, species that carry their young produce dilute milk low in energy, fat, and protein. Infants nurse on demand and ingest small amounts of milk frequently. Ring-tailed lemurs (*Lemur catta*) and true lemurs (*Eulemur* spp.) fall in this category. Species in which infants are left unattended for extended periods and nurse only upon return of the mother produce milk with higher fat, protein, and gross energy. This group includes ruffed lemurs (*Varecia variegata*), aye-ayes (*Daubentonia madagascariensis*), and many small nocturnal lemurs and prosimians. Preliminary evidence suggests that sifakas produce milk with a high fat content relative to other primates that carry their young. Fat levels in two samples of sifaka milk collected at the Duke University Primate Center and analyzed at the National Zoological Park in Washington, DC, had fat levels of 11.5 and 13.5%, respectively. If the use of artificial formulas becomes necessary, they should approximate as closely as possible the composition of normal mother's milk for the species being raised. While lemurs have been successfully raised on cow milk formulas, formulas using human infant formula or Zoologic Milk Matrix (PetAg) as a base are preferable because the balance of vitamins, minerals, and micronutrients is likely to be more appropriate for young, growing primates. It is important to note that if human or Milk Matrix formulas are used, supplemental pediatric vitamins should be avoided as the combination can lead to overdoses of certain vitamins and minerals, particularly iron (Spelman, Osborn, and Anderson 1989). Thus, when human formulas are used, low-iron varieties are preferred. For recommended formulas see Table 15.1.

Care must be given to mixing formula consistently and in a hygienic manner. Keep in mind the following points:

- Formula spoils quickly so prepare only enough to last 24 hours and keep unused portions refrigerated. Heat only the portion to be fed during a single feeding and discard heated formula that is not consumed.
- Sterilize mixing bottles before preparing formula. It is not necessary to sterilize the formula

Table 15.1. Formulas

Ring-tailed Lemurs and True Lemurs

Formula 1: 30 ml human infant formula prepared according to directions
30 ml nonfat milk
3 ml 50% dextrose
Formula 2: Zoologic® Milk Matrix 20/14—10 g powder to 100 ml water

Ruffed Lemurs

Formula 1: 100 ml human infant formula prepared according to directions
5 g nonfat dried milk powder
Formula 2: Zoologic Milk Matrix 20/20—18 g per 100 ml of water
Formula 3: 120 ml whole cow's milk
15–22 ml rice cereal *or* 7 ml 50% dextrose
1–2 drops pediatric vitamin drops per animal per day

Sifakas

Formula 1: 5 g powdered human infant formula
2 g Esbilac milk replacer powder (or Zoologic Milk Matrix 30/55).
Add water up to 40 ml
Formula 2: Zoologic Milk Matrix 23/30—20 g per 100 ml of water

Notes: Zoologic Milk Matrix and Esbilac distributed by PetAg Inc., 261 Keyes Ave., Box 396, Hampshire, IL 60140; Phone 1-800-323-0877; www.petag.com

itself. Syringes, feeding tips, and stomach tubes can be washed, soaked in dilute chlorhexidine disinfectant, and rinsed well between uses.

- The temperature of the formula is very important. Infants generally prefer formula at body temperature and may reject formula that is too hot or too cold. The person feeding the infant should always test the temperature by dropping a few drops on the inside of his or her wrist prior to feeding.
- Warming formula in a microwave or water bath may result in overheating or uneven heating (hot spots). Always mix formula thoroughly before testing the temperature.

Energy requirements of lemur infants are estimated according to those of other nonhuman primates and range from 0.15–0.25 kcal/g of body weight/day in newborns. Energy requirements increase for several weeks thereafter depending on the species.

WHAT TO FEED INITIALLY

For the first 24 hours give warmed electrolyte solution containing dextrose every one to two hours orally at a volume of 1–2 ml/100 g body weight. Saline with dextrose added to 10% is preferred but Pedialyte (Ross) alone may be used in a pinch. If after the first day nutritional support is still needed, transition infants to formula by feeding half-strength formula and electrolyte solution (or Pedialyte) for 24 hours, three-fourths-strength formula for another 24 hours, and finally full-strength formula. Normal stools and a lack of abdominal bloating indicate tolerance of the formula. Normal stools of sifaka infants are pelleted while those of most other species are semiformed and yellow to brown in color.

In most mammals there is antibody transfer in the initial milk, or colostrum, produced by the mother. Thus, infants who receive colostrum have an advantage over those that do not. If an infant is not able to nurse or is prevented from nursing by the dam, colostrum can be manually expressed from the mother and fed by syringe. Alternately, many dams will allow infants to be manually placed on the nipple to suckle if lightly sedated and gently restrained. Keeping a dam's mammary glands emptied also encourages continued milk production, which is important if infants are to be reunited with their mothers. This is preferred because mother's milk will likely continue to provide some degree of antibody protection to the infant.

NURSING TECHNIQUES

Feeding and handling techniques should approximate the natural feeding position and nipple size of the dam as much as possible. Lemur neonates may be difficult to feed initially. Weak or sick infants may have a depressed suckle reflex and will not take fluids voluntarily. Slowly dripping fluids from a syringe or eyedropper may be necessary. Many are also reluctant to suckle on artificial nipples. As feeding volumes are initially small, it is easier to control delivery rate and to track amounts consumed if infants are fed by syringe. A red rubber feeding tube can be cut to size and attached to the syringe tip to serve as a nipple. Even though a neonate may suckle on the nipple, the feeder determines the rate of the delivery of the formula with the syringe. Once the infant is larger, it can be trained to feed from a pet nurser if desired (Fig. 15.3).

Most infants come to accept an artificial nipple well. Occasionally an infant refuses the nipple altogether and must be fed by stomach tube or gavage. Size 8–12 French red rubber catheters make ideal stomach tubes. First measure the distance from the nose to the last rib to determine how far to insert the tube. Mark the appropriate length with a piece of tape or indelible marker. With one person holding the infant, a second inserts the tube in the infant's mouth and slowly guides the tube over the base of the tongue, past the gag reflex, and down the throat. Once past the gag reflex, the tube should advance easily into the stomach. If the tube does not advance easily to the measured length withdraw it and start over. Infants may not always cough or gag in response to the tube entering the trachea. Once inserted, the proper position of the tube in the esophagus can be verified by palpation of the tube in the neck just alongside the trachea. Older infants may need to be swaddled in a towel to prevent them from grabbing the tube and pulling it out of their mouth. Deliver the formula slowly by syringe. Extreme care must be taken not to overfill the stomach. Initially, feed only 75% of the volume that would be fed by bottle or syringe and increase gradually only if the infant seems to accept the increases easily. With the tube still in place, flush the remaining formula from it with a small amount of water and kink the tube before removing to prevent backflow.

Hand-fed infants are at risk of developing aspiration pneumonia if formula or fluids are fed too quickly. Give careful attention to the rate formula is fed and to using proper technique when passing stomach tubes. For consistency, limit the number of feeders if an infant requires repeated stomach tubing.

FREQUENCY OF FEEDING AND AMOUNTS TO FEED

Newborns should be fed every two hours around the clock for the first week. Once the infant is gaining weight steadily, formula quantity and the time between feedings can be gradually increased. Lemurs that normally ride on their mothers, nurse for long periods and it is important to resist the temptation to spread out feedings too quickly when

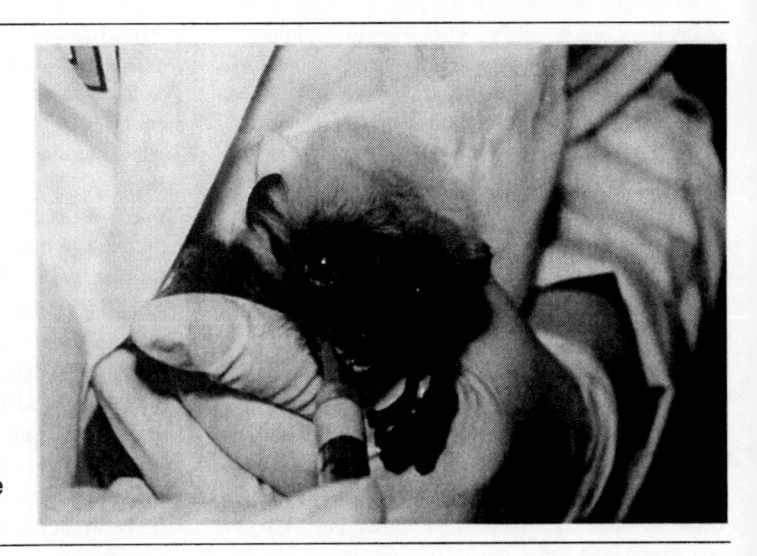

Figure 15.3. Technique for feeding a sifaka infant by syringe (photos by David Haring, Duke University Primate Center).

hand feeding. Feedings should be administered on a body-weight basis with the frequency and amount adjusted according to individual tolerance and weight gain. The amount of formula consumed daily as a percentage of body weight will vary but 25% is a good target amount. Ruffed lemurs appear to be an exception. Meier and Willis (1984) documented a consumption of 50–60% of body weight per day in formula-reared infants. Consumption peaked at three weeks then steadily declined to 25% of body weight by the third month.

EXPECTED WEIGHT GAIN

After an initial one- to two-day period of adjustment, infants should gain weight and increase formula intake on a daily basis. If a progressive increase in both is not seen, an assessment of the infant's diet and health is warranted. Expected weight gain per day varies among species. Growth rates are typically slower the first month and increase thereafter. An additional acceleration occurs when animals begin consuming significant portions of solid food around weaning. Weight gain of formula-fed infants should ideally approximate that of maternally reared infants (Figs. 15.4–15.7). The following values are for maternally raised infants through four to five months of age.

- Ruffed lemurs (*Varecia variegata variegata*) average 4–8 g/day for the first month then increase to 12–15 g/day.
- Ring-tailed lemurs (*Lemur catta*) and Coquerel's sifaka (*Propithecus verreauxi coquereli*) both average 4–7 g/day through the first four months but the rate of gain during the first two weeks is slower for sifakas averaging only 2–4 g/day.
- Among the true lemurs (*Eulemur* spp.), average birth weight and adult body weight vary with the subspecies. In blue-eyed black lemurs (*Eulemur macaco flavifrons*), weight gain is minimal the first week then increases to 5–7 g/day thereafter.

HOUSING

Because neonatal lemurs rely on their mother's body heat to keep them warm, they become rapidly hypothermic if removed from their mother. Warmth is one of the most important considerations especially during the first weeks of life. The basic requirements are a regulated heat source, a thermometer to monitor temperature, and a secure enclosure that is easy to clean. Incubators are preferable especially for very young animals. Set humidity at 50–65% and surrounding air temperatures at 96–98°F (35.5–36.7°C) for neonates, and adjust as needed to maintain body temperature between 96–98°F (35.5–36.7°C). Temperatures are gradually decreased as the infant ages and its ability to thermoregulate improves. House only one infant per incubator unless the incubator can be divided, as oversuckling of digits or other body parts may occur in group-housed neonates. For infants older than a month, a heat lamp or warm-water circulating heat blanket may be sufficient if an incubator is not available. Standard heating pads are not recommended because temperatures can become hot enough to burn infants.

It is important that clinging species be provided a soft surrogate on which to cling. Ideally, surrogates

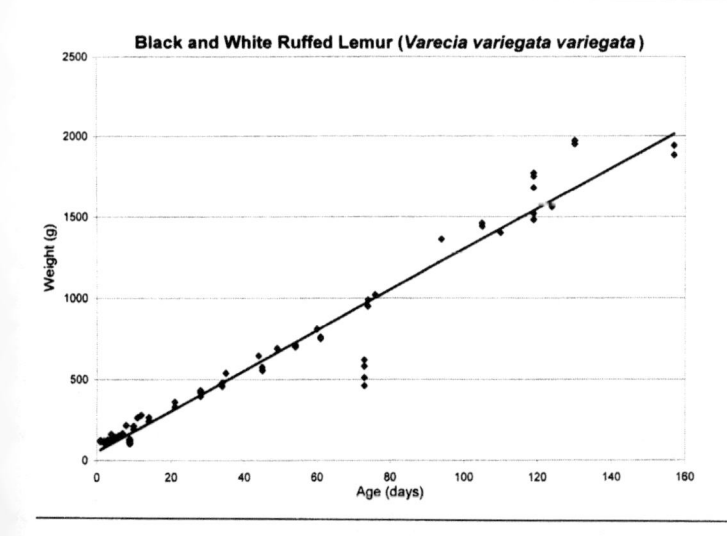

Figure 15.4. Growth of 7 maternally reared black and white ruffed lemur; 1 singleton, 1 set of twins, 1 set of quadruplets.

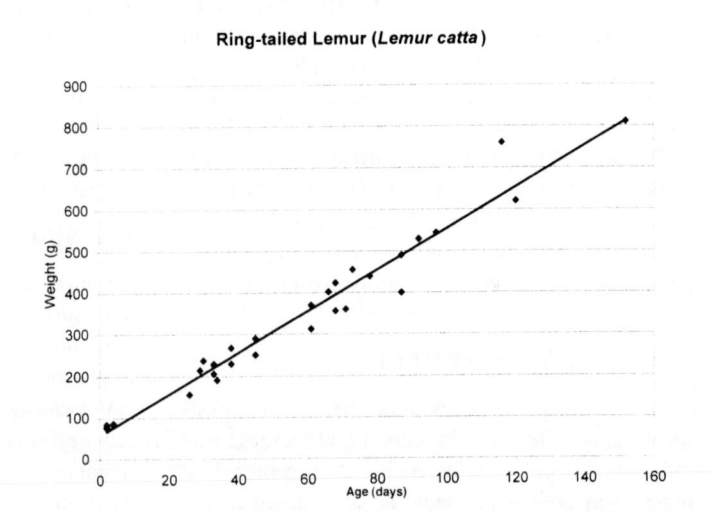

Figure 15.5. Growth of 8 maternally reared ring-tailed lemurs; 4 singletons and 2 sets of twins ($r^2 = 0.97$; $r = 0.98$).

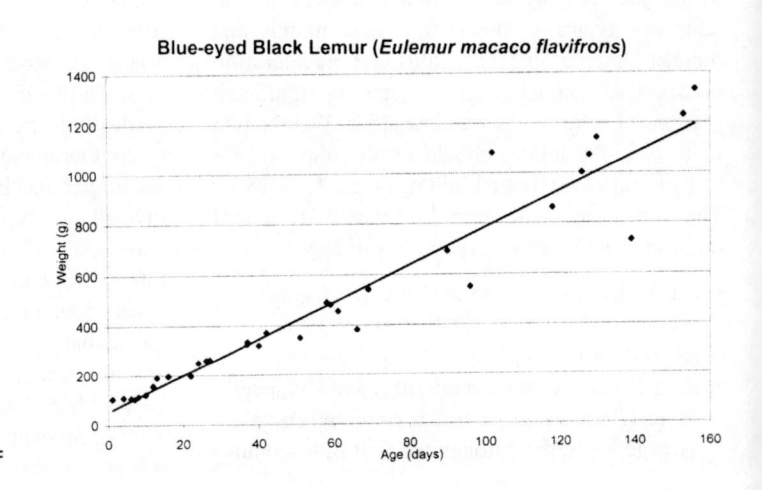

Figure 15.6. Growth of 13 maternally raised blue-eyed black lemurs; all singletons ($r^2 = 0.93$).

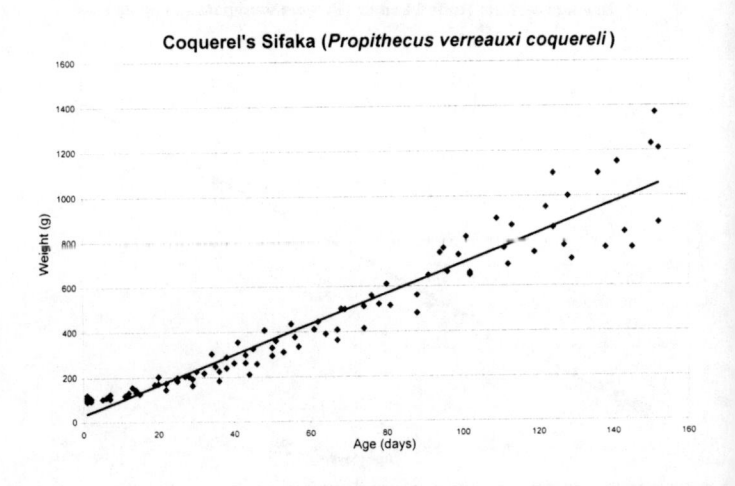

Figure 15.7. Growth of 7 maternally reared Coquerel's sifaka; all singletons ($r^2 = 0.92$).

should allow the infant to cling in a position that mimics that on the mother. While a wide variety of surrogate designs have been described for primates, washable stuffed animals are readily available and well accepted by most infants. Once infants are moved out of the incubator to a larger cage or enclosure, branches, chains, ropes, or boxes may be added to encourage jumping, leaping, and swinging behaviors.

SPECIAL NEEDS

Infants that are fed artificial formulas are not receiving antibodies normally present in mother's milk. Therefore, care should be taken to minimize exposure to potential pathogens. Personnel handling the infant should wear clothing designated for that infant including gloves and a clean lab coat or gown. Clothing should be changed between handling different infants. People with upper-respiratory infections, flulike symptoms, or active herpes lesions should not have any exposure to the infants. Clean the incubator and change towels and bedding daily.

Mothers groom the anal-genital area of neonates to stimulate urination and defecation. In hand-reared infants, gently rubbing a cotton ball dipped in warm water across the anal-genital area after feeding accomplishes the same purpose and should be done after every feeding. Mothers will provide grooming for supplemented infants that are returned after feedings.

Social interaction in the way of grooming, playing, and bonding interactions are important to normal lemur development. An ideal time to provide social stimulation and encourage physical activity in hand-reared infants is after feeding. Grooming an infant with a toothbrush not only helps keep it clean, but also provides tactile stimulation it would normally receive from its mother. If multiple infants are being raised, they can be housed together starting at one and a half to two months. Infants raised in isolation of other group members need opportunities for physical activity outside of their enclosure. Infants as young as a month can make small jumps between closely spaced branches or poles or even between the table and the handler to begin developing physical coordination.

TIME TO WEANING

Depending on the species, maternally raised infants are weaned between four and six months but tolerant dams may allow nursing for several months beyond the normal weaning time. For the purposes of hand rearing, ruffed lemurs and sifakas are weaned at five months and ring-tailed lemurs and brown lemurs at four months.

TIPS FOR WEANING FROM FORMULA TO SOLID FOOD

Finely ground old world primate biscuit (Purina Monkey Diet 5038, PMI Nutrition International) or similar substitute is added to the formula and fed by syringe or bottle similarly to straight formula starting at four weeks of age. Grinding chow with a mortar and pestle eliminates lumps but it may be necessary to increase the opening in the end of the nipple to accommodate the thicker formula. Add 2.5 g chow per 100 ml formula for infants four to eight weeks of age and increase to 5 g per 100 ml for infants eight weeks and older. Solids in the form of softened chow, fruits (bananas, grapes, apples), cooked vegetables (sweet potato, carrots, corn), and leafy greens (spinach, collards, kale) are offered starting at four weeks. Avoid fruits containing pits as they may cause diarrhea.

Sifakas possess specialized adaptations of the large bowel, including a spiral colon, which enhances their ability to derive energy from bacterial digestion of fiber. Feeding fruits and simple carbohydrates to young sifakas disrupts the balance of normal gut bacteria and should be fed only in small amounts, if at all. The inclusion of fresh leafy browse starting at four to six weeks of age helps encourage the colonization of the hindgut with beneficial fiber-fermenting bacteria.

Experience at the Duke University Primate Center shows that lemurs develop taste preferences early in life and adult diet habits result from experiences with food as a youngster. During the weaning process it is important to encourage the consumption of a nutritionally balanced primate chow over that of fruits and vegetables. Infants that obtain a majority of their caloric requirements from fruit and vegetables are at risk for developing nutritional deficiencies during weaning and adolescence. Encouraging infants to wean onto chow instead of fruit takes perseverance. Softening the chow in formula, fruit juice, or small amounts of mashed banana makes it more appealing to young taste buds. Old world primate biscuit is used initially for all species. Sifakas should be gradually changed to a high-fiber biscuit during the weaning process (Mazuri Leaf Eater #5672, PMI Nutrition International, or similar substitute).

COMMON MEDICAL PROBLEMS

Hypoglycemia, hypothermia, and dehydration are common problems in lemur infants. Lethargy and anorexia are commonly seen when one or a combination are present. Giving oral 10% dextrose is appropriate even if blood cannot be obtained to check the glucose level. If glucose cannot be given orally, 5% dextrose in fluids is an alternative. Hydration status is difficult to assess in young lemurs and prophylactic treatment for dehydration with warmed subcutaneous fluids is appropriate. Both lactated Ringer's solution and 0.9% sodium chloride are good choices

Gastrointestinal problems can result from improper feeding or formula composition. If care is not taken to remove air from syringes and feeding tubes, it accumulates in the stomach causing the infant to become fussy or refuse feedings. Gas in the stomach is easily verified on radiographs. Passing a stomach tube and using a 5–10-ml syringe to apply light suction effectively removes gas retained in the stomach. Gas can also accumulate diffusely throughout the gastrointestinal tract leading to abdominal distension and discomfort. Gas accumulation is secondary to decreased gastrointestinal motility resulting from enteritis, improper formula composition, or intestinal obstruction. Drugs that enhance gastrointestinal motility are rarely beneficial and are contraindicated in cases of suspected obstruction. Therapy is aimed at correcting the underlying problem.

Diarrhea is a common problem in hand-reared lemurs. Following strict hygiene protocols when making formula and handling infants is the best prevention against infectious causes of diarrhea. Stool cultures for *Salmonella, Shigella, Yersinia*, and *Campylobacter* help rule out diarrhea caused by pathogenic bacteria. When performing fecal parasite exams, give particular care to rule out *Cryptosporidia* and *Giardia*. Diarrhea can also be a sign that the formula or recently introduced solids are not well tolerated. To combat diarrhea, first dilute the formula or decrease the amount fed. In some cases soy-based formulas are better tolerated than one based on casein or cow's milk. Restrict solids to small amounts of those tolerated well before the onset of diarrhea. Limiting fruit alone may solve the problem.

REINTRODUCTIONS

Reintroducing lemur infants to their mother, natal group, or unrelated lemurs must be undertaken with care as both males and females will frequently kill young they do not recognize as their own. In general, longer separations are tolerated for older infants than for younger infants. Dams separated from their offspring at birth may become aggressive in as little as 24–48 hours if they are out of visual and auditory contact. During reintroductions, providing visual, auditory, and olfactory contact is a good way to assess the level of aggression directed toward a youngster by an adult. If no signs of aggression are noted contact is gradually increased until the animals have full continual contact. The rate at which reintroductions can be accomplished varies greatly depending on the species, age, and relationship of the animals being introduced. In-depth descriptions of reintroduction procedures are beyond the scope of this chapter but additional information is available in articles by Coffman (1990) and Brockman, Willis, and Karesh (1987).

SOURCES OF PRODUCTS MENTIONED

PetAg Inc., 261 Keyes Ave., Hampshire, IL 60140; 1-800-323-0877, 1-800-323-6878; www.petag.com

PMI Nutrition International, Inc., Brentwood, MO

Ross Products Division, Abbott Laboratories, Columbus, OH 43215-1724; 1-800-986-8510; www.abbott.com, www.ross.com

REFERENCES AND FURTHER READING

Anderson, J. H. 1986. Rearing and intensive care of neonatal and infant nonhuman primates. In *Primates: The road to self-sustaining populations*, edited by Kurt Benirschke New York: Springer-Verlag.

Brockman, D. K, M. S. Willis, and W. B. Karesh. 1987. Management and husbandry of ruffed lemurs, *Varecia variegata*, at the San Diego Zoo, II. *Zoo Biology* 6:349–63.

Coffman, B. S. 1990. Hand-rearing and reintroduction of a golden-crowned sifaka (*Propithecus tattersalli*) at the Duke University Primate Center. *International Zoo Yearbook* 29: 137–43.

Meier, J. E, and M. S. Willis. 1984. Techniques for hand-raising neonatal ruffed lemurs (*Varecia variegata*) and (*Varecia variegata rubra*) and a comparison of hand-raised and maternally-raised animals. *Journal of Zoo Animal Medicine* 15:24–31.

Mittermeier, R. A., I. Tattersall, W. R. Konstant, D. M. Meyers, and R. B. Mast. 1994. *The Conservation International tropical field guide series, Lemurs of Madagascar*. Washington, DC: Conservation International.

Spelman, L. H., K. G. Osborn, and M. P. Anderson. 1989. Pathogenesis of hemosiderosis in lemurs: Role of dietary iron, tannin, and ascorbic acid. *Zoo Biology* 8:239–51.

Tilden, C. D., and O. T. Oftedal. 1997. Milk composition reflects pattern of maternal care in prosimian primates. *American Journal of Primatology* 41: 195–211.

16
Tamarins

Laurie Hrdlicka and Cynthia Stringfield

NATURAL HISTORY

The average birth weight varies between species of tamarins. Examples include the cotton top tamarin (*Saguinus oedipus oedipus*) weighing an average of 53 grams at birth, the golden lion tamarin (*Leontopicthus rosalia*), which averages 60 grams at birth, and the emperor tamarins (*Saguinus imperator imperator*) or (*Saguinus imperator subgrisesans*), which weigh approximately 39 grams at birth.

Births are not usually seasonal. Multiple births are common, usually with twins or triplets born. Singletons are usually larger. It is often necessary to hand rear one infant when triplets are born.

RECORD KEEPING

Initial records are started at birth. Parent I.D. and ages, past history, litter size, and reasons for hand rearing are noted. Daily charts are maintained and include feeding times, food intake, supplements, medication, behaviors including attitude and appetite, and urine and feces production including consistency and color.

EQUIPMENT

Initially infants are fed with a 1-ml (tuberculin) syringe with the tip of a size 8 French rubber catheter/feeding tube attached to the syringe tip. At four to six weeks infants learn to take formula from a hamster-size water bottle. Formula is prepared daily and stored in 4-oz (120-ml) glass baby bottles. You will also need an artificial lamb's-wool rug and a surrogate stuffed toy (World Wildlife species-specific [tamarin] stuffed animals are best).

CRITERIA FOR INTERVENTION

Infants that have been dropped by the parents are pulled for hand rearing. In some cases one triplet will be pulled for hand rearing to ensure the survival of all three.

ASSESSMENT OF THE NEONATE

Infants should cling tightly to a surrogate. If not, this signals weakness. Hydration, body temperature, weight, and respiration are assessed upon the initial and all subsequent physical examinations.

INITIAL CARE AND STABILIZATION

The umbilicus is treated with 100% Betadine solution daily until it drops off. The infants may be placed on a warm water bottle or heating pad set on low if hypothermia is a concern, until a normal body temperature is achieved. A normal body temperature may range from 97 to 99°F (36 to 37°C). Subcutaneous fluids may be administered to a dehydrated infant and an antibiotic administered if bite or trauma wounds are present. Once initial care and stabilization are completed, the infant should be placed in an incubator to rest.

FORMULA AND SUPPLEMENTS

All tamarins are hand reared on Similac low-iron infant formula (Ross). This is a canned ready-to-use formula. Until recently a supplement called Sustagen powder was added to the formula at the rate of 1/2 tsp (2.5 ml) per 30 ml Similac to increase caloric intake and improve weight gain. Because Sustagen is no longer available, we have replaced it with canned liquid Boost at the rate of 10 ml Boost per 30 ml Similac, and have seen marked improvement in weight gain. We use vanilla-flavored Boost (Mead Johnson). Remember that:

- Prepared formula expires in 24 hours.
- Feeding equipment and storage bottles are sterilized between each use.
- Formula is heated in warm water to an approximate body temperature before feeding. Test formula temperature on wrist before feeding.
- Any formula not consumed at the feeding should be discarded.

WHAT TO FEED INITIALLY

The first feeding should be warm Pedialyte (Ross) to ensure the neonate is swallowing normally. This should help to determine if the palate is normal. Neonates are so tiny it is difficult to examine the palate. If the palate is normal, proceed with 50% formula and 50% Pedialyte for two feedings, then 75% formula and 25% Pedialyte for two feedings, then full-strength formula, barring any complications. Initially infants are fed every two hours from 6 A.M. until midnight. The only time an infant would be fed throughout the night would be if it were received late in the day, if it were weak, or if it were not nursing readily (Fig. 16.1).

NURSING TECHNIQUES

Begin feeding by placing a drop of fluid on the tongue or mouth of the infant. It should begin to swallow immediately, however sometimes it takes a few feedings before it catches on. The infants usually begin lapping formula within the first 48 hours and most will actually suck on the catheter tip. Use extreme caution at this time not to cause the infant to aspirate by putting too much pressure on the plunger of the syringe.

Animals are stimulated to defecate by wiping the perineum with a warm, moist, sterile cotton ball at every feeding initially. This is decreased as the animal begins to defecate on its own. Tamarins usually do not need stimulation to defecate after the initial 24 hours.

AMOUNTS TO FEED

Initially, infants are fed 10% of their body weight per 24 hours. For example, an infant weighing 30 grams would be fed 0.3 ml each feeding, for ten feedings in 24 hours, or 3 ml total. (At the Los Angeles Zoo, feedings begin at 6:30 A.M. and continue every two hours until 12:30 A.M.) Once an infant is readily consuming all formula offered, the amount is increased by 0.1 ml total each day. The animal's weight gain, vigor, acceptance of increases, and stool quality are all taken into account while adjusting formula amounts. Each animal should be treated as an individual. At three weeks of age solid foods are introduced and feedings are decreased in number (see Time to Weaning below).

EXPECTED WEIGHT GAIN

Infants are weighed daily before the first feeding on a gram scale that measures grams in tenths for complete accuracy. Traditionally we have experienced poor weight gains until infants begin consuming solid foods. Neonates lose weight initially and do not reach their birth weight again until the second week. We usually don't see a significant weight gain until two weeks of age and even then the weight will fluctuate until the infant is readily consuming solid foods at three to four weeks of age. As mentioned earlier, we recently amended our formula. To date, we have only raised one infant on this new formula. This infant surpassed its birth weight on day 6 and by day 21 had a 40% weight gain. This is a marked improvement overall.

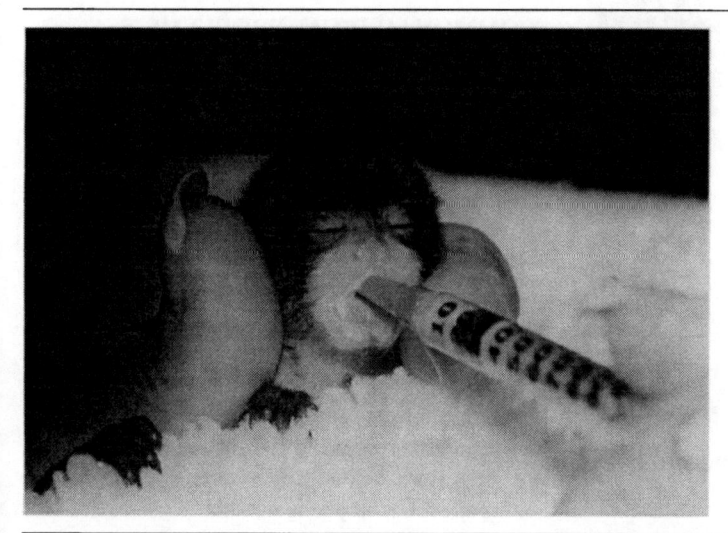

Figure 16.1. Tamarin eating from syringe.

HOUSING

All tamarin infants are housed in brooder-type or Armstrong hospital incubators (older model, Armstrong X4 baby incubator model 500: The Gordon Armstrong Co.) with an initial temperature of 90°F (18°C). The incubator temperature is gradually decreased to room temperature by four weeks of age. The incubator is kept adjacent to the adult family of tamarins that is housed in the nursery to allow the infants to socialize. When the infant reaches four weeks of age, it is slowly introduced for short periods of time to a wire cage, which is also adjacent to the adult enclosure. The time the infant spends in the adjacent cage is increased as the infant adjusts to the new environment. The infants continue to sleep in the incubator at night for approximately two more weeks. Incubators and cages are bedded with towels and artificial lamb's-wool rugs, and a stuffed animal (species-specific) surrogate is provided (Fig. 16.2). The cages have natural perches of various sizes as well.

Zoo tamarins are raised purposely with minimal human contact to enable them to be properly socialized with other tamarins.

TIME TO WEANING

Tamarin infants are weaned from formula by three to four months. At 21 days, solid food is introduced (banana) and the first morning feeding is eliminated. As solid food intake increases, formula feedings are eliminated every seven days, beginning with the night feedings, until the infant is weaned. If infants are not readily accepting solid foods or not gaining weight, feedings are eliminated at a slower rate, and weaning will take a bit longer. Guidelines at this age are 3.5 to 6 ml per formula feeding (depending on the size of the species and individual) at each of three to five feedings per day. During weaning, the infant is also encouraged to take formula through the wire cage from a water bottle or syringe to prepare for its reintroduction.

REINTRODUCTION TO FAMILY GROUP

At approximately six weeks old the infant's cage is placed inside the exhibit (assuming that the infant has had visual contact for several weeks). If no aggressive behavior is noted toward the infant, and the infant appears comfortable, the cage door is opened so it can venture out and/or other family members can go in. It is usually only a few days but can take up to a few weeks for the infant to interact and socialize with the family. Oftentimes, the infant will choose to ride on an adult or older sibling. Fuzzy rugs are tacked into the bottom of the nest boxes for security. If the infant chooses to sleep in the cage, we often bring it back to the nursery at night, but once it begins sleeping with the other family members in the nest box it will stay in the exhibit permanently. The infants are still on day formula feedings, at this point through the cage wire. Weaning is usually completed after the infant is living in the exhibit. This introduction technique has proved very successful. There have been cases in which we had to halt introduction due to aggression by certain adults, but we were later successful in introducing those infants to other families.

COMMON MEDICAL PROBLEMS

Tamarins are affected most commonly by the following medical problems.

Viral diseases of people (for example herpes simplex) can be fatal to tamarins. Appropriate precautions must be taken to prevent transmission of diseases from people to tamarins.

Animals must be exposed to full-spectrum light and/or taken outdoors to receive natural sunlight to prevent metabolic bone disease.

Animals may present with chewed fingers, toes, and tail, inflicted by the parent(s). Wound care and antibiotic coverage are important to prevent systemic infection. Enrofloxacin is one antibiotic that has been used successfully to treat appropriate bacterial infections in young tamarins.

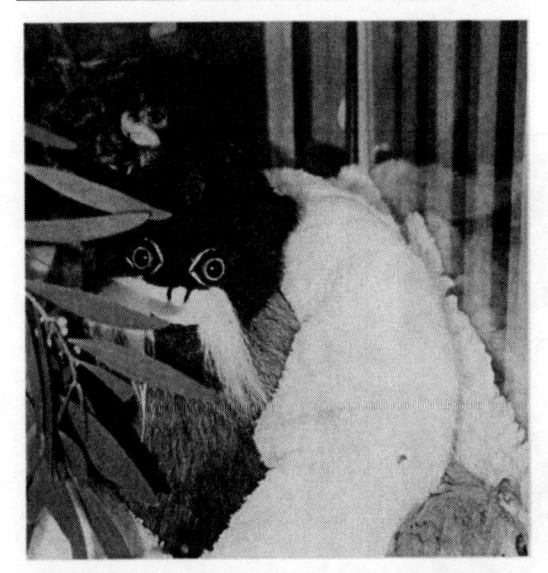

Figure 16.2. Infant tamarin with stuffed toy surrogate.

Animals are commonly presented as hypothermic, dehydrated, and weak. Systemic bacterial infection may also be present. Supportive care including fluids, warmth, and antibiotics, is needed.

Culture of feces or rectum and stool sample analysis for *Giardia*, *Campylobacter*, and others are indicated in diarrhea cases and appropriate treatment should be instituted. Enrofloxacin has been used to treat *Campylobacter*, and either fenbendazole or metronidazole have been used to treat giardiasis.

Cleft palate has been seen in only one tamarin born at our institution.

SOURCES OF PRODUCTS MENTIONED

Gordon Armstrong Co., Inc., Bulkley Building, 1501 Euclid Ave., Cleveland, OH

Mead Johnson Nutritionals, Evansville, IN 47721; 1-800-222-9123; www.meadjohnson.com

Ross Products Division, Abbott Laboratories, Columbus, OH 43215-1724; 1-800-986-8510; www.abbott.com, www.ross.com

REFERENCES

Montali, Richard J., and Mitchell Bush. 1999. Diseases of the Callitrichidae. In *Zoo and wild animal medicine current therapy 4*, edited by Murray Fowler and Eric Miller. Philadelphia, PA: Saunders.

Phone conversation with author. California Primate Research Center, University of California, Davis.

17
Macaque Species

Laura Summers, Laurie Brignolo, and Kari Christe

NATURAL HISTORY

Two species of macaques commonly raised in captivity are the rhesus macaque (*Macaca mulatta*) and the smaller cynomolgus macaque (*Macaca fascicularis*). The average birth weight for rhesus monkeys is 450–525 grams and they are generally born during the springtime months (March–June). Cynomolgus monkeys are smaller at birth with the average birth weight being 325–375 grams, and are born at any time throughout the year. Both species may be weaned at 10–12 weeks.

RECORD KEEPING

Keep a daily log of hydration, food intake, appetite, attitude, fecal production, fecal consistency, and body weight.

EQUIPMENT

The following items should be on hand:

PetAg bottles (65 ml) and nipples for small mammals
Human infant formula
Incubator (see Fig. 17.3)
Towels, cloth diapers
Stuffed plush toys
Self-feeding device (see Figs. 17.2, 17.5)
Hanging (Lixit) bottles
Small cage at time of weaning
Dextrose (5%) and Tang with electrolyte solution or Gatorade
Personal protective equipment: gloves, surgical masks, eye protection, arm protection (see Fig. 17.1)

CRITERIA FOR INTERVENTION

It is necessary to hand rear macaque infants that are failing to thrive, orphaned, or abandoned. While it is normal for neonates to lose up to one-tenth of their body weight within the first week of life, they should subsequently be steadily gaining weight. Infants should appear bright and alert and cling to their mothers with both hands and feet. The first sign of a weak infant is often failure to cling. Maternal abuse is not uncommon in the macaque species and infants need to be immediately removed from an abusive situation. First-time mothers are the most common abusers.

All macaque species are potential carriers of cercopithicine herpes 1 (simian herpes B virus). In macaques, this virus is relatively benign and causes occasional vesicles in or around the oral cavity. If a human contracts the virus it can cause a fatal neurologic disease. The virus may be present in any of the monkey's body fluids, but is most concentrated in saliva. Because of the risk of viral infection, all caretakers should wear appropriate personal protective equipment to prevent exposure to primate bodily fluids (see Fig. 17.1). It is also recommended to have established a relationship with a physician knowledgeable with the pathophysiology of cercopithicine herpes 1 prior to working with these animals.

All enteric diseases that affect nonhuman primates will cause disease in humans as well. Gloves should be worn at all times when handling infants or soiled bedding. Hand washing after handling the infant is also recommended for all caretakers.

Macaque species are highly susceptible to measles virus (rubeola). In macaque infants the disease can cause anything from a mild rash to severe immunocompromise and death. For this reason, all caretakers working with macaques should be vaccinated for measles. Caretakers with known recent exposure to measles virus (within seven to ten days) should refrain from working with macaque infants.

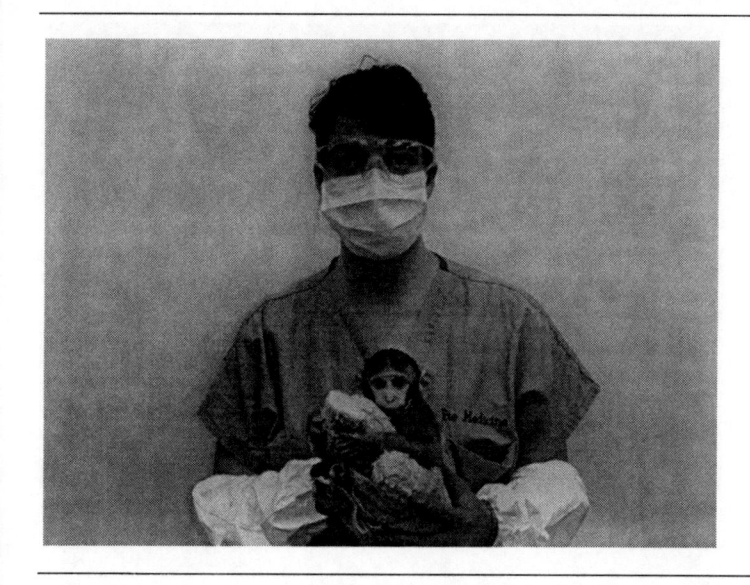

Figure 17.1. Appropriate personal protective wear for working with macaque species.

ASSESSMENT OF THE NEONATE

Newborns that require attention need a complete physical exam. Hydration status is best evaluated clinically by skin turgor and eye position. Dehydrated infants will have skin that remains tented over the forehead when pinched and will have sunken eyes. An accurate temperature, fecal culture and stool sample for parasitology, and a blood sample for electrolyte and glucose measurements should be obtained.

FORMULAS

Infant macaques generally do quite well when fed any of the commercially available human infant formulas. Enfamil (Mead Johnson) or Similac (Abbott) are good choices. Infant macaques require 200 kcal/kg/day for adequate growth to occur. Formula should be mixed in accordance with the package directions. Formula should be warm but never hot. Formula in a bottle may be used for up to two hours after warming and then must be discarded.

NURSING TECHNIQUES

Healthy infant macaques may readily be hand reared. Infants should be held upright for feeding, and wrapping the animal in a diaper or small towel is often helpful. Infants will generally nurse well from a pet nurser and with a few training sessions, can be taught to nurse from a bottle in a self-feeding device (see Fig. 17.2). Care must be taken to not allow the infants to nurse too quickly as this may lead to vomiting and possible aspiration. Making the hole in the nipple just large enough that a drop of formula forms when the bottle is inverted will minimize aspiration risk. For difficult infants that do not have a strong suckle reflex, formula may be slowly dropped onto their tongues, as they will generally swallow the formula once it is placed in their mouths.

TUBE FEEDING

Due to the risk of vomiting and aspiration, we generally do not use this method of feeding. If this method of feeding is used, it can be done using a 5 French red rubber catheter (Kendall Sovereign Feeding Tube and Urethral Catheter).

An infant macaque should be tube fed when other feeding attempts are unsuccessful. Since infant monkeys can grab with their hands, it is easiest to have one person restrain the infant, holding the arms gently next to the animal. Alternatively, the infant can be wrapped in a towel keeping the arms and hands out of the way. Size 5–8 French red rubber or silastic catheters make good feeding tubes. Measure the distance from the nose to the last rib to determine how far to insert the tube. Mark the appropriate length with indelible marker. Hold the infant's head in one hand and guide the catheter into the mouth with the other. Gently advance the catheter into the stomach. If the tube does not advance easily to the measured length, withdraw it and start over. Infants, especially those that are very weak, may not

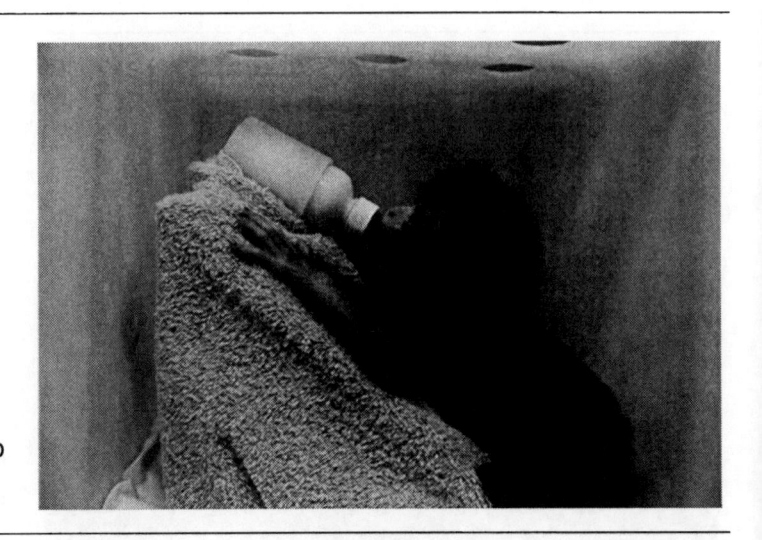

Figure 17.2. Infants may be trained to use the self-feeder by gently holding them on the ramp of the feeder and allowing them to nurse.

cough or gag in response to the tube entering the trachea. To verify proper placement, pass a small amount of water (enough to fill the catheter and an additional 1 ml) through the tube. This fluid should be easily aspirated back into the syringe, and should be clouded by stomach contents. Once placement into the stomach is verified, deliver the formula slowly by syringe. Feed only 50–75% of the volume that would be fed by bottle to prevent overdistension of the stomach and possible vomiting. Once the formula has been delivered, with the catheter still in place, flush the catheter with a small amount of water. Kink the tube to prevent backflow and gently remove it.

FREQUENCY OF FEEDING

Infants should be fed every two to four hours from morning to late evening (approximately 7 A.M. to 10 P.M.) until about five weeks of age. Food intake ranges from 50 to 150 ml/ day for the first few days but is generally 200–250 ml/ day by the time an infant reaches 14 days of age. Solid food such as formula-soaked primate chow (Purina Lab Diet), rice cereal with formula, and fruit (apple and banana) may be added into the diet starting at two weeks of age. Macaque species will generally explore their environment and begin eating whatever foods are offered to them. For infants that are not eating well on their own, rice cereal may be hand fed to them using a small spoon or tongue depressor. Water and electrolyte solution (Gatorade or Tang with oral electrolytes) may be offered in Lixit bottles attached to the side of the cage and should be added to the diet at three to four weeks of age. At four to five weeks of age, infants can begin using hanging bottles for formula. Pet nursers and self-feeders may be removed once the animal is drinking formula well from hanging bottles and eating solid food. Formula may be stopped completely at about three months of age.

EXPECTED WEIGHT GAIN

It is not uncommon for infants to lose up to 10% of their body weight during their first few days of life, but usually they are gaining weight by day five to seven. Infants generally gain from 15 to 30 grams per week.

HOUSING

For the first three weeks the infant should be housed in an incubator. A medium-sized, commercial incubator can be purchased from Petiatric Supply Company or one may be constructed from a Nalgene seven-gallon tank. The Nalgene tanks may be purchased from Cole-Parmar (catalog number U-06323-11). See Figures 17.3a and 17.3b.

To build an incubator follow these steps:

1. Place the Nalgene box on its side so the opening is facing you.
2. There will be a lip around the opening of the box. On the top side of the box, trim off the edge of the tank to allow for a door.
3. Add runner strips on the two vertical edges, perpendicular to the cut edge.

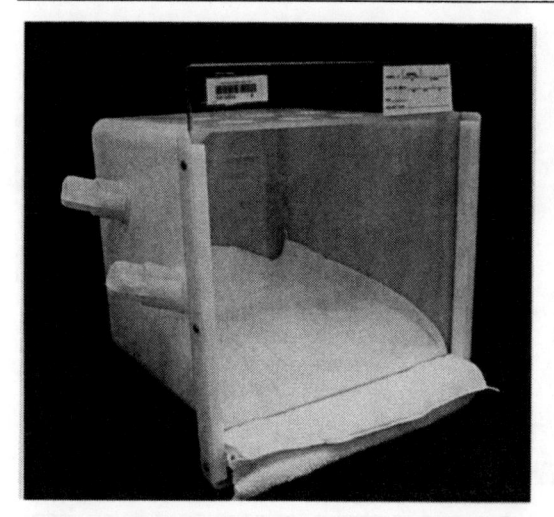

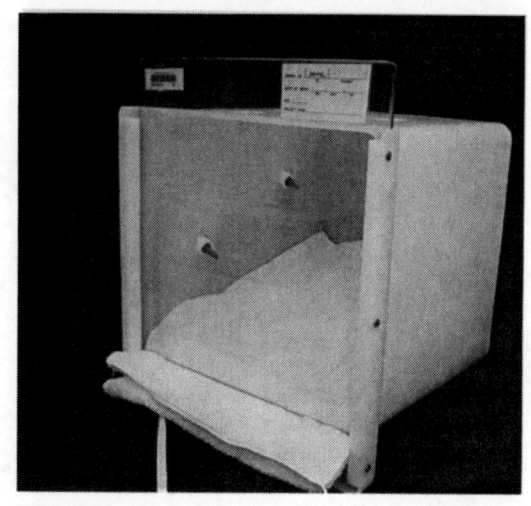

Figure 17.3. (a) Incubator made from a Nalgene carboy tank. (b) Side holes with PVC piping allow for a built-in self-feeder.

4. Use a 14 × 16 × 1/4 inch clear polycarbonate square as a door. Slide this into the runner strips.
5. Drill nine 1-in (2.5-cm) holes in the top to allow for ventilation.
6. Drill two 1-in (2.5-cm) holes on one side at two varying heights. (This will allow you to place infant bottles on the side of the incubator.)
7. Cut two 1 1/4 × 3-in (3 × 7.5-cm) pieces of HDPE or PVC tubing. Cut a 30-degree bevel at one end of each tube; affix the beveled end around the openings of the side hole. These will serve as bottle holders.

Temperature is controlled within the incubator by placing an electrical heating blanket at the bottom of the incubator. Place a thick, folded towel and a cloth diaper over the heating pad so that the infant is not in direct contact with the heating pad (see Fig. 17.3). The cloth diapers must be changed as soon as they become soiled (often several times a day). The thick towels should be changed at least daily, more often if they are soiled with feces or urine.

For the first four days, the ambient temperature in the incubator should be kept at 90–94°F (32.2–34.4°C), which corresponds to a heating pad set on "medium." For days 5 through 30, the temperature may be decreased to 80–84°F (26.7–28.9°C), which corresponds to a heating pad set on "low."

At 21 days of age, the infant may begin spending a few hours a day in a small indoor cage (ambient temperature 72–75°F (22.2–23.9°C). The cage should be about 2 × 2 × 3 feet (0.6 × 0.6 × 1 m) in size and have a tight enough mesh to prevent an animal from getting its arms and legs caught while exploring its environment. This is also the ideal time to begin socializing orphaned animals with other orphans of similar size and age. Gradually increase the time spent in the cage over seven to ten days until the infant is no longer spending time in the incubator.

Infant macaques have a natural tendency to "cling" to their mothers. It is helpful to place a plush toy (about 5 in [13 cm] tall) with the infant. The plush toy may be of any shape and will serve as a surrogate and allow natural behavior. Allow the infant to cling to the plush toy during handling (weighing, physical exams, etc.), as this will keep the infant from becoming panicked and accidentally scratching the caretaker.

Infants may be trained to use a self-feeder in their cage or incubator. Building a self-feeder is practical if several infants are being nursery reared at one time. However, if only one infant is orphaned, hand feeding may be a more suitable option. If a commercial incubator is used the self-feeder may be placed within the incubator. The self-feeder may also be placed within the cage once the infant is old enough to begin spending time out of the incubator (Fig. 17.4).

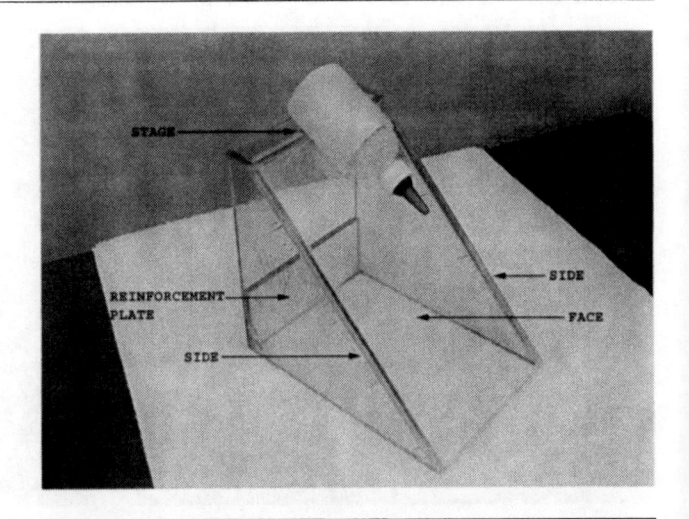

Figure 17.4. Assemble all cut pieces of the self-feeder; fasten together using clamps and polycarbonate glue.

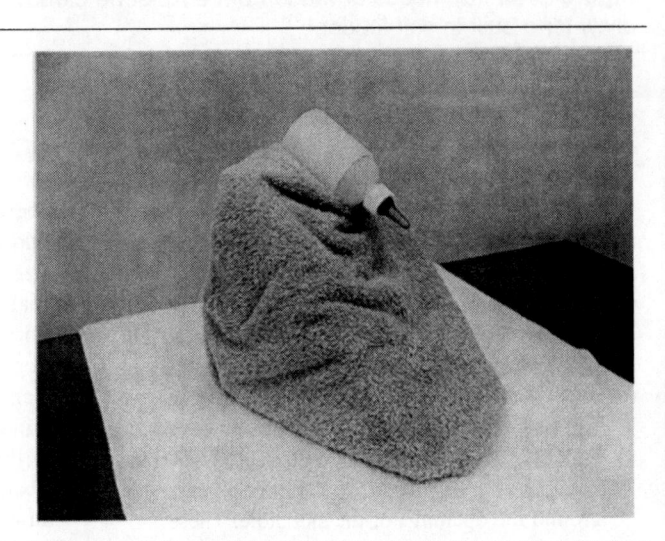

Figure 17.5. Self-feeder with a towel wrapped around it for padding.

To build a self-feeder, follow these steps:

1. Using 1/4-in polycarbonate (Lexicon), refer to the diagram and photo and cut out a total of five individual pieces.
2. Cut two side pieces.
3. Cut one face piece.
4. Cut one rectangular stage.
5. Cut one rectangular back reinforcement plate.
6. Using clamps and polycarbonate glue, affix the pieces together as shown in the diagram.
7. Cut a 1/2-in "V" shape at the center of the top edge where the face meets the stage.
8. Using 1 1/2-in-diameter PVC pipe, cut a piece that is 2 1/2 in long.
9. Now cut the pipe open by making a single, longitudinal cut down one side of the PVC pipe. (This will allow the pipe to open and close just slightly.)
10. Set the pipe into the "V" cut on the top of the device. Using a single screw, affix the pipe to the top of the self-feeder. (The opening of the pipe should face downward.)

Wrap the self-feeder in a towel and secure the towel with heavy cloth tape (duct tape). Place the bottle into the PVC pipe at the top of the feeder. There should be just enough spring in the pipe to hold the bottle securely (Fig. 17.5).

TIME TO WEANING

Weaning takes place in both species at approximately 10 to 12 weeks.

COMMON MEDICAL PROBLEMS

Gastrointestinal problems such as diarrhea are relatively common and may result from diet change from breast milk to formula, gastrointestinal viruses (rotavirus, coronavirus, parainfluenza), bacterial or parasitic etiologies. If liquid stool persists for three days, or compromises the infant's intake and hydration, a stool sample for direct examination and rectal culture should be obtained.

The most common bacterial etiology for diarrhea is *Campylobacter* (99%), which may be treated with tetracycline (20 mg/kg PO TID × 10 days) or azithromycin (40 mg/kg PO SID × 1 day, then 20 mg/kg PO SID × 4 days). *Shigella* and *Yersinia* are isolated more often from animals housed outdoors and may be treated with enrofloxacin. For *Shigella*, 5 mg/kg IM SID × 5 days is sufficient, whereas *Yersinia* requires 5 mg/kg IM BID for 10 days. Alternatively, *Shigella* may also be treated with trimethoprim sulfa at a dose of 4 mg/kg PO BID for 10 days. Different species of *Escherichia coli* may be treated with neomycin (50 mg/kg PO BID × 10 days).

Common parasitic etiologies are *Giardia*, *Balantidium coli*, and *Trichuris*. *Giardia* is treated with metronidazole (50 mgl/kg PO SID × 10 days). *B. coli* is best treated with tetracycline (20 mg/kg PO TID × 10 days) because it treats both the trophozoite and cyst forms, while metronidazole only treats the trophozoite forms. *Trichuris* is treated with fenbendazole (50 mg/kg PO SID × 3 days).

For persistent diarrhea of unknown etiology, metronidazole (50 mg/kg PO SID × 10 days) is used for its anti-inflammatory properties as well as to treat possible anaerobic overgrowth.

Maintaining adequate hydration is essential. Hydration status is most accurately determined by daily weighing; but can also be assessed by skin turgor and eye position. Skin turgor should always be tested in the same place on the animal. With normal hydration, the skin at the brow midline should return to its normal position immediately when pinched. If the skin remains tented for one to five seconds, the animal is approximately 5–10% dehydrated. If the skin remains tented for more than five seconds, the animal is greater than 10% dehydrated. If the skin does not return to normal position on the brow, the animal is likely greater than 15% dehydrated and in need of emergency care. Eye position, while helpful in determining hydration status, can be misleading. Typically, a dehydrated animal will have eyes that appear sunken in their sockets. However, animals that have lost weight will also have sunken eyes even when their hydration status is normal. Mucous membranes can also be evaluated for hydration status. A dehydrated animal will have mucous membranes that are dry or tacky to the touch.

Supportive care is indicated if the infant's hydration status begins to decline. Parental fluids may be given at any age. Foods with high water content can be used if the infant is eating solid foods. Good oral supplements include bland foods such as rice cereal with liquid high-protein drinks (Boost or Ensure) or primate chow soaked with water or fruit-flavored children's drinks (Tang) and are readily available options.

Parenteral fluids may be given several different ways. Try to select a route of administration based on clinical condition and animal temperament. If an animal is severely compromised, a continuous intravenous infusion over three hours at 30 ml/kg/hr is the most effective means of rehydration. However, infant macaques have very dexterous hands and can easily remove an IV catheter. For this reason, infants will often require temporary restraint on a padded restraint board. The fluid infusion rate should balance restraint time and gradual rehydration. For infants with moderate dehydration, a combination of an IV bolus and subcutaneous (SC) fluids is often adequate. An IV bolus of up to 10 ml/kg can be safely given, additionally SC fluids can be given up to 40 ml/kg. For mild dehydration, SC fluids are adequate. Lactated Ringer's solution (LRS) is a good choice for maintaining continued electrolyte balance. Normal electrolyte values are Na^+ 144, K^+ 4.0, Cl^- 110, Ca^{+2} 1.00, and Osmo 290. Supplemental potassium may be added if the infant is hypokalemic. If IV or SC fluids are given, the potassium may be safely supplemented up to 1 mEq/kg/hr. If an infant is severely acidotic (pH less than 7.2), bicarbonate should be added to IV fluids: 0.5–1 mEq/kg/hr is a safe rate of administration.

If an infant appears weak, hypothermia (normal temperature is 98–100°F or 36.7–37.8°C) and hypoglycemia (glucose less than 80 mg/dl) should be ruled out. A rectal temperature should be obtained for accuracy. A severely hypothermic infant (less than 85°F or 29.4°C) can be most effectively rewarmed using central core warming (warm IV, IP, or oral fluids). External rewarming (warm water bottles, hair dryer, warming blankets) is sufficient for moderately hypothermic infants (temperature at 85–95°F or 29.4–35°C). Care must be taken not to cause external burns when using external rewarming techniques. Blood glucose may easily be assessed on a stat glucometer with only one drop of blood; but assessing a response to placing a few drops of 50% dextrose on the oral mucous membranes is quick and easy. Any infant with increased activity after oral glucose administration was likely hypoglycemic. Dextrose can be easily administered orally or in IV fluids, but is not recommended in subcutaneous fluids as it may temporarily osmotically pull some fluid subcutaneously before being absorbed into the tissues. Also, an animal that is hypothermic may not appropriately absorb subcutaneous fluids.

Infants commonly develop skin rashes. Infant dermatitis may have many etiologies: contact irritation, viral (measles, parainfluenza), bacterial, or fungal. The bacterial and yeast rashes are opportunistic infections that are usually promoted by using rough diapers or towels in the incubator. Abrasions secondary to rubbing on abrasive towels are not uncommon. Use soft cotton diapers over the rougher towels to protect the infant's delicate skin from irritation. Do not use any towels or diapers with holes or frayed edges as infants can twist the strands around their fingers, toes, or tongues occluding blood supply and necessitating amputation. Infants soil incubators very quickly by urinating, defecating, and eating soft foods such as fruit and soaked chow. Perianal scalding and occasionally umbilical infections may develop if the incubator and bedding are not kept scrupulously clean. The best way to address these conditions is preventive medicine: change the diaper as often as necessary to keep the incubator clean and dry. If dermatitis does develop, keep the affected area clean by bathing the infant daily or every other day with a mild shampoo, drying the infant well, and optionally applying zinc oxide ointment.

REINTRODUCTION

For reintroducing a weanling to a stable group environment, select an adult member of the family to serve as a foster aunt or uncle. This adult should be fairly high ranking in the family hierarchy, but not critical for group stability. When the weanling is about four to five months of age, remove the adult member from the group and slowly allow him or her to become bonded to the weanling. Begin by housing the two animals in separate cages where they have visual and tactile access to each other. (Ideally, this should be a pair cage with a slide divider.) Begin by using a wire mesh divider or a clear Plexiglas divider and observe their interactions for a few days. If the adult is aggressive to the infant, select another adult to serve as the foster. If the adult is not aggressive to the infant, open the slide divider enough to allow an adult arm through. If the animals are interacting well and there is no adult-to-weanling aggression, allow them into the same cage under very close supervision. An escape route for the weanling can be made by having the division between the two cages be just large enough for the weanling, but not large enough for the adult to fit through. It is advisable to separate the two when caretakers are not available for supervision until the two are a comfortable pair. This may take up to a few weeks. Once they are established as a pair, then begin reintroduction into the group. Again careful supervision is important. The goal is that the adult will be bonded well enough to the weanling to protect it, and also be of high enough rank to keep the peace within the group.

ACKNOWLEDGMENTS

John Steele, Senior Lab Technician, California Regional Primate Research Center

Wilhelm von Morganland, Staff Research Associate, California Regional Primate Research Center

SOURCES OF PRODUCTS MENTIONED

Abbott Laboratories: www.similac.com

Cole-Parmer: www.coleparmer.com

Kendall Company, Mansfield, MA 02048; 1-800-962-9888

Lixit: www.lixit.com; 1-800-358-8254

Mead Johnson & Company, Evansville, IN 47721

PetAg Inc., 261 Keyes Ave., Hampshire, IL 60140; 1-800-323-0877, 1-800-323-6878; www.petag.com

Petiatric: www.petiatric.com

Purina: www.purina.com

REFERENCES

Ruppenthal, Gerald C. 1979. *Nursery care of nonhuman primates*. New York: Plenum Press.

18
Great Apes

Dawn Strasser

NATURAL HISTORY

The great apes seen commonly in captivity include the lowland gorilla (*Gorilla gorilla gorilla*), the bonobo (*Pan paniscus*), the common chimpanzee (*Pan troglodytes*), the orangutan (*Pongo pygmaeus abelii*), and the siamang (*Hylobates syndactylus*). Births in captivity may be any time of the year.

PROTOCOL

There have been 47 lowland gorillas born at the Cincinnati Zoo since 1961 and the zoo staff has hand raised over 30, using the protocol outlined here. Lowland gorillas will be the focus of this chapter, but the information pertains to the other species as well. The protocol was established with the assistance of Drs. Uma Kotagal and Paul Perlstein at the Cincinnati Children's Medical Hospital.

Great ape infants are kept in strict quarantine and are handled by only two nursery personnel in addition to the veterinary staff and human pediatric doctors. Surgical or dressing gowns are always worn when handling a neonate. Shoes and hair should be covered on anyone who has been anywhere in the rest of the zoo. Ideally, staff working with these animals should have no exposure to the rest of the collection, and the building where the infants are housed should be a quarantine facility. Hands and arms should be washed before and after handling the neonate. Personnel who are ill should not be allowed near the neonates. No additional staff should be added to the animal care team until the neonate is one month old, or older if the neonate is not stable. When the neonate is no longer in critical condition, night keepers may be allowed to administer feedings.

Bedding should be disinfected frequently with liquid bleach. Liquid detergent is recommended over powders because some neonates have had allergic reactions to powdered detergent.

Vaccination protocols should be followed according to recent research in human infants. The following vaccinations should be given at different intervals: hepatitis, DPT (diphtheria-pertussis-tetanus), polio, measles, and rabies. The apes should be tested for tuberculosis annually. Mother-raised infants should be vaccinated at opportune times, taking into consideration the risk of the disease to the infant. The nursery keepers should be tested for tuberculosis biannually.

RECORD KEEPING

The importance of accurate record keeping cannot be overstated. Keep a daily log of body weight and food intake. Monitor and record the frequency and consistency of the feces. Use descriptive words like pasty, seedy, loose, or watery, and note any unusual smells to describe feces. Avoid ambiguous descriptions such as "good." Monitor the temperature, pulse, and respiration every three hours around the clock for the first two weeks. Once the infant is stabilized, the body temperature should be monitored twice a day for the next two weeks, then once a day for the following month. Continue to take monthly measurements such as crown diameter and body length and record behavioral changes as they develop.

EQUIPMENT

Human baby bottles made of glass are preferred, but plastic is acceptable. Preemie or Evenflo nipples (Evenflo) are recommended. Use the same type of nipples used for a human newborn. Steam-sterilize the nipple, bottle, and formula as one complete unit for 15 minutes. Do not handle the nipple once it has been sterilized. It is crucial that bacterial exposure is kept to a minimum. Sterilize all bottles and nipples used during the first six weeks of life, and subsequently, use hot soapy water to clean feeding implements. Heat the formula in the bottle in a pan of hot water and check frequently to ensure it is not overheated. A microwave may be used but requires careful attention. Hot pockets of formula may form that could burn the infant's mouth if the formula is not mixed thoroughly after heating. The milk should be tested on the inside of your wrist prior to feeding and it should be warm, not hot to the touch.

Use the same scale every day when weighing the neonate. A scale that is accurate to one-tenth of a kilogram is adequate, but a greater accuracy of 0.01 kg is preferred. Body temperature should be taken with a rectal thermometer that has been disinfected with alcohol before and after use.

CRITERIA FOR INTERVENTION

There are several reasons intervention may be necessary. Removing a neonate from its mother at any time during its first year is a difficult decision. Reasons to intervene may be obvious within the first few days after birth, or the neonate could be as much as six months old before intervention is deemed necessary. Careful observation by the caregivers is crucial.

A 24-hour watch is recommended before and after the birth. This is especially important for first-time mothers. Observers should look for proper positioning for nursing, which we call "ventral vertical" (infant's chest to mother's chest with the infant's head up). Length of nursing sessions should be noted. Two to three minutes in a 1- to 1 1/2-hour period is normal. Too much nursing may indicate a problem. The infant may appear to be nursing for excessively long periods if there is an inadequate supply of milk. The female may be simply not producing enough milk, or she may be self-expressing milk from her mammary glands, or another gorilla could be nursing from her, which could be either an adult or an infant. Females may develop mastitis, which should be considered if one breast becomes considerably larger than the other. Whatever the cause, the infant needs to be supplemented or pulled from the mother and hand reared if it is not getting enough nourishment.

Obvious maternal neglect, such as holding the infant improperly, abusive behavior, and lack of nursing, or lack of "rooting" for the nipple by the infant in attempts to nurse are also reasons to intervene. One sign the neonate is not doing well is a limp body. Newborn infants are not able to hold their heads up very well initially, but the muscles in their necks will strengthen daily. It is important to observe this process each day and be able to compare the progress from birth to the present. It is significant if the infant's neck appears to weaken over time. Other significant signs are a "ghostly gray" color to the face, dull glassy eyes, sunken chest, and inability to grasp the hair of the mother.

Gorillas develop "suck knobs," which are knobs of tissue that resemble a small round drawer knob, on their cheeks five to ten days after birth. It is abnormal if these do not develop or develop and disappear in the first few months after birth. The knobs will disappear on their own once the infant starts to eat solids. It is unknown exactly what function the knobs serve, but in our experience, failure for them to develop or premature disappearance of these "knobs" has always indicated a problem. It is important to remember that once the infant starts to show signs of trouble, there is little time to intervene; it may be only 24–48 hours before it is too late to be able to help the infant.

When a neonate is removed from its mother, blood and stool samples should be collected to screen for various diseases. If the infant has diarrhea, the problem needs to be dealt with as soon as possible. If an infant with diarrhea is being mother-raised, it will most likely need to be pulled from its mother, as its health may rapidly decline. This will be a challenge if the infant is a six-month-old mother-raised ape, as it will be frightened and will not trust you. It takes a great deal of patience to build a bond with the infant. We have found that if we need to remove an older infant from its mother, it will struggle and try to bite even if it is severely debilitated. Sitting and rocking the infant with it wrapped tightly in a towel may help to calm it, and will keep it from struggling. Keep the infant's face well away from your body as it can and will bite you if the opportunity arises. After holding the infants, we then place them in a wire dog kennel or open floor cage so they can be close to us and watch us throughout the day. Within a few days, sometimes longer, they will be calmer and more accepting of us.

ASSESSMENT OF THE NEONATE

When the infant first arrives in the nursery, a complete physical examination should be performed. This examination should include drawing blood for a complete blood cell count, serum chemistries, electrolytes, blood culture, and blood glucose levels using a Dextrostick. A stool culture should be submitted for culture for *Salmonella, Shigella,* and *Campylobacter*. The infant's mouth should be checked and the palate should be examined for evidence of abnormalities. Auscultate the thorax and evaluate the heart and lungs. Record the heart rate and listen for murmurs. Record the respiratory rate. Palpate the abdomen and the genitals and evaluate for abnormalities. Palpate the fontanel, or soft spot, on the skull and evaluate for abnormalities. Weigh the infant and take measurements of the head circumference, chest circumference, lengths of heel to crown and crown to rump. Record the rectal temperature. Treat the umbilical cord with dilute Betadine or Nolvasan solution and treat again every three hours until it dries up and falls off. The umbilicus usually falls off at five to ten days of age. Vitamin K may also be administered during the examination. Depending on the condition of the infant, antibiotic therapy may be indicated. Establishing a relationship with pediatric physicians in your area who are willing to help with an ape infant may be very beneficial. They often will make emergency equipment available that could be useful on infant primates. Their expertise, especially if you are unfamiliar with primates, could be invaluable.

INITIAL CARE

An incubator or human isolette is used to warm the baby initially (see Fig. 18.3). Set the incubator temperature to 85°F (30°C). Rubbing the extremities helps to increase circulation and raise the body temperature. Use cotton blankets to cover the neonate rather than placing clothing on the baby. This enables the infant to self-regulate its temperature by easily removing the blanket. Materials other than cotton may cause the infant to overheat. The only time clothing is placed on ape infants at our institution is if there is a problem with the infant maintaining body temperature, such as with a premature infant.

FORMULA AND SUPPLEMENTS

Pediatric specialists have recommended the use of human formula substitutes to raise great apes. At Cincinnati Zoo and Botanical Gardens, Enfamil with Iron (Mead Johnson) has been used successfully as a base formula. Starting at one month of age, neonates may be supplemented with a baby multivitamin, Poly Vi Sol (Mead Johnson) at 1.0 ml once a day.

Monitor the serum calcium in infants regularly, at least once every two weeks. We found it necessary to supplement one infant with 100 mg/kg per day calcium gluconate 10% (Calciquid, Econolab), and do UV phototherapy 20 minutes per day in a specialized booth with UV lights.

Infants with lactose intolerance have been given soy-based Isomil (Ross Products) with calcium supplements. Mead Johnson Company has a pediatric product handbook available, which is an excellent resource for evaluating formulas, especially if you are having problems with your neonate.

NURSING TECHNIQUES

The neonates should be handled like human infants by supporting the back of the head whenever they are picked up. When feeding, let them rest in the cradle of your arm at about a 45-degree angle. Place the nipple gently into the infant's mouth. Never force the nipple. Rubbing its chin will stimulate it to take the nipple if it doesn't accept it initially. It will probably have several short suckling spurts of a few seconds each during each feeding for the first week. It is important to allow the infant to have rest periods of a few minutes between the suckling attempts until it develop a strong suckling reflex (Fig. 18.1).

FREQUENCY OF FEEDING AND WEANING

The larger great apes (1.5 kg or larger) may be started on 60 ml every three hours (eight times per day) around the clock. At two weeks of age feed 70–90 ml every three hours from 8 A.M. to 2 A.M. (seven times per day). These infants are fed on a "semidemand" basis, whereby they are given the formula 30 minutes before a scheduled feed if they are awake and hungry; or if sleeping the feed time will be extended as much as 30 minutes after the scheduled feed time before waking the infant to feed it. They seem to eat better if they wake up on their own before the feed. Once on a schedule, the infants will usually wake up prior to each feeding. The increases in formula amounts offered depend on the demand of the infant.

Between four and five weeks increase the feed amount to 120 ml and feed every four hours (six times per day). At two months of age eliminate the

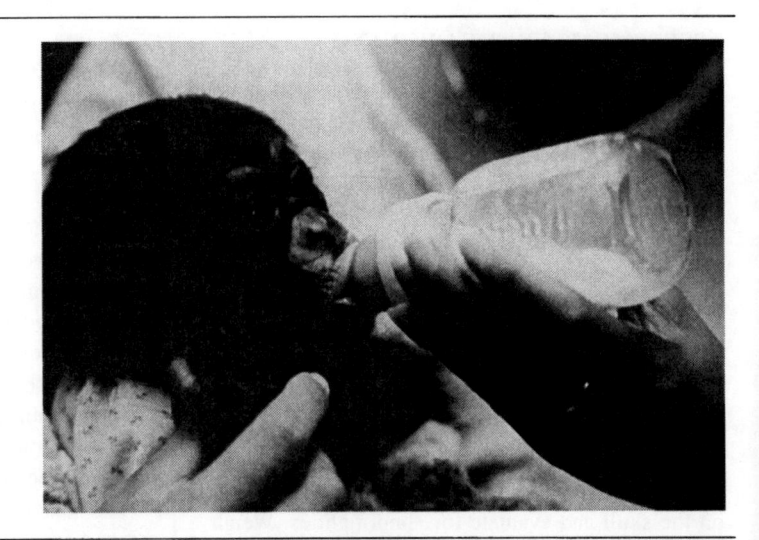

Figure 18.1. Holding infant while bottle-feeding (photo by Steve Castillo, courtesy of Six Flags Marine World).

night feeds after midnight and feed 150 ml per feed, five times per day from 9 A.M. to 11 P.M. At three months feed 180 ml five times per day. At four months feed 240 ml four times per day (three day feeds and one night feed). Between five and six months, feeds are increased to 360 ml and only offered twice each day. Between six and nine months, gradually replace the formula with homogenized whole cow's milk. The switch should take five to seven days as long as no problems are encountered. Start by adding 25% volume of homogenized milk to the regular formula, then increase the percentage daily until the infant is nursing 100% homogenized milk. We begin using a cup instead of the bottle at this point. It is typically difficult to convert the infant from nursing from a bottle to drinking from a cup. It will take time and patience to make the final transition to having the infant accept drinking from a cup.

When the infant reaches 90 days of age, we begin to introduce solids. As the solid-food intake increases, the formula intake is decreased. The items offered first are celery sticks, raw carrot strips, apple slices, and green beans. Food that is easy for them to hold and easily put into their mouths is best. Once they begin to eat these items, we hand feed soft or cooked food. Cooked carrots or sweet potatoes, and bananas are fed by hand at this time. The midday milk feeding is discontinued as the infant consumes more solids. By now the infant will start to pick out favorite foods. Offering vegetables during the day and the favorite fruit at night works well. Gradually, the remaining items in the adult diet are added as the infant's eating skills improve. Between ten months and one year the maximum amount of milk offered to large great apes such as gorillas and chimpanzees is 360 ml two times a day. Primate biscuits are added to the diet at this time, the vitamin drops are eliminated, and any brand of quality chewable children's multiple vitamins are introduced.

Smaller animals such as siamangs should follow a similar feeding regimen except at a lower volume. Siamangs larger than 600 grams are fed 30 ml six times per day between 7 A.M. and 10 P.M. If smaller than 600 grams, they are given 15–20 ml every three hours around the clock. At one month of age offer up to 45 ml five times per day. Continue to increase the feed amounts until the infants are eating 70 ml per feed five times per day. The smaller species are fed five times per day until about four months of age, when they begin to pick up and eat solid foods. The feeds remain at 70 ml but are decreased to four times per day. At five months of age the feeds are increased to 100 ml but only offered three times each day. At six months of age the formula is gradually replaced with homogenized milk and offered at 120 ml twice each day. They are given this amount of milk in addition to solid food for one year.

The appetite of the neonate determines the amounts that are given. Increases are made if they are eating everything and appear to want more. Avoid making sudden changes in their diet.

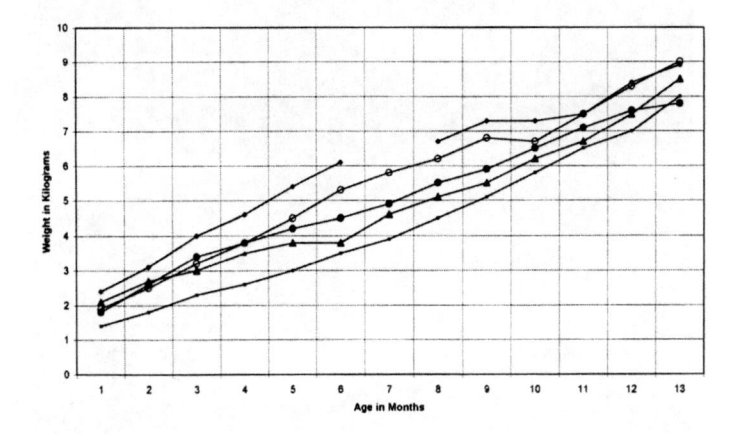

Figure 18.2. Lowland gorilla growth curve.

EXPECTED WEIGHT GAIN

Figure 18.2 shows the growth over a year's time for five lowland gorillas.

HOUSING

Keep neonates in an incubator at 85°F (30°C) until the neonate can maintain a rectal temperature of 98°F (36–37°C) (see Fig. 18.3). At that time decrease the temperature in the isolette or incubator by 2°F per day until the isolette reaches room temperature of 75–78°F (24–26°C). The infant must be able to maintain its body temperature at each change and maintain its body temperature outside of the isolette. This process is usually done between 7 and 14 days of age. When this is accomplished and the infant can maintain its body temperature, move it to a 2 × 3-ft (0.6 × 1-m) Formica box with a window viewing area. This enclosure needs to be kept warm, and not drop below room temperature of 78°F (26°C). It is important to ensure there are no drafts around the infant. Blankets are used so the infants are able to crawl out and away from them. The use of diapers is recommended to keep them clean until they are able to crawl away from feces. Pampers brand work well as they are small enough for a snug fit. One tip for urine collection is to put the disposable diapers on inside-out.

As the infant becomes more mobile, move it into a larger holding area. Remember that even though apes are similar to human infants, their strength will develop at a faster rate, so the housing for them must be very sturdy.

Use brightly colored children's toys to aid in stimulation. Trapezelike items allow the infants to grasp and pull themselves up, and are very useful to aid in developing muscle tone. Holding the infants and spending quality time with them is very important for their mental development.

COMMON MEDICAL PROBLEMS

Sepsis in newborns has been reported. Common bacterial diseases seen include infections with *Streptococcus B, Campylobacter* spp., *Salmonella* spp. and *Shigella* spp. The clinical signs are usually diarrhea and/or lack of appetite. These diseases may occur in newborns but also later in life during stressful times such as when the animal is being weaned.

Diarrhea is fairly common. Formula or clear fluids may be offered during periods of diarrhea if the neonate will drink them. Oral electrolytes are the preferred treatment. Some of the items great ape infants will drink include Kool-aid or flavored electrolytes such as Pedialyte (Ross). Pay close attention to the infant's hydration status. If the condition persists and the infant refuses to drink formula or fluids, medical attention will be required. Diarrhea needs to be treated as soon as it is noticed. The neonate may become dehydrated in 24–48 hours if it does not receive IV fluids or oral electrolytes. Blood gasses and electrolytes should be monitored when the diarrhea is severe or persistent. Pediatric specialists are very helpful in assistance with treatment plans for neonates with diarrhea.

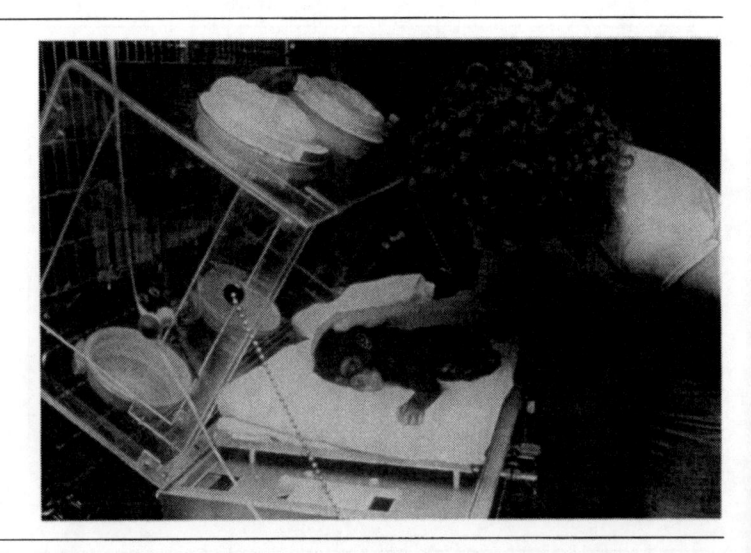

Figure 18.3. Infant chimpanzee in Isolette (photo courtesy of Six Flags Marine World).

Malnourishment is another common problem. The infant may be nursing but not getting enough calories. Poor body condition, reduced muscle tone, and listlessness are typical clinical signs. This can happen at any time during infancy. Tube feeding will be necessary if there is no nursing response.

Lactose intolerance, while not common, has been seen at our facility in several infants from the same mother. Diarrhea occurs in infants with this condition within 24 hours of receiving a cow's-milk-based formula. There are no other clinical signs; the body temperature and appetite may be normal. We rest the gastrointestinal tract for 24 hours by feeding only electrolyte solutions, such as Pedialyte. Then the neonate is started on a soy-based formula like Isomil (Ross). It is important to include a daily calcium supplement to avoid a bone density problem. Routinely submitting blood for serum chemistries to monitor calcium levels is important.

Scrotal and umbilical hernias are not common but do occur. They are usually surgically repaired between six and nine months of age unless there is a complication requiring emergency surgery.

An unusual condition occurred at our facility when an infant stopped breathing while nursing. If this problem occurs, it is important to remain calm. All infant caretakers should be trained in cardio pulmonary resuscitation (CPR) for infants. We have found no medical reason for this condition.

REINTRODUCTION

It is crucial that primates have other primates to interact with when growing up (Fig. 18.4). Other primates that are not related, such as lemurs, may be raised with gorillas or other great apes as long as they are carefully observed, and there is no aggression between them. Great apes may be allowed to interact with nonprimates while in the nursery being carefully supervised (see Fig. 18.5). Such contact with other animals is helpful in developing the groundwork for reintroduction. Reintroduction of hand-raised great apes into a display or family group is a complex task that requires much research before being attempted. It is beyond the scope of this chapter to go into the details, but I recommend the reader contact zoos where these animals have been raised and successfully reintroduced to gather important tips and information from experienced, qualified staff.

COMMENTS

I cannot emphasize enough how important it is to contact facilities where great apes have been raised, and to consult with pediatric physicians for advice. We have learned a great deal from our mistakes, but there would have been more losses if it were not for the doctors who have assisted us. Good communication among local pediatric medical facilities, the veterinary staff, and the caregivers is of utmost importance in successfully raising great apes. In addition, critical observation by the daily caregivers while the neonates are with their mothers is essential to monitoring their condition, and often facilitates making the decision of when to intervene.

ACKNOWLEDGMENTS

Special thanks to the human medical community members who have willingly shared their time and

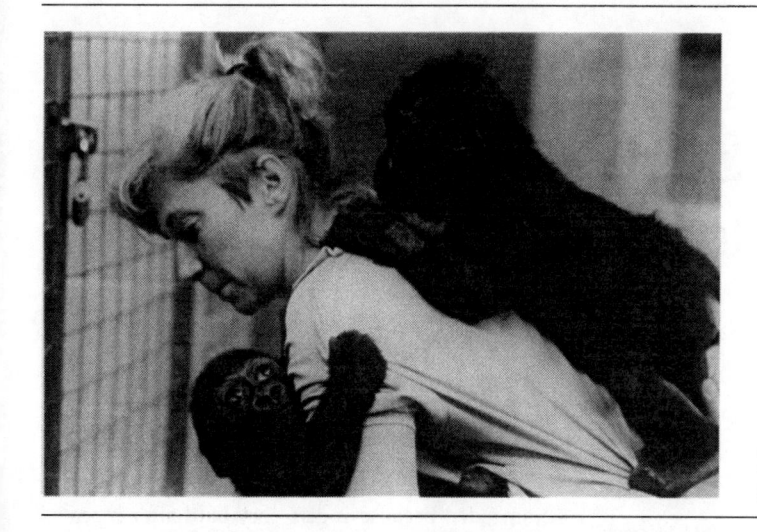

Figure 18.4. Author with infant gorillas.

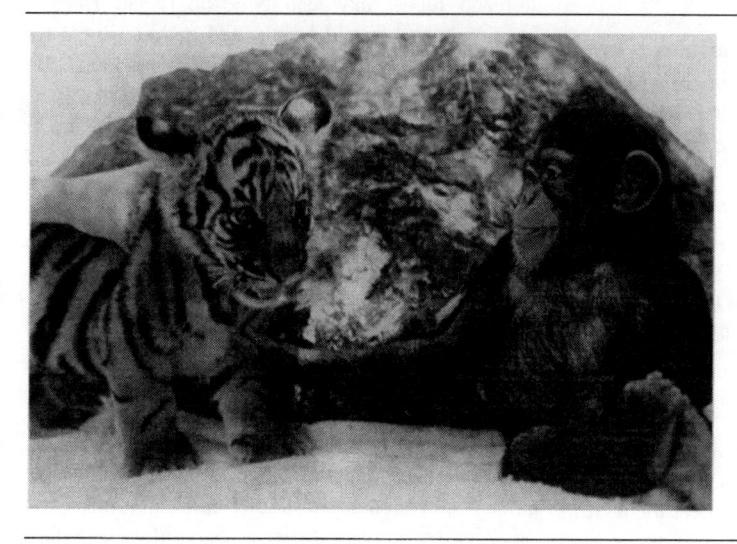

Figure 18.5. Chimpanzee and tiger cub (photo by Steve Castillo, courtesy of Six Flags Marine World).

expertise. My admiration and respect to Lynn Krammer, D.V.M., Uma Kotagal, M.D., and Paul Perlstein, M.D., for all their years of dedication to the gorillas. To Carol Schottelkotte for her friendship, devotion and years of patience to teach me, I will be forever thankful. Thanks also to the staff at the Cincinnati Zoo: Mark Campbell, D.V.M., Ken Cameron, D.V.M., and Jenny Kroll.

SOURCES OF PRODUCTS MENTIONED

Evenflo Company, Inc., 1801 Commerce Dr., Piqua, OH 45356; 1-800-233-5921; www.evenflo.com

Mead Johnson & Company, Evansville, IN 47721

Ross Products Division, Abbott Laboratories, Columbus, OH 43215-1724; 1-800-986-8510; www.abbott.com, www.ross.com

19
Harbor Seals and Northern Elephant Seals

Rebecca Duerr

NATURAL HISTORY

The average birth weight for harbor seals (*Phoca vitulina*) is 8 kg (17.6 lb). Pupping season for harbor seals is February through July off the west coast of the United States, May through June in the western Atlantic, and June through July in the eastern Atlantic. Pups are usually born later in higher latitudes. Harbor seals are usually weaned between four and six weeks of age.

Northern elephant seal (*Mirounga angustirostris*) pups have an average birth weight of 35 kg (77 lb). Pups are born with a black pelage between January and March. The black coat is shed and replaced with a tawny-to-gray colored coat when they are weaned at approximately four weeks of age.

RECORD KEEPING

Keep a daily log of food intake, fecal production and consistency, and behavioral notes including attitude and appetite, in addition to a complete medical record. Pups should be weighed at least twice a week.

EQUIPMENT

You will need a blender, a food processor or meat grinder (if using fish-based formula), a microwave or other method of heating the formula, suitable stomach tubes, and several large syringes. The 400-cc syringes work well for either species, and are available from Jorgensen Laboratories. The 140-cc Monoject catheter tip syringes from Sherwood Medical also get the job done, but require changing syringes midfeeding. For harbor seals, 0.5-in (1.3-cm) diameter (OD) vinyl tubing (Ryan Herco) may be used. For elephant seals, use the larger 0.75-in (1.9-cm) diameter tubing. Plastic tubing is not recommended because it gets very hard after repeated boiling and can irritate the esophagus. Large canine stomach tubes may also be used (Ryan Herco). Feeding tubes should be cleaned and sterilized by boiling before each use. Cut tube ends must have the sharp edges removed by grinding and/or burning.

An alternative to using large syringes is to attach a soft rubber "milker" tubing section to the end of the stomach tube and place a large funnel at the other end of the milker. The formula is then manually milked into the animal, rather than injected via syringe.

CRITERIA FOR INTERVENTION

Wild pups require hand rearing for a number of reasons, including premature separation of mother-pup pairs (e.g., after storm conditions at rookeries), maternal abandonment, sickness or injuries, and human interference. Variations in the natural histories of different phocid species may influence when a pup needs to be rescued.

Northern elephant seal females usually nurse their pups only at the birth rookery; therefore, a pup that is washed away from its natal beach is on its own, with a vanishingly small chance of being reunited with its mother. If the pup nursed long enough to acquire a significant blubber layer before being separated from its mother, it may survive premature weaning on its own. Therefore, it may only require monitoring or relocation. Elephant seals are born with a black, curly coat that is shed during their one-month nursing period (see Fig. 19.1). If a pup has this coat or an umbilical cord and is not on a rookery beach, it probably needs to be rescued to

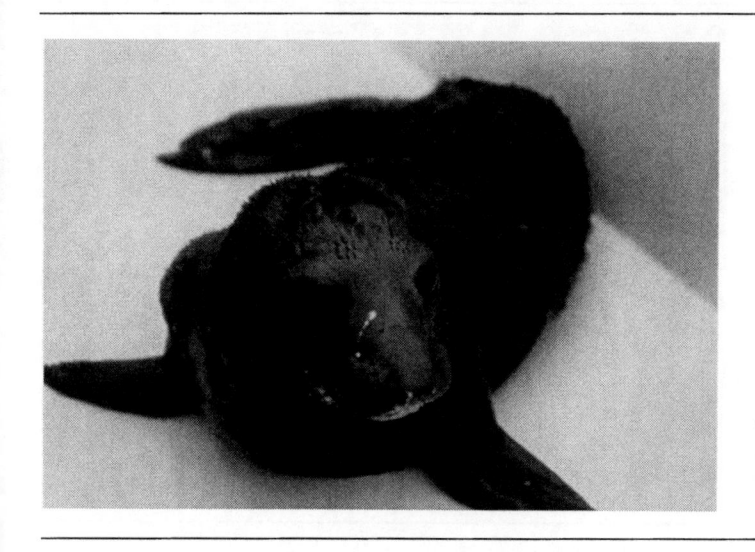

Figure 19.1. The black curly coat of a neonatal northern elephant seal (photo by Frances Gulland, courtesy of The Marine Mammal Center).

survive. The decision of whether or not to intervene is best made by a judgment of body condition. If the animal appears thin (ribs and hips obvious), dehydrated (sunken eyes with thick ocular discharge), or otherwise debilitated (injured, unresponsive, pale mucous membranes), intervention is indicated.

Harbor seal females, however, can travel with their pups, and leave them on the beach while they forage. All solitary, uninjured pups should be given the opportunity to be reclaimed by their mothers. At The Marine Mammal Center (Sausalito, California), we institute a 24-hour watch on any apparently healthy pups and keep the public away. We have frequently facilitated the reunion of separated pairs. Well-meaning people may scare a harbor seal mother off before they even see her and then mistakenly assume the pup is abandoned. A pup that is still alone after the watch period should be rescued. Harbor seals are occasionally born with a lanugo coat of fine white fur that is usually shed in utero, but it is unclear whether this can be used as an indicator of premature birth.

INITIAL CARE

Upon admission, each pup should have a physical examination, be weighed, and have blood drawn for a complete blood count and serum chemistry analysis. All pups should be assumed to be significantly dehydrated. Rehydration fluids are all a new pup should be given for at least the first 12 hours, longer in some cases, with a transition to full-strength formula occurring slowly over the first 36 to 72 hours. Vomiting and gut impactions may occur if formula is administered before adequate rehydration has occurred. Sand impactions are sometimes seen (caused by the pup nursing on sand before rescue). If a large amount of sand is noted in the mouth or feces, the veterinarian should be notified. A new pup's umbilicus should be cleaned with dilute Betadine and inspected for signs of infection.

Most phocid pups will seek out and use heat sources when available. Hypothermia often affects thin, debilitated animals. Pups that are ambulatory may have access to a wet/dry heating pad (Osborne Industries) (see Fig. 19.2), but they must have access to unheated substrate as well. Pups that are unable to move easily off the hot pad, or new pups of uncertain or unstable conditions, should not have access to hot pads. With these pups it is best to mount a hot pad on a wall in the vicinity of the pup, to provide radiant warmth. Care must be taken to not overheat pups, as brain damage and death can occur.

FORMULAS AND SUPPLEMENTS

Milk-replacement formulas for phocid seal pups should be similar to mother's milk and have a high fat content (40–60%), moderate amounts of protein (5–13%), and a very low percentage of carbohydrates. Commercially prepared powder such as MultiMilk or Zoologic 30/55 (PetAg) have been successfully used as formula ingredients for harbor seals and newborn northern elephant seals. Harbor seals may be expected to gain 0.12–0.3 kg/day on the neonatal phocid formula below. Raising harbor seal pups on blended fish without significant added fat may result in the pups gaining weight as slowly

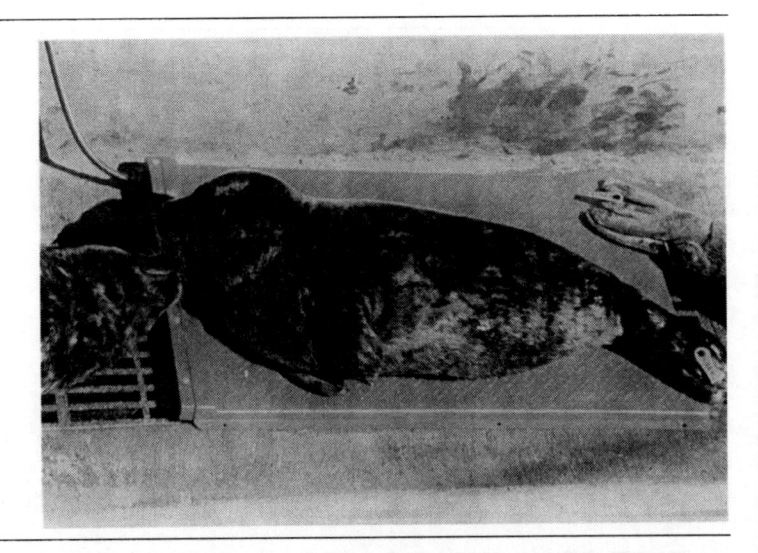

Figure 19.2. Harbor seal pup utilizing a wet/dry heating pad (photo by Frances Gulland, courtesy of The Marine Mammal Center).

as 0.05 kg/day (Wilson, Johnston, and Corpe 1999). Elephant seals may be expected to gain 0.4–0.6 kg/day, when fed the neonate formula given below. Individual animals' responses to milk-replacement formulas may vary.

Formula should be warm but never hot or cold, and must be thoroughly mixed after heating in the microwave to ensure there are no hot spots. Overheating the formula in the microwave may cause the consistency to change and may result in digestive problems. Formula in excess of what is needed should be kept properly refrigerated until the next feed and should be discarded after 24 hours.

Supplements

Harbor seal pups should be supplemented daily with 1 g salt (if kept in fresh water), plus 400 IU vitamin E (one gelcap or liquid drops), and one multivitamin such as the Vita-Zu Marine Mammal tablets (Mazuri). Elephant seal pups should be supplemented daily with 2 g salt (if kept in fresh water), plus 400 IU vitamin E, and two marine mammal multivitamins. Supplements may be broken up in a mortar and added to formula, or when the animal is weaned, the supplements may be inserted into fish.

The following formulas have worked well for us:

Neonate Phocid Formula (NPF)

450 ml water (filtered or boiled, preferably)
450 ml Milk Matrix 30/55 powder (approximately 202 g)
350 ml sardine, salmon, or other fish oil

Blend by hand with a wire whisk or spoon to avoid the addition of large amounts of air into the formula. Excessive air introduction may cause consistency changes that may encourage the addition of too much water. Formula is easily mixed in small batches. One batch yields approximately 900 ml, is 44.5% fat and 6.4% protein, and provides 4.6 kcal/ml.

Elephant Seal Weaning Formula (ESF)

0.34 kg (0.75 lb) whole ground fish (e.g., herring)
225 ml water
5 ml fish oil
250 ml whipping cream (treated with lactase at 0.75 ml per half gallon)

Grind the fish in a meat grinder or food processor and add to the other ingredients, except whipping cream, in a blender. Blend until smooth, and pour blender contents into large container. Add whipping cream with a wire whisk (do not put whipping cream in the blender). This diet is intended for weaned pups that are making the transition to whole fish. Newborn northern elephant seal pups ("blackcoats") should be fed the neonate phocid formula for the first month of life. One batch makes 825 ml and supplies approximately 19% fat, 6.5% protein, and 2 kcal/ml (values will vary depending on species of fish used and time of year).

Blended Fish Mash

0.45 kg (1.0 lb) whole ground fish (e.g. herring)
450 ml water
5 ml fish oil

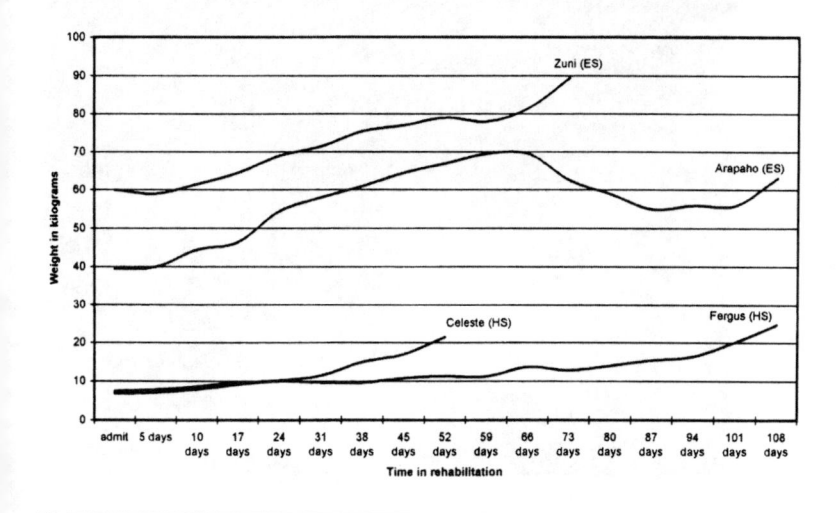

Figure 19.3. Two typical weight-gain patterns for each species. Harbor seal Fergus required twice as long as Celeste to reach 20 kg. Blackcoat elephant seal Zuni was admitted at a much heavier weight than Arapaho and did not experience the weaning process weight loss illustrated here by Arapaho.

Grind the fish in a meat grinder or food processor, add to the other ingredients in a blender, and blend until smooth.

EXPECTED WEIGHT GAIN

The expected growth chart for two blackcoat elephant seals and two harbor seals raised on neonatal phocid formula is shown in Figure 19.3.

TUBE FEEDING

Due to the short duration of nursing in phocid pups, bottle-feeding is not recommended for pups raised for wild-release. Tube feeding is quick and easy, and provides minimal contact with the animal. One person is sometimes able to simultaneously tube and restrain a pup, but this may be difficult. Two-person teams where one person restrains the animal and the other performs the tubing tend to be more efficient (see Figs. 19.4a, b, and c). Bottle-feeding is labor-intensive, and as such, may be impractical when large numbers of pups require feeding, however, it may be useful for raising permanently captive animals.

Restraint involves straddling the animal with the front flippers tucked inside the restrainer's knees, and the necessary amount of movement restriction applied via the restrainer's hands at the base of the skull. Covering the pup's head with a towel may decrease the incidence of bitten restrainers. With harbor seals, it is helpful for the restrainer to place the thumbs at the back of the skull and the fingers at the posterior curvature of the lower jaw. It is best to use as little force as necessary to accomplish the feeding, so as to inflict a minimum of stress on the animal. Be careful not to apply too much body weight force to the pup. Be gentle and try to avoid having tubing time become a stressful event for all involved. Before many teeth have erupted, the jaw may be opened on uncooperative harbor seal pups by inserting a finger at the very back of the mouth, between the jaws. This can be more challenging once the pup has a full set of teeth. Some animals will take their tubing with little or even no restraint, where the restrainer need only apply guidance against head shaking.

When the animal is restrained, the person tubing then inserts the tube down to the length of the posterior end of the sternum (about two-thirds the length of the body; see Fig. 19.5). Phocid pups very rarely allow the tube to pass down the trachea, and often vocalize during tubing, which assures the handlers that the tube is in the esophagus. Listening for stomach sounds through the tube may also be helpful in verifying tube placement. If it is still unclear whether the tube is placed correctly, a small puff of air into the tube may elicit stomach sounds. Formula should be inserted at a slow pace to discourage regurgitation, which may also occur if the tube does not reach the stomach and the formula is placed in the esophagus. The person tubing should crimp the tube when removing it from the esophagus to additionally discourage regurgitation (see Fig. 19.6). Elephant seals sometimes like to roll over and get the tubing while lying on their backs; tubing may continue without problems when this happens.

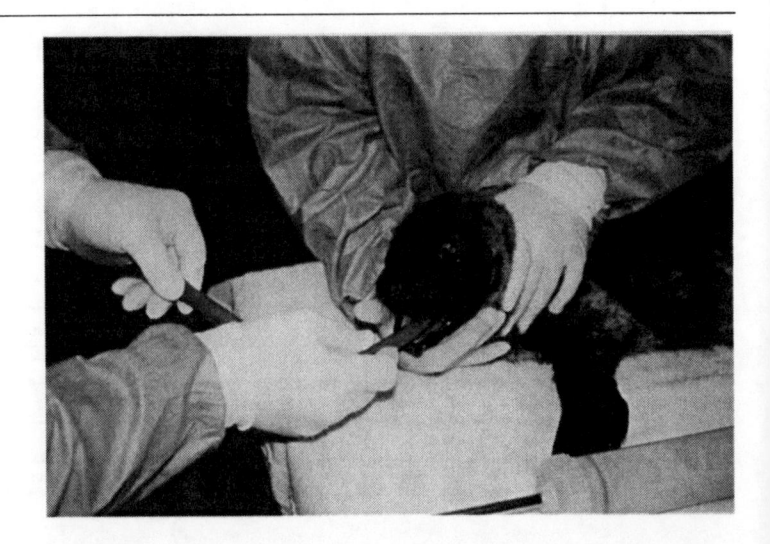

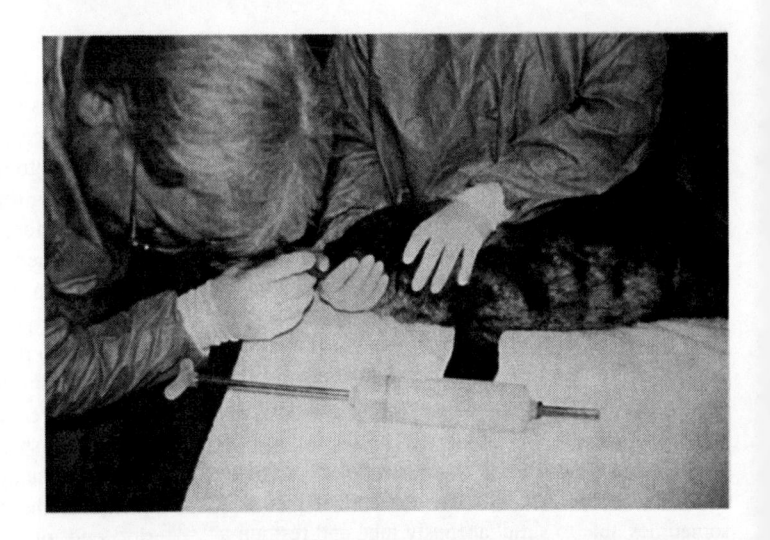

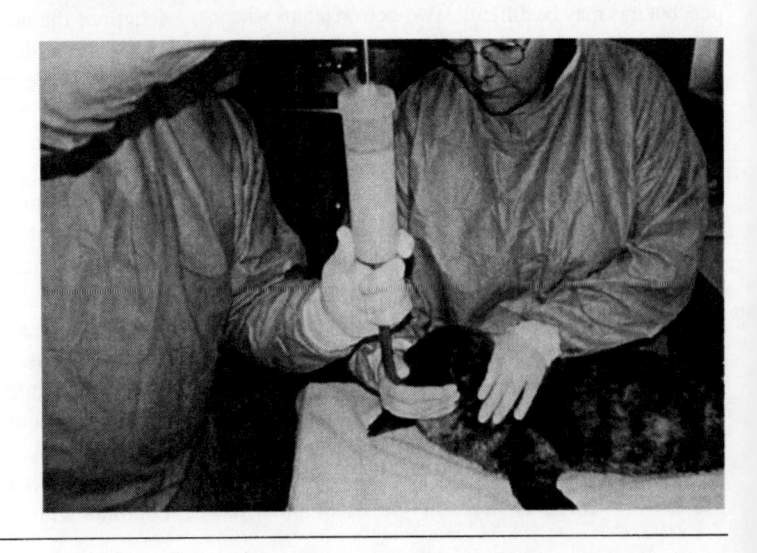

Figure 19.4. (a) Inserting the stomach tube in a harbor seal pup; (b) listening for stomach sounds; (c) delivering the formula slowly. (Photos by Bob Wilson, The Marine Mammal Center).

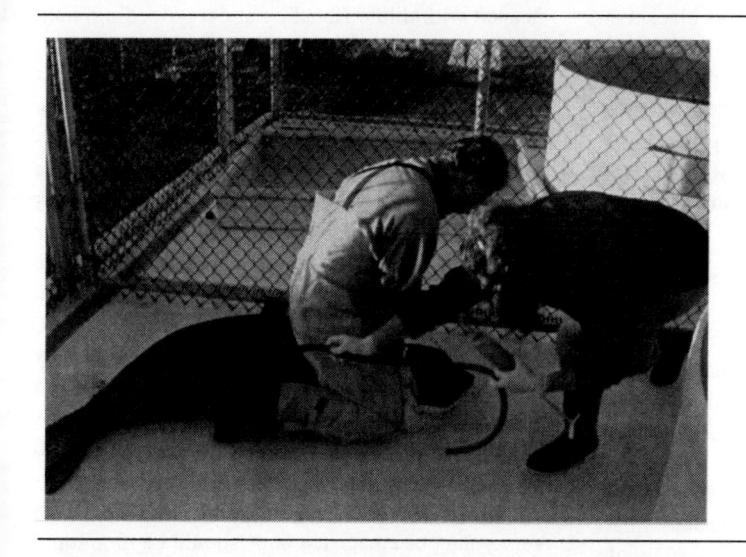

Figure 19.5. Measuring the stomach tube (photo courtesy of The Marine Mammal Center).

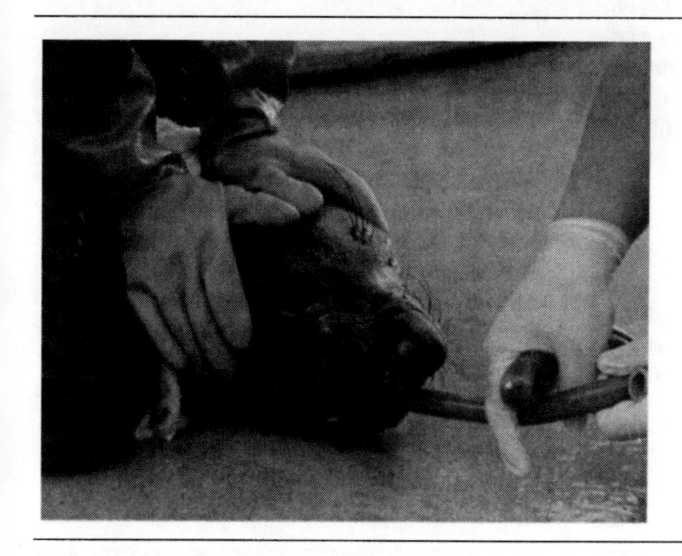

Figure 19.6. After feeding the animal, crimp the tube as you pull it out (photo by Bob Wilson, The Marine Mammal Center).

FREQUENCY OF FEEDING

During the first 24 hours, pups should be given 100 ml/kg lactated Ringer's solution (LRS) by a combination of oral and subcutaneous administration. Subcutaneous fluids are best administered beneath the skin between the scapulae. Over the first 36 hours, pups should be slowly introduced to full-strength formula by raising the relative proportion of NPF over eight or more feedings. Harbor seal pups less than 6 kg may be started on an oral volume of 150 ml, pups 6–7 kg on 170 ml, pups 7.5–8 kg on 190 ml, and pups over 8.5 kg on 220 ml tubings at four-hour intervals. Elephant seal pups less than 30 kg may be started on an oral volume of 300 ml, and pups over 30 kg may be started on 500 ml, also with a feeding interval of four hours. It is acceptable to feed the pups at midnight, then not again until 8 A.M. (i.e., 0800, 1200, 1600, 2000, 2400). Quantities of feeds may be increased by 20 ml/day for harbor seals and 50 ml/day for elephant seals, as the pup's ability to digest the formula is demonstrated (no vomiting), up to a maximum of 380 ml/feed for harbor seals and 750 ml/feed for elephant seals. If there are signs of indigestion or other problems at any stage, the case should be referred to the veterinarian.

Once an elephant seal pup has shed its blackcoat, it should be gradually switched to ESF, over a period of a day or more. Any elephant seal pup that has not reached 50 kg should be kept on the high-fat NPF formula a while longer on a case-by-case basis. Some blackcoat pups may arrive at weights well over 50 kg, but should still be fed NPF until they shed their coat.

HOUSING

Harbor Seals

In many areas of the world, harbor seal pups can suffer large mortality rates from viral infections such as morbillivirus (Duignan et al. 1995) or harbor seal herpesvirus (Borst et al. 1986; Gulland et al. 1997a) or other contagious diseases. Due to this, it is recommended that rehabilitation centers quarantine all incoming harbor seals. Procedures should be followed to prevent the caretakers from becoming vectors between pups, or to a facility's main collection, and should utilize separate clothing for each pup, such as disposable gowns and gloves. Pups should not be placed with conspecifics until such time as the pups are determined to be free of infectious disease, as determined by laboratory tests. Handling should be kept to a minimum to reduce stress, as stress may play an important role in immune function. Towels, stuffed animals, and other comfort items are not recommended due to hygiene issues and the accompanying risks of umbilical infections. The umbilicus should be cleaned with dilute Betadine at every feeding, until it is fully healed.

Large, indoor steel cages with internal, plastic-coated grates for the pups to rest upon are ideal for newly admitted pups that are receiving fluids, oxygen, or other medical care. The grates allow urine and feces to drop through, thereby decreasing contamination of the umbilicus. Clear Plexiglas door covers with gas ports may then be hooked onto the cage door to facilitate oxygen administration when necessary.

Pups should be housed outdoors as soon as they are in stable condition, and pups that are not forced to swim may experience less stress. If possible, pups should have unlimited access to shallow (4 in or 10 cm) water during the day, with a haul-out area offering heated and unheated substrate (see Fig. 19.7). Very young or emaciated pups should be monitored for hypothermia or other problems while swimming.

Once pups have been determined to be ready for conspecific companionship, they may be moved into larger pens. Ground-level pools are easiest for the animals to get into and out of, although most pups will adapt to the use of ramps. Ramped pools must have a step or ramp on the inside of the pool in order for the pup to get out of the water. Ideally, pools should be at least 3 ft (1 m) deep so that the pups can bob vertically. Wet/dry heating pads and doorless plastic pet kennels may be used in outdoor pens to provide on-demand shelter or warmth, especially at night. Pups must have adequate access to

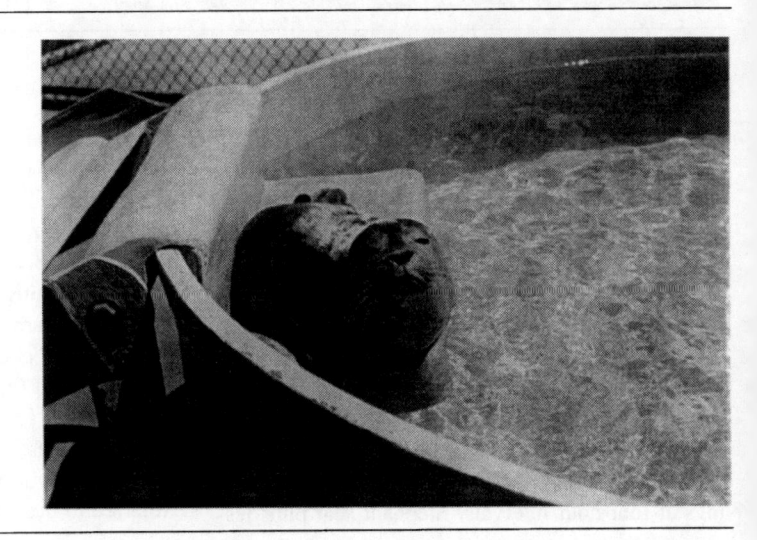

Figure 19.7. Harbor seal on shallow shelf of pool (photo by Frances Gulland, The Marine Mammal Center).

haul-out areas in the pen. Pools need to have filtration systems sufficient to maintain high water quality standards, or eye and ear infections may be a problem. Harbor seal pups are ready to wean when their teeth have significantly erupted.

Elephant Seals

Elephant seal pups should be kept in large outdoor pens, with wet/dry heating pads available. In the wild, blackcoats do not swim during their one-month nursing period. Therefore, there is no need to force the pups to swim before they shed their natal pelage. Pools for young elephant seals should be at least 8 ft (2.3 m) in diameter and 4 ft (1.2 m) deep. Older pups approaching release should have pools 12–15 ft (3.6–4.6 m) in diameter and 4 ft (1.2 m) deep. Pens should be of sufficient size to accommodate the pools, plus have ample space for the animals to rest out of the water. Pens should have surfaces that can be easily disinfected, and should be cleaned daily and disinfected frequently, particularly when animals change pens.

When pups have been weaned and are fully self-feeding, it is recommended that they have as large a pool as is available, and that human contact be kept to a minimum if the pups are to be released into the wild.

TIME TO WEANING

Elephant seal weaners (pups that have teeth and have already shed their blackcoats) should also be given 100 ml/kg LRS over the first 24 hours, by a combination of oral and subcutaneous routes. Pups less than 30 kg may be started on an oral volume of 300 ml, pups 30–35 kg on 500 ml, and pups over 35 kg on 750 ml at four-hour intervals. Elephant seal weaners frequently have problems with vomiting. This may be alleviated by introducing pups to blended fish mash first, then to ESF over the first 12 feedings, phasing in each change slowly. By the end of the third day, the pups are on full-strength ESF, and quantities may be increased by 50 ml/day up to a maximum of 750 ml/feed. If there are signs of indigestion or other problems at any stage, the case should be referred to the veterinarian.

Pups ready to begin weaning have shed their blackcoats and have well-erupted teeth. Once the animal reaches 50 kg, the tubings should decrease in frequency to encourage hunger and interest in fish. Discontinuing the 4 P.M. tubing so that the pup can be offered fish, or "fishschooled," instead, stimulates hunger during the middle of the afternoon.

TIPS FOR WEANING FROM FORMULA TO SOLID FOOD

First, offer fish or fish pieces to the pup in the water and do not give up immediately if the pup seems disinterested. Offer a fish piece under water and another above water. Tie a string with a loose knot on the tail and pull it across the pool in front of pup to imitate a live fish. Injecting air into the fish so it floats also may be helpful. You can try tossing a fish in the pool and leave it there to see if the pup will investigate it on its own. Sometimes, a ripped piece with some of the guts hanging out will be more interesting to a pup than a cut piece. Live fish, if available, are a very natural stimulant that often works; we have used anchovies or sardines to good effect. The fishschooling process takes patience, but is well worth the effort.

Often elephant seal pups are not comfortable in deep pools when they are first learning to eat. Shallow plastic pools simulate the tide pools a pup would play in on a beach. Sturdily built children's pools have been used with great success. These should be low enough that the pups are able to easily see over the edge and climb in, and large enough for the pup to comfortably crawl around in. After their agility has improved, pups may be placed in deeper pools for fishschool.

If elephant seal pups have reached 60 kg or harbor seals pups have reached 20 kg, and have not responded to fishschool, they may be fasted until they are eating. Strict monitoring of the pup should be maintained for hydration and body condition, and the pup should not be allowed to lose over 10% of its body weight.

When a pup takes a fish from your hand, make the pup chase after the next fish and before it grabs it, let go. If the pups are eating fish under water, it is time to push them to free feeding. Throw fish into the water and move away from the pool. If you are visible, many pups will play helpless since they know they can get you to feed them by hand. Instead, watch from a distance where the pups are not aware of your presence. Leave the pups alone for at least 15–20 minutes before giving up on their ability to eat on their own. Once a pup is eating on its own, the amount of fish fed may be raised by 1/8 kg per feed up to 10% of body weight, divided up into two or three meals per day. Be sure to monitor individual weights at this stage to verify that each pup is eating his share.

Elephant seal pups often lose weight during the weaning process if they do not learn to eat solid food quickly, but this is not necessarily of major concern. In the wild, weaned northern elephant seals associate in groups on their natal beaches and do not eat for a month or more. They slowly learn to catch shallow-water fish and invertebrates while depending on the body reserves laid down during the lactation period. It is difficult to mimic this natural history in a rehabilitation setting. The procedures set forth here, however, have resulted in a high success rate for wild-released pups.

COMMON MEDICAL PROBLEMS

Table 19.1 shows common medical problems and describes treatment options for handling conditions such as hypoglycemia, dehydration, hypo and hyperthermia, abscesses, and parasites. Several commonly seen diseases will be briefly described here. For a more thorough discussion of the diseases of pinnipeds, see Dierauf and Gulland (2001).

Viral infections affect harbor seal pups, especially those that strand in poor nutritional condition. Clinical signs of phocine herpesvirus (PhHV-1) include severe electrolyte and blood glucose abnormalities (Gulland et al. 1997a). In addition, PhHV-1 has been reported to cause pneumonia in harbor seal pups undergoing rehabilitation (Borst et al. 1986). Pneumonia may also be caused by other viruses, such as influenza, phocine distemper virus, and canine distemper virus. Affected pups should be treated with supportive care and quarantined.

Table 19.1. Common Medical Problems in Phocid Pups

Problem	Clinical signs	Treatment
Dehydration	Dry, sunken or mucousy eyes, dark urine, dry mucous membranes, curly vibrissae	Rehydrate with 100 ml/kg LRS via oral and subcutaneous routes
Hypothermia	Lethargy, shivering, pale mucous membranes, cold flippers	Provide heating pad or warm-water bottles, administer warm fluids
Hyperthermia	Lethargy, open mouth breathing, dry mucous membranes, hot flippers ometimes held away from body	Wet animal, administer fluids, place ice near but not on animal
Hypoglycemia	Lethargy, pale mucous membranes, dull or nonresponsive, vibrissae sometimes held forward, may present as seizure activity or shaky movements	If a pup is "shaky" but still responsive, subcutaneous fluids such as 0.45% NaCl, with 2.5% dextrose may be administered. If animal is seizuring, a rectal bolus of 25% dextrose or an IV bolus of 10% dextrose may be administered. If an IV bolus is given, a blood sample should be taken prior to administration to determine the initial blood glucose level. After the pup is stable, it should be referred to the veterinarian for further treatment.
Umbilical abscesses	Swelling or hardness around umbilicus, discharge from umbilicus or its scar	Flush area with dilute Betadine or Nolvasan (chlorhexidine), refer to veterinarian for appropriate antibiotic therapy
Bite wounds/ other injuries, such as fishery interactions, gunshot, boat strikes	Visible wounds or swelling	Flush area with dilute Betadine or Nolvasan (chlorhexidine), refer to veterinarian for appropriate antibiotic therapy
Parasites	Fecal tests and/or visible worms	Appropriate anthelminthics

Animals with bacterial pneumonia may present with tachypnea, dyspnea, lethargy, and cough, and may be treated with appropriate antibiotics. Viral infections may often be accompanied by bacterial infections, so treatment of respiratory disease with antibiotics is recommended.

Harbor and elephant seals are vulnerable to infestation with the nematode *Otostrongylus circumlitis*. These parasites grow to be quite large, and in harbor seals, reside in the bronchi and bronchioles, where they may cause obstructive bronchitis and bronchiolitis. Treatment of affected animals may include fenbendazole, antibiotics for secondary bacterial infection, and corticosteroids such as dexamethasone to reduce inflammatory responses to dead worms. Diagnosis may be based on fecal analysis, however, the infestation may be quite severe before larvae are present in feces. In some individual elephant seals, *O. circumlitis* may not able to complete its life cycle, and animals may develop plugs of worms obstructing the heart and pulmonary vessels (Gulland et al. 1997b). *O. circumlitis* infestation in northern elephant seals has been associated with disseminated intravascular coagulation, which is characterized by bleeding from the nares, extended clotting times, and other blood abnormalities (Gulland et al. 1996). Treatment of suspected affected animals is as above for harbor seals.

Phocid pups may develop skin nodules characteristic of seal pox virus. Lesions begin as small (0.5–2-cm diameter) raised nodules, often on the foreflippers, hind flippers, and chin, and may become enlarged and ulcerated. Nodules persist for four to eight weeks and the virus is quite contagious to other pinnipeds (Hastings et al. 1989). This condition has not been shown to be life threatening to the pups, but may require antibiotic therapy to control secondary bacterial infections. This virus has also been suggested to have zoonotic potential, so gloves should always be worn when handling affected animals (Hicks and Worthy 1987).

ACKNOWLEDGMENTS

Many thanks to Deb Wickham and Lisa Phoenix for feeding and weaning information, to Dr. Frances Gulland for medical information, and to Guthrum Purdin and Denise Grieg for reviewing the chapter. Thanks to Bob Wilson for photographic assistance.

SOURCES OF PRODUCTS MENTIONED

Jorgensen Laboratories, 1450 N. Van Buren Ave., Loveland, CO 80538; 1-800-525-5614

Mazuri, 1050 Progress Dr., Richmond, IN 47374; 1-800-227-8941; Mazuri.com

Osborne Industries, 120 N. Industrial Avenue, Osborne, KS 67473; 1-800-255-0316

PetAg Inc., 261 Keyes Ave., Hampshire, IL 60140; 1-800-323-0877, 1-800-323-6878; www.petag.com

Ryan Herco, 1819 Junction Ave., San Jose, CA 95131-2101; 1-800-848-1411

Sherwood Medical, Ballymoney, N. Ireland

REFERENCES

Borst, G. H. A., H. C. Walvoort, P. J. H. Reijnders, J. C. van der Kamp, and A. D. M. E. Osterhaus. 1986. An outbreak of a herpesvirus infection in harbor seals (*Phoca vitulina*). *Journal of Wildlife Diseases* 22(1): 1–6.

Dierauf, L., and F. Gulland, eds. 2001. *Handbook of marine mammal medicine*. Boca Raton, FL: CRC Press.

Duignan, P. J., J. T. Saliki, D. J. St. Aubin, G. Early, S. Sadove, J. A. House, K. Kovacs, and J. R. Geraci. 1995. Epizootiology of morbillivirus infection in North American harbor seals (*Phoca Vitulina*) and gray seals (*Halichoerus grypus*). *Journal of Wildlife Diseases* 31(4): 491–501.

Gulland, F., L. Lowenstine, J. Lapointe, T. Spraker, and D. King. 1997a. Herpesvirus infection in stranded Pacific harbor seals of coastal California. *Journal of Wildlife Diseases* 33(3): 450–58.

Gulland, F. M. D., K. Beckmen, K. Burek, L. Lowenstine, L. Werner, T. Spraker, and E. Harris. 1997b. *Otostrongylus circumlitus* infestation of northern elephant seals (*Mirounga angustirostris*) stranded in central California. *Marine Mammal Science* 13(3): 446–59.

Gulland, F. M. D, L. Werner, S. O'Neill, L. J. Lowenstine, J. Trupkiewicz, D. Smith, B. Royal, and I. Strubel. 1996. Baseline coagulation assay values for northern elephant seals (*Mirounga angustirostris*), and the diagnosis of a case of disseminated intravascular coagulation in this species. *Journal of Wildlife Diseases* 32: 536–40.

Hastings, B., L. Lowenstine, L. Gage, and R. Munn. 1989. An epizootic of seal pox in pinnipeds at a rehabilitation center. *Journal of Zoo and Wildlife Medicine* 20(3): 282–90.

Hicks, B., and G. Worthy. 1987. Sealpox in captive grey seals (*Halichoerus grypus*) and their handlers. *Journal of Wildlife Diseases* 23: 1–6.

Wilson, S., T. Johnston, and H. Corpe. 1999. Radiotelemetry study of four rehabilitated harbor seal pups following their release in County Down, Northern Ireland. *Journal of Wildlife Rehabilitation* 22(3): 17–23.

FURTHER READING

Goldstein, T., S. P. Johnson, L. J. Werner, S. Nolan, and B. A. Hilliard. 1998. Causes of erroneous white blood cell counts and differentials in clinically healthy young northern elephant seals, *Mirounga angustirostris*. *Journal of Zoo and Wildlife Medicine* 29(4): 408–12.

Gulland, F. M. D., M. Haulena, S. Elliott, S. Thornton, and L. Gage. 1999. Anesthesia of juvenile Pacific harbor seals using propofol alone and in combination with isoflurane. *Marine Mammal Science* 15(1): 234–38.

Thornton, S. M., S. Nolan, and F. M. D. Gulland. 1998. Bacteria isolated from California sea lions (*Zalophus californianus*), harbor seals (*Phoca vitulina*), and northern elephant seals (*Mirounga angustirostris*) admitted to a rehabilitation center along the central California coast, 1994–1995. *Journal of Zoo and Wildlife Medicine* 29(2): 171–76.

Trupkiewicz, J. G., F. M. D. Gulland, and L. J. Lowenstine. 1997. Congenital defects in northern elephant seals (*Mirounga angustirostris*) stranded along the central California coast 1988–1995. *Journal of Wildlife Diseases* 33(2): 220–25.

20
Sea Lions and Fur Seals

Laurie J. Gage

NATURAL HISTORY

The most common species of sea lion and fur seal presented for hand rearing are the California sea lion (*Zalophus californianus*), and the northern fur seal (*Callorhinus ursinus*). The average birth weight of a California sea lion pup is 6.0–9.0 kg while northern fur seal pup birth weights average 4.5–5.4 kg.

Births are seasonal for both species, with the majority of California sea lion births seen in May and June while the northern fur seal pups are typically born in June and early July.

Wild California sea lion pups generally are weaned at four to eight months of age, between the months of September and February. Captive sea lion pups often will nurse for a year or more. Weaning may not take place until they are physically removed from the dam. Northern fur seals usually are weaned at four to five months of age, in October or November.

RECORD KEEPING

Keep a daily log of feed intake, fecal and urine production, fecal consistency, body weight, and behavioral notes including attitude and appetite.

CRITERIA FOR INTERVENTION

Sea lion or fur seal pups may be orphaned or abandoned and will by necessity need to be hand reared. In captive situations, especially with primiparous females, new mothers may initially reject or ignore their pups. If the mother is not aggressive toward the pup, removing the two from the exhibit and placing them in a holding area may force the female to accept her pup and allow it to nurse. Sometimes it seems the discomfort of giving birth makes the female irritable and resistant to letting the pup nurse. Giving the female 20 to 30 mg diazepam three to four times daily seems to help the situation. As long as the pup is strong and shows normal suckling behavior, intervention may not be necessary. The pup should be weighed daily, and if there is a loss of weight, it should be tube fed. If the pup is not nursing, or trying to nurse but not allowed, give it 10–12 ml/kg body weight Pedialyte or an electrolyte solution via gavage (tube feed) after 24 hours, and place it back with the dam. If insufficient nursing has taken place after 36 hours and the pup has lost weight, tube feed it formula and place it back with the dam. Only if the pup seems weak and shows no attempts at nursing, or the dam is overly aggressive towards it, should it be removed completely to be hand reared. The pup should be tube fed as often as necessary to keep it hydrated and to keep weight loss to a minimum. If the pup is making good attempts at nursing, tube feeding once a day usually will be sufficient. Try any reasonable method to keep mother and pup together. Usually, after three days to a week of confinement and diazepam, the mother will accept and successfully rear her pup, however this result could take several weeks to achieve.

FORMULAS

Sea lions have been successfully raised on a variety of formulas. The formula should be similar to mother's milk by being high in fat, moderate in protein, and low in carbohydrates.

It is important to include daily supplements of 200 mg thiamin, 400 IU vitamin E, 1.5 g salt, and 100 mg taurine when using powdered formulas. Failure to include these supplements may lead to severe health problems. The easiest formulas to use are commercially available powdered formulations.

PetAg's MultiMilk or Zoologic 30/55 (PetAg) both have been used successfully in these species by this author. Another tried and true formula appropriate for sea lions and fur seals is the Marine Mammal Center Fish-Based Formula (Table 20.1).

When using a powdered formula, care must be given to making the formula consistently. A rule of thumb for making the formula is to mix 2 parts water to 1 part powder initially. If this mixture agrees with the pup, and no diarrhea or constipation is noted, the strength of the formula may be increased gradually to 1.5 parts water to 1 part powder. The consistency of the formula may vary from batch to batch of powdered product. Pay attention to the thickness of the formula when preparing it, and be careful when making formula from a new batch of powder. When the consistency in a new batch of powdered formula is different from the previous batch, adjustments of the powder-to-water ratio may need to be made.

Making the formula too thin will result in poor weight gain and often frantic, hungry pups. Making the formula too thick results in gastrointestinal problems such as diarrhea, vomiting, constipation, or inappetence. Keep the following guidelines in mind:

- Powdered commercial formulas must not be overblended. Use a wire whisk to mix; or if using a blender, three to four seconds of blender mixing at the high setting are usually sufficient. Over ten seconds in the blender adds too much air to the formula and may cause the pups to have indigestion.
- Temperature of the formula is very important and pups will often be very particular about accepting formula that is consistently the right temperature. This varies between individuals and requires some experimentation to find the most ideal formula temperature for each individual. Some pups will only accept formula that is over a certain temperature.
- Formula should always be temperature tested by placing a few drops on the inside of your wrist. Formula should be warm but never hot. Overheating the formula in the microwave may cause the consistency to change and may result in digestive problems.
- Bottles must be thoroughly mixed after heating in the microwave to ensure there are no hot spots within the bottle.
- Formula may be reheated in the bottle up to three times in a thirty-minute period, but then should be discarded. Formula that was heated and not consumed during a feed should be discarded. Formula that is over 24 hours old should be discarded.

Table 20.1. Marine Mammal Center Fish-Based Formula

1. Start with 0.68 kg of high-quality herring. Remove heads tails and fins. Do not debone the fish any further.
2. Cut fish into small pieces, add 200 ml water, and grind into a smooth paste in a food processor. Transfer paste to a rice strainer to remove the larger bone fragments.
3. Place 0.45 kg fish paste into a blender with the remaining ingredients:
   300 ml Pedialyte or 5% dextrose in lactated Ringer's solution
   1 multiple vitamin ground into a powder
   2 g salt
   200 mg vitamin B1
   400 IU vitamin E
   280 mg calcium gluconate
   500 mg vitamin C
   10 ml safflower oil (or the preferred salmon oil, which is sometimes hard to find)
   10 ml lecithin
4. Blend all ingredients to an even consistency. Pour contents into a clean container and add 400 ml treated whipping cream.[1] Rock the container until ingredients are mixed.
5. Label the container with the date and time prepared and refrigerate. *Discard after 24 hours.* Recipe makes approximately 1280 ml formula.
6. Invert container several times during a 24-hour period before use.

[1]Treated whipping cream: Add 0.75 ml lactase to 1 quart whipping cream.

WHAT TO FEED INITIALLY

Start newborns initially on straight Pedialyte (Ross) or any balanced electrolyte solution such as lactated Ringer's solution. Pups should be well hydrated before starting them on formula. Start with a dilute formula: 25% formula to 75% electrolyte solution. Gradually increase the strength of the formula over the next 24 to 36 hours. See the Formulas section for how to make up the formula.

NURSING TECHNIQUES

Sea lion and fur seal pups are generally uncomplicated to hand raise, but getting pups to suckle from a bottle may be a challenge. One tip to encouraging pups to accept you as a surrogate and to become comfortable suckling is to wear the same clothing whenever handling the pup. The familiar smell, which will be pungent to you after a few days, seems to comfort the pup (Fig. 20.1).

Healthy pups usually have a good suckle reflex and will nurse on clothing, fingers, and often everything but the nipple. It helps to boil the nipples or wash them thoroughly in hot soapy water, rinsing well to remove any latex or rubber flavor. To get pups accustomed to the flavor of the formula put a small amount on their lips wherever they start to suckle. Try to slip the nipple into the pup's mouth as it is suckling on something else. This must be done gently and requires much patience. Have a variety of nipples on hand as individual pups prefer different nipple types. Pups are often particular about the nipple they select. Have several nipples of each brand on hand so when one wears out it can be replaced with a new one of the same type. Two of the more commonly accepted nipples are the NUK nurser (Gerber) or a rubber lamb's nipple (available from most feed stores or from Jeffers Livestock). It may take several days to a week or longer for pups to accept the bottle and nurse consistently. Therefore, newborns may need to be fed via gavage (tube fed) three to four times each day for days to a week or longer. Occasionally pups never accept the bottle and must be gavaged several times each day for two or more months until they are weaned and eating a fish diet.

TUBE FEEDING

Pups being fed via gavage, or stomach tube, will not tolerate the same amounts of formula that bottle-fed pups are able to nurse in one feeding session (Gage 1993). Formula amounts tube fed to pups must be reduced by 25% to 30% of what nursing pups will suckle each feed.

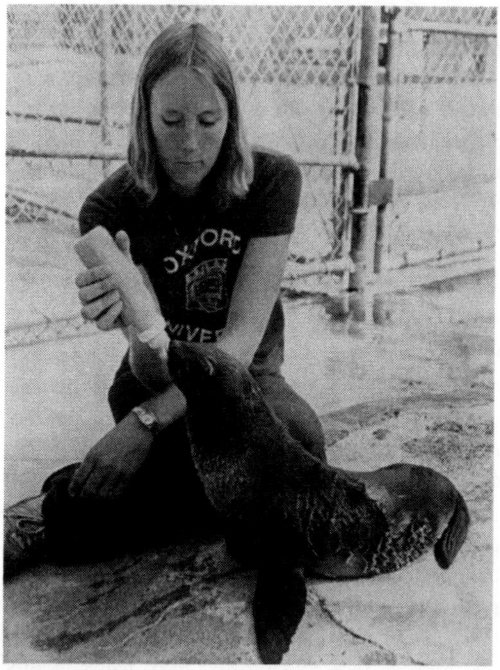

Figure 20.1. Northern fur seal nursing on a bottle.

An ideal tube for sea lion or fur seal pups is a 1/2-in (1.3 cm) diameter (OD) large canine feeding tube (KI 700) custom cut to 3 ft (90 cm) in length (Kalajian Company). Half-inch (1.3 cm) diameter (OD) vinyl tubing (Ryan Herco) may also be used. If the animal is smaller than 6 kg, the 3/8-in (0.95 cm) diameter (OD) small canine feeding tube (KI 600, Kalajian Company) cut to about 90 cm may be used. Red rubber stallion catheters have also been used with good success. The clear vinyl tubes are preferred because the formula can be visualized in the tube, and the cleanliness of the inside of the tube is more easily evaluated. The tube is laid out alongside the pup to the area of the stomach, just past the last rib, and a mark is made with an indelible marker at the tip of the snout to indicate how far to pass the tube. Gently open the pup's mouth and insert the tube to the back of the throat. Push gently until the pup swallows the tube. You should be able to feel the tip of the tube advancing down the esophagus on the left side of the neck as you pass it. If the tube is in the trachea you will not be able to feel it pass, and you will not be able to advance the tube as far as your mark. You may or may not hear breathing through the tube if it is in the trachea by mistake, so do not depend on that factor for confirmation of its location. If you have never passed a stomach tube, ask for help from a veterinarian or experienced rehabilitator.

Formula may be delivered by gravity through a funnel attached to the feed tube, or by using a catheter-tip 60-cc syringe. If the syringe is used, the formula must be delivered very slowly, allowing 30 to 40 seconds for the delivery of formula from each 60-cc syringe.

FREQUENCY OF FEEDING

Newborns weighing less than 7 kg (15.4 lb) should be fed every four hours. Once pups begin gaining steady weight the feed amounts may be increased gradually. Once the pup weighs over 7 kg, the feeding frequency may be decreased to five times each day, eliminating the 4 A.M. feed, and gradually increasing the amounts of the other feeds. Once the pup weighs over 10 kg, the frequency of feeds is then decreased to four feeds per day. Bottle-raised pups may limit the amount they eat at some feed times. They may choose to nurse large amounts at one time of day, and refuse entire feeds at other scheduled feed times. If this happens consistently, a feed may be eliminated, and the amounts offered at the other feeds may be increased accordingly.

AMOUNTS TO FEED

In general, pups may be bottle-fed 15 to 25 ml per kg per feed (7 to 12 ml per lb), totaling 75 to 125 ml per kg (34 to 57 ml per lb) per day initially.

If you must tube feed the pup, start with 15 ml per kg (6.8 ml per lb) and increase the amount by 0.5 to 1 ml per kg every other feed until you are tube feeding 20 ml per kg. If at any time during the feeding process the pup regurgitates, the amount per feed must be reduced.

Pups may chose to nurse less than what they are offered. If pups are consistently finishing off the offered amount and seem hungry, feed amounts may be gradually increased. Pups tend to nurse up to 250 ml of formula per feed by the time they are three to four weeks of age. By the time they are six weeks old, expect them to suckle between 250 to 300 ml per feed, four times each day. Be aware that if the formula amount is increased too quickly, pups may vomit or refuse the next several feeds. Similarly, if the formula is powdered and made up too rich, pups may suffer with digestive upsets, such as diarrhea or constipation.

EXPECTED WEIGHT GAIN

Expect sea lions to gain 0.08 to 0.125 kg per day the first two weeks (Fig. 20.2). Fur seals may gain slightly less weight per day. Pups should be weighed daily. Once pups are nursing well on a bottle, a gain of approximately 0.2 to 0.5 kg per day is expected. It is not unusual for pups to gain weight steadily for a few days and then have one or two days per week with no significant gains.

HOUSING

Full-term sea lion and fur seal pups are prone to hyperthermia. They should be housed at temperatures between 65 and 78°F (18.3 to 25.5°C). An extra source of heat, such as a radiant heat lamp, or

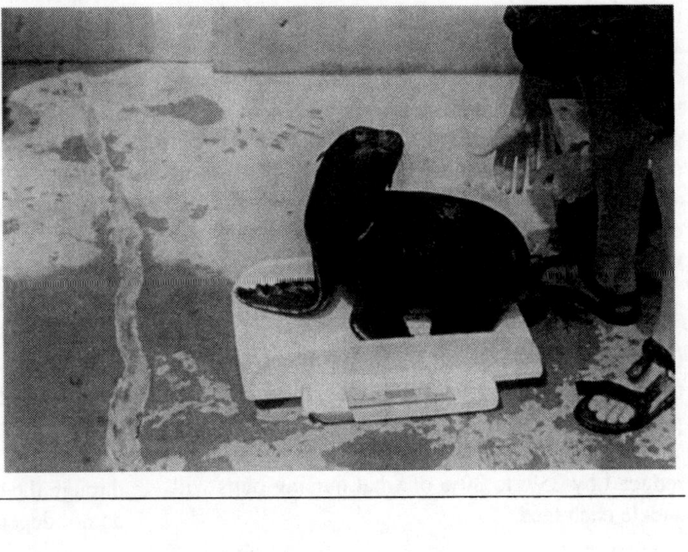

Figure 20.2. One-week-old California sea lion pup on a scale.

a wet/dry heating pad (Osborne), should be used only if the pup is underweight or is seen shivering, or if the ambient temperature falls below 65°F (18°C). When using heat sources, ensure the pup always has an unheated area available to it. If the ambient temperature exceeds 78°F (25°C), ensure the pup has access to a shallow pool, or a place a water spray in the vicinity of the pup.

Pups should be exposed to a shallow-water pool within 72 hours of birth and will need assistance with swimming at first. A pool with a gradually sloping bottom from the beach into shallow and then deeper water is ideal because it enables the pup to easily get out of the pool on its own. Pups quickly learn to swim but their front flippers are weak and they cannot pull themselves out from a deeper pool with a lip or an edge at the perimeter.

Most pups need to be supported for their first few attempts at deep-water swims. This is done by holding the scruff of their neck and lightly pulling them into the deeper water. They usually will not venture to deeper water without encouragement and support. They need to be closely supervised when swimming for the first few weeks until they develop sufficient strength in their front flippers. Allowing them to play in shallow water is advised and they should have several hours of supervised water time each day for the first few weeks. They should be housed in a secure, dry area when unsupervised until they have demonstrated good swimming ability and are able to haul out onto dry ground on their own.

IMMUNE STATUS AND SPECIAL NEEDS

Newborn pups that have not nursed may have decreased immunoglobulins and must be handled with care. There should be no exposure to other animals unless the pup can be reintroduced to its mother. Personnel handling the pups should wear clothes designated for that pup. Clothing should be changed between handling different individuals. Cleanliness is a must and all bottles, nipples, or tubes should be boiled or steam sterilized between each feeding. Frequent water changes or a quality filtration system for pools is necessary, and haul-out areas or dry enclosures should be cleaned and disinfected several times daily.

TIME TO WEANING

Sea lions and fur seals may be weaned off formula and started on a fish diet as early as six weeks of age, however it is preferable to feed them formula for at least three months before starting the transition to whole fish. Once sea lions and fur seals are eating fish, they should be receiving one marine mammal vitamin (Mazuri Vita-Zu Mammal Tablet) for every 5 to 7 lbs of fish consumed each day. In addition to that, supplementing with 400 IU vitamin E daily is recommended.

TIPS FOR WEANING FROM FORMULA TO SOLID FOOD

There are many clever ways to wean pups from formula to fish. One method is to begin adding small chunks of fish guts and muscle to the formula and enlarging the nipple hole enough to allow the clumps to be nursed along with the formula. Over a period of several weeks, the size of the chunks is increased until the pup is nursing cherry-sized clumps of fish from the bottle. Once the pup is accustomed to swallowing the larger chunks, whole fish may be introduced to the pup in the dry area or while it is in the pool. Allowing the pup to play with whole fish and fish pieces while in the pool may also entice it to begin to eat fish. Wiggling the fish under water may help to entice the pup to focus on the food item.

One other successful method is to allow the pup to play with ice cubes in the pool. Small chunks of fish are frozen into the cubes, and as the pup accepts those, the chunks of fish are enlarged. Soon the pup will accept ice-cube-sized chunks of fish. Not every method works with every pup so experimentation must be done to find the least stressful way to entice a pup to accept fish.

As a last resort, pups may need to be force-fed fish each day. This involves restraining the pup, prying open its mouth, and introducing small whole or cut fish. Herring is a good choice. This must be done with care as sea lion and fur seal pups are inclined to bite their handlers. We have found the crude method of taping tongue depressors or using heavy tape on the handler's index finger (to prevent bite wounds) works better than using tongs to insert the fish past the gag point. When force-feeding, ensure the fish you are using is stiff. It may help to have it still partially frozen, but only cold enough to add some "stiffness" to the fish. Do not force-feed frozen fish. Small fully thawed fish may be too soft and are difficult to push past the gag point. Usually after a week or two of being force-fed at least one feed per day, with bottle or tube feedings making up the rest of the feeds, pups will begin to eat fish on their own. It may be necessary to decrease the number of daily feeds offered to heighten the pup's appetite. Weigh the pup daily to ensure there is no significant weight loss during this transition period.

COMMON MEDICAL PROBLEMS

Gastrointestinal problems such as diarrhea or constipation are generally associated with improper feeding techniques or changes in the formula. Pups fed formula normally have yellow to tan soft-formed feces that dissipate easily in water. If the feces are chalklike or too hard, one to two pinches of any psyllium product (Equi-Aid) or Metamucil and 1–3 ml of vegetable oil may be added to each bottle. If too much oil is added, the feces will appear slick or oily. The amount of oil should be reduced accordingly.

Inappetence is usually an indicator of the gastrointestinal problems relating to the formula, but may also be a sign of another illness. Taking blood once in the first week with a follow-up at one month of age is recommended, however blood samples may be difficult to obtain and are sometimes more stressful to the animal than they are useful.

Anemia has been seen in hand-reared fur seals and other young otariids (Gage et al. 1996; Gulland, Haulena, and Dierauf 2001). It is important to obtain a complete blood count every four to six weeks to screen for this. If anemia is diagnosed, ensure the pup is parasite-free and is getting at least 400 IU vitamin E and 200 mg thiamin daily. Be aware that pups may be able to detect and selectively reject fish with supplements. Anemic pups have been treated with erythropoietin with good success.

Parasites are reported in wild stranded fur seal and sea lion pups. Especially important in young wild pups is hookworm (*Uncinaria* sp.), which may cause severe anemia. Infected fur seals and sea lions have been successfully treated with fenbendazole at a dose of 10 mg/kg orally for three consecutive days.

Pneumonia is another common medical problem. Pups have been treated with appropriate antibiotics and nebulization, and regain their appetites quickly once the problem is diagnosed and properly treated.

Proper hydration is a must and if a pup is not eating well it should be given subcutaneous fluids to maintain hydration. Lactated Ringer's with 5% dextrose is a good choice as the glucose is absorbed quickly and may help to prevent hypoglycemia. There have been no ill effects from giving these fluids subcutaneously.

If pups are limp or unresponsive, hypoglycemia should be considered. Blood should be drawn and a blood glucose test run to determine if this is the problem. If the blood glucose is under 80 mg/dl, a 10% to 25% glucose solution should be given IV to effect. A 5% glucose solution may be given subcutaneously and 50% glucose solution may be given via gavage to help to stabilize the pup.

It is difficult to draw blood from otariids. The caudal gluteal vein is a good choice for experienced handlers. The jugular vein is another choice in well-restrained pups. For those inexperienced in handling otariid pups, trimming a toenail is sometimes the most expedient way to obtain a blood sample for testing blood glucose.

Pups housed in fresh water have an absolute requirement for sodium, which must be included in their daily formula at a dose of no less than 1.5 grams NaCl per individual per day. Clinical signs of hyponatremia are vague neurologic signs; primarily muscle fasciculation or seizures. Normal serum levels of sodium should exceed 140 mEq/l. If serum levels are lower than 140 mEq/l, sodium chloride must be increased in the diet. Sodium levels below 130 mEq/l are life-threatening. Administering 3% sodium chloride intravenously may reverse this condition.

RELEASE: CAPTIVE VERSUS WILD

Sea lion and fur seal pups imprint readily on people and if they are being raised for release to the wild they must have very little exposure to humans. This may be accomplished by using a puppet or a padded box with a hole through which the nipple is secured. Stuffed animals or sturdy pillows the pup can snuggle against for comfort are used to replace human contact. Talking within earshot of the pups must be avoided. Getting a pup to nurse on a bottle without having it imprint on its caregiver is a challenge, but with patience and ingenuity, it can be accomplished. If more than one pup is being hand reared, they can be housed together for companionship. Imprinted sea lion pups are poor release candidates, and tend to seek out human companionship after returning to the wild. Imprinted fur seal pups may have a greater chance of reverting to a suitable wild disposition.

SOURCES OF PRODUCTS MENTIONED

Equi-Aid Products, Inc., Phoenix, AZ 85027

Gerber Products Company, c/o Consumer Affairs, 445 State Street Fremont, Michigan 49413-0001; www.gerber.com; 1-800-443 7237

Jeffers Livestock, www.jefferslivestock.com; 1-800-533-3377

Kalajian Company, Long Beach, CA; 1-562-424-9749

Mazuri:1-800-227-8941; mazuri@purina-mills.com

Osborne Industries, 120 N. Industrial Avenue, Osborne, KS 67473; 1-800-255-0316

PetAg Inc., 261 Keyes Ave., Hampshire, IL 60140; 1-800-323-0877, 1-800-323-6878; www.petag.com

Procter and Gamble: www.metamucil.com; 1-800-686-7139

Ross Products Division, Abbott Laboratories, Columbus, OH 43215-1724; www.abbott.com

Ryan Herco, 1819 Junction Ave., San Jose, CA 95131-2101; 1-800-848-1411

REFERENCES

Gage, L. J., K. Beckmen, D. Wickham, and D. M. Smith. 1996. Transfusion of a Guadalupe fur seal (*Artocephalus townsendi*) with California sea lion (*Zalophus californianus*) blood. *Proceedings IAAAM 1996 Conference.*

Gage, Laurie J. 1990. Hand rearing pinniped pups. In *Handbook of marine mammal medicine*, edited by Leslie Dierauf. Boca Raton: CRC Press.

———. 1993. Hand rearing pinnipeds. In *Zoo and wild animal medicine*, edited by Murray E. Fowler. Philadelphia, PA: Saunders.

Gulland, F., M. Haulena, and L. Dierauf. 2001. Seals and sea lions. In *Handbook of marine mammal medicine*, edited by Leslie Dierauf and Frances Gulland. Boca Raton: CRC Press.

21
Walrus Calves

Laurie J. Gage and Terry S. Samansky

NATURAL HISTORY

There are two subspecies of walrus: the Pacific walrus (*Odobenus rosmarus divergens*), and the Atlantic walrus (*Odobenus rosmarus rosmarus*). The average birth weight of walrus calves is 45–80 kg (99–176 lb). Births are seasonal, from mid-April to mid-June, but occur primarily in May. In the wild, calves may nurse for as long as two years; some may nurse longer if the cow does not give birth to a new calf (Fay 1982).

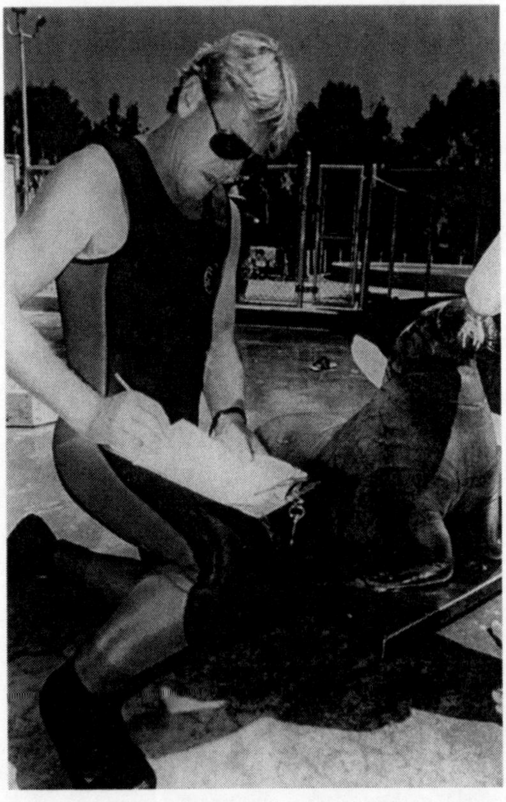

RECORD KEEPING

Keep a daily log of food intake, fecal production, consistency, and appearance, body weight, and behavioral notes including activity, attitude, and appetite. Keep careful records on formula adjustments (Fig. 21.1).

EQUIPMENT

The following items should be available:

Blender: Heavy duty commercial blender (i.e., Waring Commercial One Gallon Blender)
Large calf bottles and a variety of calf and lamb nipples
Microwave or other method of heating formula
Large diameter vinyl stomach tube (1.9 cm OD)
60-cc or 140-cc syringes

CRITERIA FOR INTERVENTION

Wild walrus pups may be abandoned or orphaned. Captive walrus calves that are rejected by the cow, or are unable to nurse either due to poor milk production in the cow or because the calf is weak, by necessity will need to be hand reared.

FORMULAS

Walrus calves have been successfully raised on a variety of formulas. The formula should be similar to mother's milk by being high in fat, have moderate amounts of protein, and have trace amounts of carbohydrates.

The easiest formulas to use are commercially available powdered formulations. PetAg's Multi-

Figure 21.1. Charting the weight of a walrus calf.

Milk or Zoologic Milk Matrix 30/55 (PetAg) have been used successfully by these authors. Another formula made from readily available ingredients is the Walrus Formula in Table 21.1.

When using a powered formula, ensure that the consistency of the formula is maintained for every new batch. A rule of thumb for making the formula is to mix by volume, 2 parts powdered Milk Matrix 30/55 to 5 parts water initially. After one month of age, if this mixture agrees with the calf, and no diarrhea or constipation is noted, the strength of the formula may be increased gradually to 1 part powder to 2 parts water; which will increase the caloric value (kcal/liter) by about 50%. The consistency of the formula will vary from batch to batch of powdered product. Pay attention to the thickness of the formula when preparing it, and be careful when making formula from a new batch of powder. Adjustments of the powder-to-water ratio may need to be made. If the weight gain of the calf dips or levels out, the ratio may be again increased gradually to 1.25 parts powder to 2 parts water.

Making the formula too thin will result in poor weight gain. Making the formula too rich results in gastrointestinal problems such as diarrhea, vomiting, constipation, or inappetence. The following tips will aid in use of formula:

- Powdered commercial formulas must not be overblended. When blending, several bursts of four to six seconds of blender mixing at the high setting are usually sufficient. Overblending adds too much air to the formula and may cause the pup to have indigestion.
- Temperature of the formula is very important and calves may be particular about accepting formula that is consistently the right temperature. This varies between individuals and requires some experimentation to find the most ideal formula temperature for each individual. In our experience, the preferred formula temperature ranges between 95 and 102°F (35 and 39°C).
- Formula should always be temperature tested by placing a few drops on the inside of your wrist.

Table 21.1. Walrus Formula Ingredients

Clams	1 kg
Herring	1 kg
Safflower oil	100 ml
Cod liver oil	10 ml
Isomil	150 ml
Marine mammal vitamin	1 tablet
Dicalcium phosphate	250 mg
Vitamin B_{12}	125 mcg
Vitamin C	250 mg
NaCl	5 g
Nutrical	20 ml
Lecithin	10 ml
Yogurt	200 ml
Bottled water	500 ml
Bottled water	1200 ml
Whipping cream	300 ml

Instructions for Preparation

Weigh out clams and place in a heavy-duty commercial blender. Weigh herring, remove loose scales, and place in blender. Add all vitamins, dicalcium phosphate, NaCl into a mortar and grind to a powder. Place in blender. Measure safflower oil into a beaker and add Nutrical to the beaker until 40 ml of liquid has been displaced (Example: 100 ml of oil will read 140 ml after 40 ml of Nutrical has been added). Add cod liver oil, Isomil, and lecithin. Put mixture into blender. Add 500 ml water and mix in blender on high for 30 to 45 seconds. Add remaining 1200 cc water. Mix 10 seconds. Add the whipping cream and mix for exactly 3 seconds; no more. Label and date the container. Refrigerate formula, and discard unused formula after 24 hours.

Formula should be warm but never hot. Overheating the formula in the microwave may cause the consistency to change and may result in digestive problems.
- Bottles must be thoroughly mixed after heating in the microwave to ensure there are no hot spots within the bottle. This is done by securing the nipple on the bottle and shaking vigorously.
- Formula may be reheated in the bottle up to three times in a 30-minute period, but then should be discarded. Formula that was heated and not consumed during a feed should be discarded. Formula that is over 24 hours old should be discarded.
- Crushed, powdered, or liquid vitamins are added to the bottles and mixed thoroughly after they are heated.
- Care should be taken to maintain a steady and controlled weight gain. Artificial formulas too high in fat and too low in calcium have been associated with seizures, weak bones, and fractures (Walsh 1990).
- Clams and fish must be pureed before adding to the formula. It is highly recommended that an industrial blender be used for this reason.

At 10 weeks of age, add 115 g ground clams to each liter of formula. At 16 weeks of age, increase the clams to 230 g/liter of formula. At five months of age, add 70 g ground herring per liter to the formula.

SUPPLEMENTS

Supplements change and are increased as the animals grow. The following protocol is based on our experience raising four healthy walruses at our facility.

- Give initial daily supplements of one multiple marine mammal vitamin (Vita-Zu Marine Mammal tablets; Mazuri), 1 g thiamin, 800 IU vitamin E, 600 mg dicalcium phosphate, and 250 mg taurine.
- At 2 weeks of age, increase the calcium supplement to 500 mg dicalcium phosphate twice a day.
- At 3 weeks of age, increase taurine to 250 mg BID. Add 2 ml cod liver oil to each liter of formula. Increase this amount gradually over the next week to a total of 8.7 ml cod liver oil per liter of formula. This will increase the caloric value of the formula.
- At 6 weeks of age, increase the dicalcium phosphate to 1000 mg BID, and gradually increase the cod liver oil to 13 ml/liter of formula fed.
- At 8 weeks of age, add one additional marine mammal vitamin daily.
- At 10 weeks of age, gradually bring the cod liver oil to 17 ml/liter of formula.
- At 14 weeks of age, increase the cod liver oil to 22 ml/liter.
- At 4.5 months of age, increase the marine mammal vitamins from two to three per day, and decrease the thiamin from 1 g to 500 mg/day.
- At 9 months of age, when the animal is beginning to eat clams consistently, eliminate the taurine from the formula.

WHAT TO FEED INITIALLY

Start newborns initially on 50:50 bottled water:Pedialyte (Ross) or any balanced electrolyte solution such as lactated Ringer's solution. Give 20 to 40 ml/kg per day divided into four to five feeds initially. This will likely need to be given via gavage (tube fed). Calves should be well hydrated before starting them on formula. Dehydrated calves should receive up to 80 ml/kg per day of electrolyte solution by a combination of oral and subcutaneous administration. When introducing the formula, start with it diluted—10% formula: 90% electrolyte solution. Gradually increase the strength of the formula over the next 48 hours. At that point we used a ratio of one part MultiMilk to two parts water (PetAg). PetAg has replaced MultiMilk with Milk Matrix 30/55, which has a higher caloric density. Based on that change, we recommend starting with a 2:5 ratio of Milk Matrix 30/55 powder to water. All ratios mentioned in this chapter are by volume. These ratios are only guidelines. If using the Milk Matrix product, be sure to check with PetAg for any recent formulation changes.

NURSING TECHNIQUES

Walrus calves often will not accept the bottle and formula at first and must be tube fed. Healthy neonates usually display a very strong suckle reflex and will try to nurse on fingers, elbows, and other available objects, however, they often reject an artificial nipple and bottle when first offered. Have a variety of types, shapes, and sizes of human and animal baby bottles and nipples available, as individual calves will have different preferences. It helps to boil the nipples or wash them thoroughly in hot soapy water, rinsing well to remove any latex or rubber flavor. We found the calves that we raised would accept warm water from the bottle before accepting the formula. This may be due to the difference in taste, temperature, and/or consistency of the formula versus mother's milk. Once the calves were comfortable with the equipment and consistently taking water from a bottle, we added a small amount of dilute premade formula to the water to allow the calf to get used to the taste and consistency. Slowly the concentration of formula was increased until the calf was readily accepting the formula at full strength. Temperature of the formula seems to be critical to each individual, and most calves seem to prefer the temperature to be between 95 and 102°F (35 and 39°C). The calves we reared ultimately accepted the large calves' nipples attached to one-liter plastic calf bottles (see Fig. 21.2). Some calves may prefer the smaller lamb's nipple attached to the larger bottle. These are available from most feed stores or from Jeffers Livestock. It may take several days to a week or longer for pups to accept the bottle and nurse consistently. Therefore, newborns may need to be fed via gavage three to four times each day for several days to a week or longer.

TUBE FEEDING

Vinyl tubing with an outside diameter (OD) of 0.75 in (1.9 cm) (Ryan Herco) may be used. Plastic tubing is not recommended because it gets very hard after repeated boiling and may irritate the esophagus. Equine stomach tubes may also be used (Kalajian).

Be careful when passing the stomach tube. We found it is very easy to accidentally pass the tube into the trachea. Formula or fluids delivered through the trachea into the lungs would probably result in death. To avoid this, follow these guidelines:

- It will take one person, possibly two, just to restrain the calf.
- Lay the tube out alongside the calf to the area of the stomach, just past the last rib, and mark the tube with an indelible marker at the tip of the snout to indicate how far to pass the tube.
- Gently open the calf's mouth and insert the tube to the back of the throat. Push gently until the calf swallows the tube. You will probably not be able to feel the tip of the tube advancing down the esophagus on the left side of the neck as you pass it. You may need to use your hands and fingers to depress the calf's tongue so that the tube can enter the esophagus.
- When the tube is passed correctly down the esophagus, you may hear the crackling sound of stomach gasses or see stomach contents reflux back up into the tube.
- If the tube passage stops short, and does not pass easily to the indelible mark, you may have passed it into the lungs. For this reason, never force the tube; when it is in the esophagus, it should always pass smoothly to the stomach.
- Listen for sounds of breathing through the tube. Often, but not always, when the tube is in the

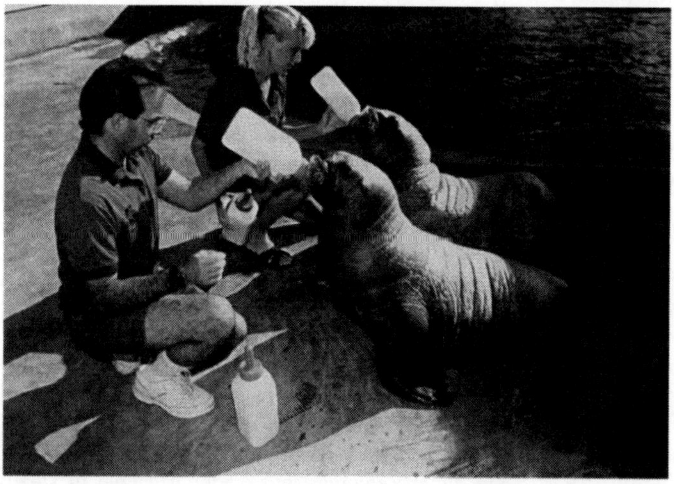

Figure 21.2. Bottle-feeding walrus calves (photo by Charlotte Fiorito, courtesy of Six Flags Marine World).

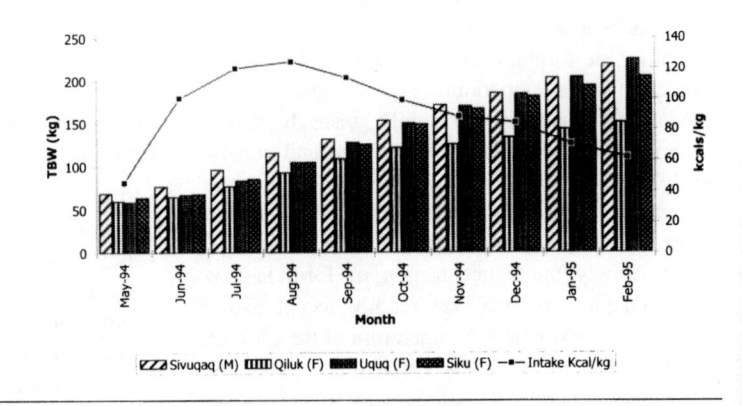

Figure 21.3. Pacific walrus calves at Marine World Africa USA; Average total body weights and daily caloric intake.

trachea, breathing sounds may be heard through it. If you suspect the tube is in the trachea, remove it and restart the tubing process.
- When the tube placement is in doubt, blow a puff of air into the tube while someone else is listening to the stomach area with a stethoscope. This produces gurgling sounds, which will be heard when the tube is in the stomach. This is not recommended to perform frequently, as it introduces gas into the stomach and may cause discomfort.
- If you have never passed a stomach tube, ask for help from a veterinarian or experienced rehabilitator.

Formula may be delivered by gravity using a funnel, or by using catheter-tip 60-cc or 140-cc syringes. Gravity feeds are preferred. If the syringe is used, the formula must be delivered slowly, allowing about 20 seconds for each 60 ml delivered.

FREQUENCY OF FEEDING

Newborns up to one month of age should be fed every four hours from 8 A.M. until midnight (five times per day). If they are doing well, gaining weight, and have normal feces, the midnight feed may be discontinued at four to five weeks of age, and the extra volume divided into the remaining four feeds.

AMOUNTS TO FEED

In general, calves may be fed 30 to 40 ml per kg per day (13 to 18 ml per lb), divided into five feeds (6 to 8 ml per kg per feed) until two weeks of age. The amounts may then gradually be raised to 40 to 50 ml per kg per day for the next month. The goal is to achieve steady and controlled growth and weight gain. During the first six months of life the formula's average caloric value should be about 100 kcal/kg body weight/day. While the total amount of food and calories consumed will increase steadily, the ratio of calories consumed compared to total body weight (kcal/kg body weight/day) will probably rise for a few months and then gradually decrease as the calves grow and mature (see Fig. 21.3). The concentration of the formula may gradually be increased to increase the caloric density of the diet. At one month of age, the concentration may be increased gradually over several days from a ratio of two parts (by volume) Milk Matrix 30/55 powder to five parts water; to a concentration of one part Milk Matrix 30/55 powder to two parts water. If at any time during the feeding process the calf regurgitates or has abnormal feces, the amounts per feed or the concentration of the formula must be reduced. Also note the consistency of the formula with each new batch of powdered product. Occasionally the formula will be much thicker or thinner when made with a new batch of powdered diet, and must be adjusted accordingly.

CALORIC VALUE DETERMINATIONS

It is important to know the amount of fat, protein, and carbohydrate present and the total caloric value of any formula fed. Daily caloric intake, along with daily body weights, appetite, activity level, and fecal appearance are important factors in determining dietary changes and reaching a goal of steady and controlled growth and weight gain. Each formula component and food item should be analyzed for fat, protein, and carbohydrate composition utilizing the product labels, supplier's laboratory analysis, or literature search. Approximate caloric values may be determined by multiplying each macronutrient by its average energy coefficient: fat = 9 kcal/g, protein and carbohydrates = 4 kcal/g. The caloric density of the formula is adjusted primarily by varying the ratios of the Milk Matrix to water. Volume and caloric density of the formula are increased gradually to allow the calves sufficient time to adjust to each successive change.

Here are some examples of caloric values of formula ingredients:

Milk matrix 30/55 2:5 ratio: Fat = 6.8%, Protein = 3.8% (percentages taken from the label)
Calculation of calories: 1 liter = 1043 g (by weight)
Note: One liter of water weighs 1000 g, once the powdered formula is added, one liter of formula weighs approximately 1043 g.

Fat = 6.8% (0.068) × 1043 g = 70.9 g × 9 kcal/g = 638.3 kcal
Protein = 3.8% (0.038) × 1043 g = 39.6 g × 4 kcal/g = 158.5 kcal
Total caloric value = 638.3 + 158.5 = 796.8 kcal/liter.

We contacted PetAg and were able to obtain the protein, fat, and carbohydrate values for a 1:2 ratio of Milk Matrix 30/55. One part powder to two parts water had nutritional values of 18.2% solids, 6.06% protein, 10.33% fat, and 0.64% carbohydrates with a total caloric value of 1217.2 kcal per liter.

When Milk Matrix is mixed in a 3:4 ratio (1.5 parts powder to 2 parts water), it yields 1373.7 kcal per liter.

The caloric value of 1 ml of cod liver oil is 7.83 kcal. One gram of clams contains approximately 0.6 kcal.

Figure 21.3 illustrates the average total body weights and average daily caloric intake of four orphaned Pacific walrus calves successfully hand raised at Marine World Africa USA from May 1994 through February 1995. During this period the approximate caloric value of the formula varied between 921 and 1370 kcal/liter and fat content ranged between 7.9% and 11.9%. Total protein rose from 4.3% to 8.2%. At their peak, the calves were gaining approximately 0.5–0.7 kg (1.1–1.5 lb) of total body weight (TBW) per day and were consuming about 125 kcal/kg (TBW) per day. Note that the ratio of calories consumed versus total body weight (kcal/kg TBW) decreased substantially after the fourth month while total body weights continued to rise at desirable rates. Solid food (clams, squid, white bait, and herring) was first introduced at 8 months and within several days became an increasingly important source of nutrition. The introduction of solid food raised the total volume of food fed, while lowering the ratio of fat to protein (thus lowering the ratio of kcal/kg body weight). At 10 months of age, the calves were consuming between 5 and 6 liters of formula and 2.5 to 6.5 kg of solid food per day. The weaning process extended over a period of about 10 months and was not completed until the calves were approximately 18 months of age.

EXPECTED WEIGHT GAIN

Calves may lose 1–5 kg in the first 7–10 days during the transition to bottle-feeding but should gain weight steadily once they are consistently nursing. Expect calves to gain 0.5 to 0.7 kg (1–1.5 lb) per day. Calves should be weighed daily. It is common for calves to gain weight steadily for a few days in a row and then have a day or two per week with no significant weight gains. If the weight plateaus for several days or begins to drop it is a good indicator that it is time to increase the total caloric intake by increasing the volume of formula, the concentration of formula, or both. Calves should increase their body weight by about 300% in the first ten months (see Fig. 21.3).

HOUSING

Initially, walrus calves should be housed only with their own mothers or other calves. Walruses are easily startled and large adult animals may accidentally injure young ones as they rush to escape a perceived danger. Design of a walrus facility is an important part of maintaining the health of the animals. Holding facilities must be strong, secure, and easy to clean. Plenty of haul-out space should be provided to allow the mother the ability to move about freely without crowding the calf. The facility should provide a saltwater pool to allow the animals the opportunity to bath and cool off. Pools should be designed with steps and/or gradually sloping sides to allow the calf the ability to easily exit the pool if the water level fluctuates to any depth. Some institutions have constructed special birthing areas with shallow (6-in deep) "splash pools" as an added precaution to prevent accidental drownings. Mother and calf remain in this area until it is determined that the new mother is relaxed and the calf is strong enough to swim and get out of a deeper pool on its own.

Walruses are highly prone to mouth and swallow any small loose objects that they can find. They are also notorious for their ability to tirelessly investigate their exhibits and find, break, and swallow any weak or flawed structural components. Special care must be taken to ensure that all fixtures, equipment, fasteners, facades, and rock-work are "walrus proof." Regular inspections of the facilities and inventories of all toys and equipment should be made to ensure that no items are missing and perhaps swallowed. Underwater viewing windows should have a barrier covering all window seals, as walruses may ingest the sealant material. Exhibits should be designed so the public is not able to drop or throw any objects into the pool.

IMMUNE STATUS AND SPECIAL NEEDS

Newborn pups that have not nursed may have decreased immunoglobulins and must be handled with care. Cleanliness is a must and all bottles, nipples, or stomach tubes should be thoroughly washed in hot soapy water, using a bottle brush each time to scrub the inside of the bottle. Stomach tubes should be soaked in disinfectant or boiled between each feeding. Rinse thoroughly before the next use. Use boiled, filtered, or bottled water for hydration or making the formula.

Frequent water changes or a quality filtration system for saltwater pools is necessary, and haul-out areas or dry enclosures should be cleaned frequently and disinfected daily.

WEANING FROM FORMULA TO SOLID FOOD

Solid food such as clams, herring, white bait, and squid are introduced at six to eight months of age. At ten months of age walrus calves will consume 5 to 6 liters of formula and 2.5 to 6.5 kg of solid food per day. Even though the calves are eating well, bottles of formula are offered for several more months. The weaning process is gradual, and the animals are not completely weaned off of the bottles until they are about 18 months of age. From a medical standpoint, it is beneficial to continue the bottles intermittently for some time after that, as it is an easy method to rehydrate and/or give animals oral medication. For this purpose water is well accepted and may be substituted for the formula.

COMMON MEDICAL PROBLEMS

Gastrointestinal problems such as diarrhea or constipation are generally associated with improper feeding techniques or changes in the formula. Inappetence may be an indicator of the gastrointestinal problems relating to the formula, but may also be a sign of another illness. Cultures of feces should be submitted to the laboratory. Taking blood once in the first week with a follow-up at one month of age is recommended. Blood samples may be obtained from the epidural intravertebral sinus.

Salmonellosis has been reported in walrus calves. Clinical signs include acute onset of partial to complete anorexia, diarrhea, regurgitation, lethargy, and weight loss (Calle 1995).

Foreign body impactions are common and a serious concern. Walrus calves explore and orally manipulate everything in their environment. Caution should be taken when designing a walrus facility to ensure the public is not able to drop or throw anything into the enclosure. Exhibits should be designed so there is no public contact with the young animals. Some facilities may require netting over the entire exhibit, or an attendant present whenever the public is present. Exhibits with underwater viewing should be designed with protective barriers around the windows so the walruses cannot access and suck out the underwater window sealant material.

As young walruses mature and begin to grow tusks, some may develop a habit of rubbing their tusks on hard surfaces. If this behavior continues the animal may develop an ascending infection into the sinus, requiring the surgical removal of both tusks. Because walrus calves like to manipulate objects with their mouths, offering safe swallow-proof toys, blocks of ice, and other enrichment items may avert the negative behavior of wearing down their tusks (Fig. 21.4).

Walrus calves should be housed in salt water. Calves housed in fresh water have an absolute requirement for sodium, which should be included at a level of 2 g NaCl/liter in their daily formula. Clinical signs of hyponatremia are vague neurologic signs, primarily muscle fasciculation or seizures. Administering 3% sodium chloride intravenously may reverse this condition.

SOURCES OF PRODUCTS MENTIONED

Jeffers Livestock: www.jefferslivestock.com; 1-800-533-3377

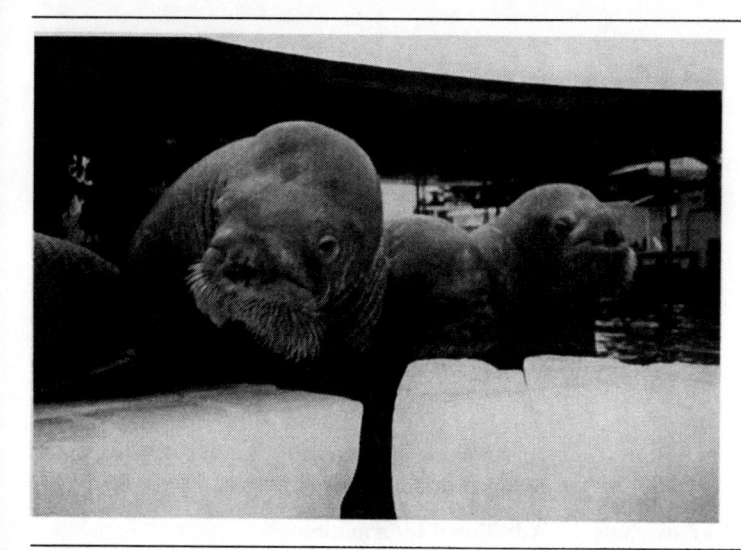

Figure 21.4. Walrus calves playing with blocks of ice.

Kalajian Company, Long Beach, CA; 1-562-424-9749

Mazuri, 1050 Progress Dr., Richmond, IN 47374; 1-800-227-8941; Mazuri.com

PetAg Inc., 261 Keyes Ave., Hampshire, IL 60140; 1-800-323-0877, 1-800-323-6878; www.petag.com

Products Division, Abbott Laboratories, Columbus, OH 43215-1724; www.abbott.com

Ryan Herco, 1819 Junction Ave., San Jose, CA 95131-2101; 1-800-848-1411

Waring Products Division, Dynamics Corporation of America, New Hartford, CT 06057

ACKNOWLEDGMENTS

We wish to acknowledge the marine mammal trainers and veterinary staff of Six Flags Marine World (formerly Marine World Africa USA) for their help raising these animals. Special thanks to Scott Rutherford, Joanne Chappel, Sonny Allen, Patrick Turley, Sue Negrini, and Kimberlee Beckmen.

REFERENCES

Calle, P. 1995. Enteric salmonellosis of captive Pacific walrus (Odobenus rosmarus divergens). In *Proceedings of the 26th International Association for Aquatic Animal Medicine*, Mystic, CT. IAAAM.

Fay, F. H. 1982. Ecology and biology of the Pacific walrus *Odobenus rosmarus divergens*. *North American Fauna* 74:1.

Samansky, T., S. Rutherford, et al. 1995. Hand raising orphaned walrus calves at Marine World Africa USA—the first year. In *Proceedings of the 26th International Association for Aquatic Animal Medicine*, Mystic, CT. IAAAM.

Walsh, Michael T., Eddard D. Asper, B. Andrews, and J. Antrim. 1990. Walrus biology and medicine. In *Handbook of marine mammal medicine*, edited by Leslie A. Dierauf. Boca Raton: CRC Press.

22
Fox Kits

Jennifer Convy, Darlene DeGhetto, and Sophia Papageorgiou

NATURAL HISTORY: RED FOX

The red fox is of the order Carnivora, family Canidae, genus *Vulpes,* and species *vulpes.* Its status is nonnative to the United States.

Description/ID

The haircoat color of the fox is usually a deep reddish-brown but a red fox can also be grayish, tannish-yellow, pale yellowish-red and black. They have black feet and legs, large, pointed ears, elongated sharp muzzles, and rounded bushy tails with a white tail tip. The pupils of the eyes are elliptical and they have a musky odor from their scent glands. Length of the head and body range from 15 to 34 inches (38 to 86 cm) and tail length is 9–22 inches (23–56 cm) (Macdonald 1995; Nowak 1991).

Reproduction

These small wild canids breed from January through February. Females sexually mature at ten months. Some foxes mate for life. Gestation is 49–56 days after which time one litter of four to five young is born (Macdonald 1995; Nowak 1991).

Habitat and Activity Period

They are primarily nocturnal or crepuscular and prefer mixed woodlands and farm lots or inhabit meadows and fields. They den in sides of hills during breeding season to rear kits (Macdonald 1995; Nowak 1991).

Natural Diet and Foraging Techniques

Foxes are omnivorous and, as opportunistic hunters, feed on small mammals, birds, eggs, fruits, reptiles, fish, insects, and carrion. Food caches for future consumption are secured by burying them in leaves or dirt (Macdonald 1995; Nowak 1991).

Additional Information

The tail is used as a blanket in colder climates protecting the nose and feet from frostbite. In very cold climates, reconsider releasing a red fox with an amputated or very short tail. Female foxes are called vixens (Macdonald 1995; Nowak 1991).

Behavior Characteristics–Wild and Captive

Foxes have a keen sense of sight, smell, and sound. They vocalize often in the wild and kits vocalize in captivity. They growl and scream sometimes when handled. Foxes walk on their toes digitigrade, do not hibernate, and are very quick and cunning. Because of their proficiency at digging, an escape-proof enclosure is a necessity.

Adults weigh 6 to 15 pounds (2.7 to 6.8 kg) (Macdonald 1995; Nowak 1991).

NATURAL HISTORY: GRAY FOX

The gray fox *(Urocyon cinereoargenteus* and *U. littoralis)* is also classified in some texts as genus *Vulpes* with species name *vulpes cinereoargenteus.* Its order is Carnivora, family Canidae, genus *Vulpes* or *Urocyon,* and species *cinereoargenteus* and *littoralis.* Its status is native to the United States.

Description/ID

Gray foxes have a gray head, tail, and body. They have white areas inside their legs and at their throat and ventral abdomen. The back and tail tip have black accents and they also have some rust at their neck and lower flanks. The gray fox has a head to body length of 19–26 inches (48–66 cm) and a tail length of 10–17 inches (25–43 cm) (Nowak 1991).

Reproduction

Gray foxes mate from December to March in the western United States and from January to May in the Northeast. Gestation is generally nine weeks (61–63 days). Vixens have one litter per year and usually give birth to four young, but litter size varies from one to ten young. Foxes tend to be monogamous and the young stay with their parents for their first year (Macdonald 1995).

Habitat and Activity Period

These animals are found in "wooded and brushy country." They often den in crevices and trees. They are primarily nocturnal or crepuscular and prefer mixed woodlands and farm lots or inhabit meadows and fields. They den in sides of hills during breeding season to rear kits (Macdonald 1995; Nowak 1991).

Natural Diet and Foraging Techniques

Foxes are omnivorous and, as opportunistic hunters, feed on small mammals, birds, eggs, fruits, reptiles, fish, insects, and carrion. Food caches for future consumption are secured by burying them in leaves or dirt (Macdonald 1995; Nowak 1991).

Additional Information

Gray foxes are excellent tree climbers. The species *U. littoralis* is considered rare by the California Department of Fish and Game and thus is fully protected (Macdonald 1995).

Behavior Characteristics–Wild and Captive

Foxes have keen senses of sight, smell, and hearing. They vocalize often in the wild and kits vocalize in captivity. They growl and scream sometimes when handled. Foxes walk on their toes digitigrade, do not hibernate, and are very quick and cunning. Because of their proficiency at digging, an escape-proof enclosure is a necessity.

RECORD KEEPING

Detailed records must be maintained as in all captive animal situations. Ensure accurate daily recording of attitude, weight, temperature, heart and respiratory rate (if possible), food fed (measured), and amount eaten (measured). Any procedures, physical examinations, medications provided, or other information must be written in the animal's individual record file. Case number/tag numbers should be placed on all sheets of the animal's permanent record for identification purposes.

Age Determination

The following guidelines can be used to determine age (Convy 2001; Hanes 1991):

Newborn: Weighs 100 g, blind, deaf, 10 cm long, covered with short black fur and look very unfoxlike, with blunt noses and sealed ears. They are unable to control body temperature.

11–14 days: Eyes open and are milky-blue in color; sight poor; begin to move around.

4 weeks of age: Emerge from den with fur colored rich chocolate brown, beginning to molt their juvenile pelage.

5–6 weeks: Weighs 600–700 g; molt complete; fur is short and completely reddish–orange in color.

8–10 weeks old: Completely weaned; snout and ears become long and pointed; learning to hunt with parents.

6 months: Weighs 3.5 or more kg; ready for complete independence from parents.

INITIAL CARE AND STABILIZING

Perform a complete physical examination either by manual restraint or with sedation. The animal should only be immobilized if it is in stable condition and only if necessary to perform a physical examination or do a diagnostic workup (blood panel, radiographs, etc.).

Blood (CBC and chemistry panel) and a fecal sample should be submitted for analysis. The veterinarian should be present or called in if necessary depending on the condition of the animal. Check the packed cell volume (PCV), total solids (TS), and blood glucose (BG) in order to initiate treatment for any immediate problem. If the BG is low, less than 60 g/dl, give subcutaneous or intravenous fluids (lactated Ringer's solution [LRS] or Normosol-R with a 2-1/2% dextrose solution SQ or higher percentage dextrose if given IV). Prepare blood slide smears for review by the veterinarian. Be sure to make at least two slides if possible. Prepare equipment for IV catheter placement, fluid therapy, skin scrape, and possibly X rays. Be sure to provide the animal with an external heat source for warmth, fluids, and appropriate medications based on physical examination findings.

Once the initial exam has been performed, formulate a treatment plan for any problems the animal may have. Remember, these animals are not domesticated puppies, but most of their medical problems may be treated similarly to those of domestic canine puppies. If you do not have access to a veterinarian with wildlife experience, a small-animal practitioner should be quite helpful in caring for these species. Keep in mind these are still wild animals and must function in a harsh, unforgiving environment in nature. If they have fractures, they must heal well enough that they can catch prey items for food and protect themselves as necessary. The fox must be able to leap and pounce in order to catch prey.

RESTRAINT AND HANDLING

Several things should be kept in mind when restraining and handling fox kits (Convy 2001).

Always wear gloves when handling any carnivores as a precaution against *Baylisascaris* sp. parasite worm, ringworm, and other diseases.

Young kits under 2 lb (1 kg) (fewer than eight weeks old) may be handled by wearing latex gloves with work gloves over the latex gloves. Use a thick towel or blanket to trap and catch the kit. Wrap it entirely (like a burrito) with its head visible. Depending on the procedure/plan for the animal, you may not need to anesthetize it. If you are planning a long procedure or the animal is extremely difficult to restrain, use Isoflurane inhalant anesthesia with oxygen (O_2) via a face mask. Remember that these animals are very young and you should give them fluids (LRS or Normosol-R with 2 1/2% dextrose subcutaneously) before you wake them up from the sedation or anesthesia. For longer procedures, an intravenous catheter should be placed in a cephalic (foreleg) vein to facilitate fluid-therapy support.

When the animals are less than 4 lb (2 kg), they may be caught via manual restraint and bundled in a large towel while wearing thick work gloves. At this point sedate using either Isoflurane inhalant gas anesthesia using a facemask, with or without endotracheal intubation, or injectable Telazol at approximately 1 mg/kg delivered intramuscularly. These animals should be restrained/handled with a veterinarian performing the immobilization or supervising a trained staff member during the procedure. Immobilizations without a veterinarian present should only be undertaken only in an emergency situation.

With smaller animals weighing 3–4 lb (1.4–2 kg), the sedatives may be delivered via a hand injection. Once the foxes increase in size, the drugs are delivered (1) by cornering and restraining the animal with a rabies catch pole or a net and injecting them (as outlined above), (2) by trapping them in a crate and injecting, or (3) via pole dart or dart gun. Once immobilized the animal should be supported with O_2 or a gas inhalant agent combined with O_2 via facemask or endotracheal tube. Intubation and anesthetic support will depend on the procedure(s) being performed and length of time necessary for the animal to be immobilized (Convy 2001).

FORMULAS: REHABILITATION DIET

We have had good results with the following rehabilitation diets (Convy 2001).

Infant Formula: Use dilute Esbilac (PetAg), which may be purchased from feed stores, high-end pet food stores, many veterinary hospitals, or emergency clinics.

Mix one part Esbilac and two parts water. Gradually increase the strength of the formula by thirds from the rehydrating solution (Pedialyte or LRS) to formula until they are three to four weeks old.

Start with rehydrating solution orally—LRS or Pedialyte (Ross).

Day 1: full rehydrating solution
Day 2: 2/3 rehydrating solution, 1/3 formula
Day 3: 1/3 rehydrating solution, 2/3 formula
Day 4: 100% formula (1 part Esbilac : 2 parts water).

FORMULAS: WEANING DIET

At three weeks, follow the weaning diet: Add soaked high-quality puppy chow to dish of formula (see above) for four to eight weeks. Once they are eating the dish formula, decrease the amount of formula until only soaked puppy chow remains. Then add some hard puppy chow along with fruits, feline diet, and any small dead prey animals except opossum. Add miscellaneous items sparingly to decrease chances of diarrhea. As soon as the pup is four to six weeks old, introduce small live prey such as mice.

NURSING TECHNIQUE

Feed via a baby bottle with a premature-sized human baby nipple with the kit in a sternal position (Convy 2001). The kits will lap food/formula from a dish as soon as their eyes open although you may have to point them in the right direction. After each feeding, stimulate kits to defecate/urinate by gently rubbing their anal area with a warm water-soaked towel during the time their eyes are still closed. This may be discontinued once they start to urinate and defecate on their own. Minimize human contact as they are easily humanized. Once they can be moved to an outside cage, place food into the enclosure with limited human contact by using visual blinds or guillotine doors, a self-feeder for puppy food, and PVC pipes for dead or live prey to decrease human contact. No one should talk within hearing distance of the animals during the time the animals are being rehabilitated (Convy 2001).

TUBE FEEDING

This procedure should be reserved for debilitated animals that are not eating (Convy 2001). Although not an ideal or safe situation, tube feeding may be the only solution to providing nutrition to orphans and have them strong enough to begin suckling/feeding on their own.

Equipment

The following items should be available for tube feeding:

Red rubber catheter (Kendall Sovereign Feeding Tube and Urethral Catheter)
Lubricant (KY Jelly)
Light source (flashlight or ophthalmoscope)
Syringe (3, 6, or 12 ml)
Joint to attach the syringe to the red rubber catheter (Christmas Tree Connector or Barbed Connector: Barbed Connector is distributed by Jorgenson Laboratories).
Formula as described above

Tube feeding requires one to two people, one to restrain the fox and one to pass the red rubber catheter and gently deliver the formula into the catheter. Make the length of the catheter (feeding tube) equal to the distance from the tip of the nose to the last rib. Mark this length on the tube with an indelible marker. This is how far the tube will need to be passed to reach the stomach. The catheter should pass easily into the stomach. If the tube stops short of the mark you made, do not force it; it could be down the trachea. Use the light source to double check and visualize the glottis/trachea. Another method to check that the tube is in the stomach, and not the trachea, is to palpate the neck. You should feel two firm, tubular structures, one is the trachea and the other is the tube within the esophagus. If you do not palpate two tubes or cannot visualize the glottis, then remove the feeding tube, visualize the trachea, and reinsert the tube. Be sure to once again check that the red rubber catheter is properly placed. Once the formula has been delivered, kink the tube and gently remove it.

Be very careful to check that the tube has been passed into the stomach and not the trachea (leading to the lungs). If tubed improperly (into the trachea), the animal will die very quickly as a result of having its lungs flooded with fluid causing drowning. Only trained personnel should do this procedure.

See Table 22.1 for a red and gray fox feeding guide.

HOUSING

These guidelines will help you to create optimal housing for your animals (Convy 2001). Whenever possible, house kits with conspecifics (other members of the same species).

Housing by Age and Development Stage

Newborn: Place in neonatal incubator if they are hypothermic, otherwise house in a small airline kennel lined with newspaper and towels, at 85°F (29.4 °C), with 60–70% humidity. When the kits are very small, place them in a towel-lined cardboard box inside of the kennel. Kits will cry when orphaned at a very young age and just need to be ignored. Place a stuffed animal in with them for comfort. Place a heating pad (a recirculating hot-water blanket is best) with a towel between the heating pad or blanket and the kennel. Keep the heating pad on the lowest setting with only half of the kennel over the heating pad. This allows the animal to move away from the heat source if it gets too warm in one spot. When their eyes are still closed do not give them any water in the enclosure. House kit(s) in an isolated area for decreased human contact.

Age 14+ days: Once kit(s) can walk fairly well, remove the heating pad and house them in a medium-sized airline kennel.

Age 3–4 weeks: Move kits into an enclosed outdoor exhibit with a large airline kennel or a large enclosed tub.

Table 22.1. Red /Gray Fox Feeding Guide

Weight (grams)	Amount per feed (cc)	Number of feedings per day
100	5.0	8 (night feeds)
150	7.5	7 (night feeds)
200	10.0	7 (night feeds)
250	12.5	6
300	15.0	6
350	17.5	6
400	20.0	6
450	22.5	5
500	25.0	5
550	27.5	5
600	30.0	5
650	32.5	5
700	35.0	5
750	37.5	5
800	40.0	5
850	42.5	5
900	45.0	5
950	47.5	4
1000	50.0	4

Source: Hanes (1991).

Age 6–8 weeks: Move kit(s) to a large fully enclosed outdoor pen once completely weaned. Provide an abundance of foliage and logs for privacy along with airline kennel(s) for hiding spots. Place water in a shallow pan with rocks so that kit(s) do not drown.

Age 8+ weeks: Same housing as 6–8-week-olds, except you may introduce a baby pool for water when they are 12 weeks old. Also use a self-feeder for puppy food and PVC pipes with plugs for introducing dead or live prey in order to decrease human contact/visualization. In addition provide shelving or stacked crates to offer high spots for foxes to lie on and jump up to.

A concrete enclosure/run enclosed on all six sides (preferably a combination of concrete with chain link, with a concrete floor partially lined with clean dirt at least 6–8 in deep for digging) with airline kennels and plenty of towels and blankets to provide warmth and a "denlike" environment is necessary for the kits after they are 8 weeks old. This space should be free from direct drafts and inclement weather conditions until the kits are much older (three months). Provide an external heat source if the animal is young, weak, or not thermoregulating well.

Under no circumstances should the animal be exposed to or raised with any species other than foxes. Dogs and other domestic species are not appropriate companions, and should not be introduced to the fox. The animals should not be exposed to excessive human contact and care, especially if they are to be released back into a natural habitat.

As the kits grow and age, the airline kennels may be removed, and the animal can be placed in a fully enclosed outdoor pen that allows natural light/sunlight to enter the space. Various cage furnishings such as logs can be added for climbing (be sure they can't hurt themselves if they fall off), small pools of water for play, and culverts (large steel cylinders, both ends open) to simulate den structures. Indestructible toys that can be properly sterilized (i.e., boomer balls, bowling balls, etc.), may be added as the animal matures. Trapdoor systems to provide food and water from the outside should be included in the enclosure design.

If possible, assign two enclosures to the animals so that they can be shifted to facilitate cleaning and food placement without visualizing humans. It is important that the animal does not associate people with food. Access to the fox area should be limited to essential staff only for daily care. No talking in the area should be permitted.

Be sure to have padlocks on the doors to the enclosure. Enclosures should have double door systems and if possible a perimeter fence around them.

RESTRAINT OF OLDER PUPS

In restraining foxes, do not scruff because they are able to turn their mouth around to bite you while you are holding their loose skin (Convy 2001). A fox can be confined easily by herding it into an airline kennel within a larger enclosure. If that does not work, you can either use a net or make use of a rabies control pole to restrain the fox in a large enclosure. When using a rabies pole, ensure the loop of the pole is around the neck and one foreleg when you tighten the noose. As they mature you may need to cover the animal's head with a large towel or blanket when attempting to restrain it. Wear leather gloves while working to restrain the animal. Slowly bring one hand up the animal's back and grasp the fox around the back of its neck while also holding the tail. Remove the net or control pole from the animal. While you have a firm hold on the animal's neck, use your knee to hold the torso down. Have a second handler muzzle the fox. Then grasp the neck with one hand and support the body with the other hand while moving the animal, holding the animal's body under your arm for leverage. Do not position the fox's legs toward your abdomen, as it can kick at you and get free of your hold. To restrain a fox already in an airline kennel, turn the kennel up on end with the door facing the ceiling. Slowly open the door and place a towel over the fox's head. With a gloved hand reach in and pin the animal to the bottom corner of the crate while you locate the back of the animal's neck and grasp it. Use two hands to hold the neck and lift the fox from the crate, try to support the body with your arms, or have a second person support the torso. Muzzle the fox and continue your procedure (Convy 2001).

IMMUNE STATUS AND SPECIAL NEEDS

In the wild, kits should nurse from the dam until five to six weeks old when they begin to take in some solid foods. Ideally they would have had colostrum within 24 hours of their birth, which should provide them with maternal antibodies for immunity until their own immune systems are mature. Unfortunately it is difficult to know if kits have had this first milk when they initially present.

A kit that is unthrifty, or just doesn't seem right, may not have had colostrum as a neonate or its mother may have had a weakened immune system and was not been able to pass appropriate antibodies to the kits. If a kit has had colostrum, it should do well with supportive care appropriate for its age. If you suspect a kit did not receive appropriate colostrum, keep it warm, away from all other animals (except its own littermates), and ensure it is nursing/eating well enough for its age. Such kits may require supplemental fluids (66 ml/kg/day divided in two to three daily doses), additional feedings, and judicious use of broad-spectrum antibiotics (i.e., amoxicillin, 10 mg/kg PO BID for 7–10 days). Be aware that these kits have a high mortality.

Vaccination Protocols

All vaccines may be purchased from your local veterinary drug distributor (Convy 2001). If you do not have a local contact, call your local veterinarian and get the information from him or her.

Note: Vaccination protocols apply only to the red fox species. Do not vaccinate any gray foxes with this vaccine.

Red foxes can be inoculated against distemper using modified-live virus (MLV) canine distemper vaccine. Use of MLV vaccines in gray foxes is contraindicated. Gray foxes are more likely to develop clinical distemper if a modified-live vaccine is used, and the efficacy of killed-virus vaccines in wildlife species is not well documented (White 1983).

Begin vaccines at 6 weeks and continue vaccinating every 3–4 weeks until the animal is 20–24 weeks old. Give booster yearly.

COMMON MEDICAL PROBLEMS

Parasites

Endoparasites

Fecal analysis will determine therapy. A fecal examination by direct smear and a float to determine worm infestation is part of a normal workup. The direct smear may be stained with lugol (iodine) stain for identifying giardia. If giardia is suspected and not seen on direct float, a fecal sample may need to be submitted to a veterinary diagnostic laboratory for analysis. Roundworms are treated with fenbendazole (Panacur, 50 mg/kg orally once a day for three days and repeated in two weeks for another three-day course). Coccidia are treated with sulfadimethoxine (Albon [Pfizer]) at an initial dose of 55 mg/kg once, then at a dose of 27 mg/kg once a day for ten days. Giardia is treated with metronidazole (Flagyl) at a dose of 15 mg/kg once a day for five to seven days. If tapeworms are noted, give a dose of praziquantel (Droncit [Bayer]) based on current weight and recommended dose on the bottle of the drug (Bowman 1999; Plumb 1998).

Ectoparasites

Fleas, when seen, are treated at this facility with diluted Permectrin II (Boehringer Ingelheim). Dilute it by using 3.5 ml Permectrin II to 1500 ml water.

Ticks can be found on debilitated animals and should be removed using a hemostat clamp while animal is sedated (or can be sedated safely). The animal may need to be dipped with a veterinary-approved tick dip to eliminate all ticks (Bowman 1999).

If the animal has an adverse reaction (respiratory distress, bluish gums) to any of these products, immediately bathe the animal and remove the flea product. With animals that react to a product, use a flea comb to remove fleas.

Ringworm is uncommon in kits under eight weeks of age, but it is contagious to humans. Always wear gloves when handling/treating an animal suspected of having ringworm. It is a fungal disease and the lesions are characterized by a reddish ringed worm appearance on the skin in an area of alopecia. Diagnosis is by clinical signs and doing a DTM (dermatophyte type medium) culture, which can be obtained from a local veterinary diagnostic laboratory. Consult a veterinarian for treatment. Griseofulvin ultramicrosize has been used successfully at an oral daily dose of 5–10 mg/kg for a minimum of three weeks (Bowman 1999; Plumb 1998).

Sarcoptic mange is caused by sarcoptes mites, small arthropods visible by microscope. This disease is not uncommon in foxes, but kits under eight weeks of age with sarcoptic mange are generally so debilitated they rarely survive. Clinical signs are diffuse alopecia +/- patchiness of the fur. Diagnosis is accomplished by having your veterinarian do a skin scraping. Treatment is with ivermectin injections (0.300 mg/kg SQ) repeated every 14 days. It may take up to five treatments to resolve. Discuss dosages with a veterinarian if you have any questions (Bowman 1999; Plumb 1998).

Demodectic mange is caused by a mite in primarily immunodeficient animals. Clinical presentation may be focal or diffuse and is seen as areas of alopecia with crusty scabs. Diagnosis is by skin scraping and viewing under the microscope. The mites appear like small cigar-shaped creatures with eight waving arms. Treatment is with Goodwinol topical ointment or dips with amitraz (Mitaban, Pharmacia & Upjohn, Kalamazoo, MI). Ivermectin injections may also be used in the treatment (see dose mentioned above). Diffuse demodecosis is difficult to treat, and if incurable may lead to euthanizing the animal (Bowman 1999; Plumb 1998).

Infectious Diseases

Canine Distemper Virus

Canine distemper virus is a paramyxovirus. It is transmitted via aerosolization (respiratory secretions) and invades epithelial cells, entering via the respiratory tract. This is a very serious disease, generally with a grave prognosis. Young, unvaccinated animals between three to six months old are most susceptible and affected. The "virus can be excreted for 60–90 days." It is susceptible to most veterinary disinfectants (Ettinger and Feldman 1995; Greene 1998).

CDV causes a variety of clinical signs including weakness, lethargy, inappetence, diarrhea, respiratory signs, mucopurulent oculonasal discharge, hyperkeratosis of the foot pads, and, as the disease progresses, neurological signs with characteristic retinal abnormalities in the eye. Initial nonspecific clinical signs begin two to four days postinfection with more severe signs occurring within a week. If you suspect the kit has distemper, it should be isolated and evaluated by a veterinarian for diagnosis and treatment. Treatment is often unrewarding and recovered animals may shed the virus, thereby infecting other animals. Usually, animals diagnosed with canine distemper are humanely euthanized (Convy 2001; Ettinger and Feldman 1995; Greene 1998; Morgan 1992).

Towels, blankets, kennels, food bowls, enclosures, toys, or other items should be completely disinfected before being used for any other animal. Allow the enclosure/kennel space to air out for 48–72 hours before putting another animal into the enclosure (Greene 1998).

Prevention is vaccination. See schedule under Vaccination Protocols above.

Parvovirus (Canine Viral Enteritis)

Parvovirus is a DNA virus that "requires rapidly dividing cells for replications" (Greene 1998). The virus is quite resistant in the environment and is spread from contact with feces or oronasal secretions of infected animals. The virus will also attack lymphoid tissue causing decrease of white blood cells. Clinical signs include severe lethargy, foul smelling hemorrhagic diarrhea, and vomiting. The clinical signs have a rapid onset and the animals can fail quickly. The myocardium of the heart may also be affected causing cardiac disease. Depending on the level of cardiac involvement, the kit may die suddenly from this virus. Kits exhibiting any of these signs should be treated by a veterinarian (Ettinger and Feldman 1995; Greene 1998; Morgan 1992).

Diagnosis is via a canine parvovirus CITE snap test using a fecal sample. The test is specific and sensitive for this virus. The test is available through most veterinary drug distributors. If an animal is positive on the CITE test, isolate the animal from other carnivores in a warm temperature-controlled room and consult with a small-animal veterinarian to establish a treatment plan and assess the animal periodically (Ettinger and Feldman 1995).

Animals can be treated successfully if therapy is started early in the disease process or as soon as the diagnosis is confirmed. If the animal improves and recovers, it should be isolated from other foxes as well as carnivores for at least two weeks. The kit will continue to shed the virus for that amount of time and can transmit the virus to other vulnerable animals (Ettinger and Feldman 1995).

All towels, blankets, kennels, food bowls, enclosures, toys, or other items should be completely disinfected before being used for any other animal. Allow the enclosure/kennel space to air out for 48–72 hours before putting another animal into the enclosure.

Prevention is vaccination. See schedule under Vaccination Protocols above.

Rabies Virus

Rabies is an RNA virus that is easily killed by a variety of disinfectants used in animal and veterinary facilities (Ettinger and Feldman 1995; Greene 1998). This virus is transmitted via saliva from bite wounds of infected animals. The virus affects the central nervous system (CNS) and causes aberrant neurological behavior usually exhibited as severe aggression.

If rabies is suspected, the animal is euthanized and the head submitted to a special lab for rabies testing. If rabies is suspected and the animal bites someone, it should be immediately humanely euthanized and the head submitted for special lab testing (Ettinger and Feldman 1995; Greene 1998). If someone was bitten or in contact with the animal's saliva, the person should see a physician immediately and begin prophylactic shots for exposure. This is a fatal disease if not treated immediately once someone has been exposed. Your local public health office should be informed immediately if you suspect an animal is rabid and you plan to euthanize it.

All staff members at a facility that accepts mammals to raise and/or release should have prophylactic rabies vaccinations done per instructions from your local public health office.

Rabies virus lives in wild mammal populations throughout the United States (except in Hawaii). There are different wildlife reservoirs of the virus in different areas of the United States. Raccoons, skunks, foxes, dogs, and bats (migratory) are the primary wild and domestic animals that carry rabies in this country. A level of enzootic infection is maintained in various wild animal populations. Problems arise in an area when an epizootic or epidemic occurs in an area. When this occurs, it's possible to see an increase in the carnivores presenting to wildlife centers (Greene 1998).

While most of the young neonates that you may see will not have rabies, there is a chance a juvenile fox that is positive for rabies may present to your facility and may have signs of a rabid animal. There are two forms of rabies: the furious form, with which most people are familiar, and the dumb/paralytic form that seems to allude many individuals, including many practitioners. Clinical signs of the furious form are change in demeanor/personality, excessive licking of the bite wound site, and anxiety, which lasts for approximately a week. Animals exhibit a fear of water because they cannot swallow and therefore cannot drink. They drool excessively for the same reason. The paralytic form is seen as a lower motor neuron paralysis from the site of the bite and progresses along the nerve until it reaches the CNS and lasts about two to four days. Animals occasionally exhibit choking during this phase, but it is actually a paralysis of the laryngeal nerves. Do not place your hand in the animal's mouth without protective gloves if you attempt to relieve a choking situation (Greene 1998).

For safety purposes, any towels, blankets, toys, or other items should be disinfected and thrown away. Kennels and food bowls should be completely disinfected before being used for any other animal. Allow the enclosure/kennel space to air out for at least 48 hours before putting another animal into the enclosure.

Diarrhea

Diarrhea is defined as "an increase in the frequency, fluidity, or volume of feces" (Ettinger and Feldman 1995). Diarrhea can be characterized as acute or chronic and must be differentiated as originating in the small versus the large bowel. Most of our patients with diarrhea have the acute form, which is caused by problems in either the small or large bowel. Initial treatment of diarrhea, until it can be further characterized, is fluid therapy, diet change, and gastrointestinal protectants (see treatment section below). It is best to hold off on antibiotic therapy initially, and attempt supportive care and diet change to correct the diarrhea. Most therapies suitable for young domestic dogs would be appropriate in young fox kits as well (i.e., Pepto-Bismol at 1 ml/10 lb [4.5 kg] orally two to three times a day, and cimetidine 7–10 mg/kg PO, SQ, IV two to three times daily) (Ettinger and Feldman 1995; Plumb 1998).

Causes: Acute diarrheas in young animals generally are caused by parasites, inappropriate formula or feeding methods, medications, and toxins. Chronic diarrheas may be caused by uncorrected acute diarrhea problems and rectal anatomical abnormalities (strictures, masses) and can be seen in our younger patients with infections (salmonella, clostridial), ulcers (due to stress or trauma), or toxins. Clinical signs include dehydration, bloated abdomen, loose/runny stool, fever, pain on abdominal palpation with gaseous bowel loops, weight loss, and tenesmus (Ettinger and Feldman 1995; Morgan 1992).

Diagnostics: Fecal analysis (direct and float), hemoccult fecal tests, CBC, radiographs, fecal cytology, and fecal cultures may be necessary to determine the cause and characterize the type of diarrhea (Ettinger and Feldman 1995).

Treatment: Treatment should be targeted at the underlying cause of the diarrhea. Young and baby animals should have diets reviewed and corrected and be given SQ fluids—crystalloids at appropriate dehydration/shock/maintenance until they can be placed on the appropriate diet and clinical signs resolve. A veterinarian should calculate the amount of fluids necessary to treat the fox, but approximately 60–90 ml/kg/day of crystalloids (Normosol-R or lactated Ringer's solution) delivered via IV catheter is reasonable. The young foxes may require broad-spectrum systemic antibiotics (Clavamox 13.75 mg/kg PO BID for seven to ten days or metronidazole at 15 mg/kg PO SID for five to seven days) if they are compromised and appear debilitated (Plumb 1998). Fecal examinations should be done on all patients with diarrhea and appropriate anthelminth therapy instituted (see Endoparasites above). Fluid therapy and correction of formula are the primary mechanisms to correct most of the acute diarrheas we see in babies and juveniles at the wildlife center.

Chronic diarrheas are more difficult to treat. Abdominal radiographs should be done. If parasites and dietary problems/indiscretion have been ruled out and the diarrhea is persistent, the veterinarians should reassess the patient and decide on the next course of diagnostics and therapy. Maintaining fluid balance and correcting for dehydration and ongoing losses should continue in the patient (e.g., ongoing fluid therapy IV, PO, SQ at appropriate fluid rates) (Ettinger and Feldman 1995).

Hypoglycemia

Young animals have higher glucose requirements than most adults of their species (Ettinger and Feldman 1995; Morgan 1992). The increased requirement is important as a source of energy for maturing metabolic functions, growth, and maintenance of normal blood glucose (BG) levels. They utilize all nutrients faster because of accelerated growth rates at young ages. It is important to restore and continue to meet their BG needs.

Clinical signs of hypoglycemia may be noted if the blood glucose (BG) is less than 60 gm/dl. Animals may appear hungry, show signs of ataxia, or have small seizures that may escalate and lead to loss of consciousness. Initial therapy is to quickly apply Karo syrup to the gums and then give dextrose via gavage tube (orogastric tube), subcutaneously, or intravenously. If giving dextrose SQ, remember to give only a concentration of 2.5% dextrose. In most wildlife neonatal patients, it can be difficult to place an IV. An intraosseous catheter may be placed by a veterinarian, if the animal is severely dehydrated or hypoglycemic, in order to deliver fluid therapy. Once a catheter is placed, administer 5–10 ml/kg of a 20% dextrose solution, which may be diluted from a 50% solution using a ration of 2-ml sterile saline to 1.5 ml 50% dextrose. Give this amount IV at a steady pace. Begin an IV drip of LRS or Normosol-R with an appropriate amount of dextrose added to the fluid bag to make a 2.5–10% or even up to a 20% solution of dextrose. Remember you can only give up to a 2.5% dextrose SQ but it is acceptable to give higher concentrations of dextrose intravenously if warranted. Initially recheck the BG level within the first two hours of therapy (using a different vein than the one with the catheter) and modify the amount of dextrose in the fluids to accommodate the change in BG levels. If the dextrose drip is not maintaining and/or increasing, or normalizing the BG level, give another bolus of the 20% dextrose solution as outlined above. Once the BG has been corrected and the animal is stable, proper management with environmental control, nutrition, and additional SQ fluid therapy can normalize the patient. Young fox kits will generally normalize with a minimal therapy/intervention and maintain their BG level once placed on a well-balanced diet. If simple intervention does not bring them to a normoglycemic state, then a veterinarian should be involved in establishing a treatment plan (Ettinger and Feldman 1995; Morgan 1992).

Septicemia

Septicemia is a problem manifested as a systemic infection generally carried throughout the body via the bloodstream. Animals may or may not be febrile. Generally they are lethargic, weak, inappetent, may have difficulty breathing, and have pale mucous membranes. Animals will need aggressive care and veterinary evaluation. We have not seen this as a common problem in fox kits, but if you suspect this problem be sure to have a veterinarian evaluate the animal immediately and formulate a treatment plan for the individual animal (Ettinger and Feldman 1995).

Shock/Dehydration

Shock is usually a result of trauma, disease, hypoglycemia, or severe malnutrition in wildlife patients. The animals present with severe hypovolemia and possibly hypoglycemia (see Hypoglycemia above). Animals have pale mucous membranes, glazed/glassy appearing eyes, may be recumbent, and may have an elevated temperature and a prolonged capillary refill time. If animals present with head trauma, they may have seizures, slip into a coma, or have problems thermoregulating (Ettinger and Feldman 1995; Murtaugh 1994).

If you suspect your kit is in shock or severely dehydrated, it should be treated by a veterinarian. If a veterinarian is not available, initiate treatment with shock dose fluids (60–90 ml/kg of crystalloids, Normosol-R or LRS) delivered via IV catheter if possible, or an intraosseous catheter (Ettinger and Feldman 1995; Murtaugh 1994). After shock dose fluids have been administered, fluids with 5–10% IV dextrose may be required. However, if the animal is having seizures, IV dextrose may need to be given in lieu of shock dose fluids until the animal stops seizing, then shock dose fluids may be resumed. It is important to get a small amount of blood and evaluate the animal's blood glucose levels. Intravenous antibiotics (cephalosporins, 10 mg/lb IV TID) and IV short acting steroids (Solu-Delta Cortef, 0.2–1 mg/kg IV or 1–4 mg/kg IV) should be administered (Ettinger and Feldman 1995; Plumb 1998). If the body temperature is greater than 106°F (41.1°C) apply alcohol to the foot pads or cold soaked towels to the animal until you begin to see a drop in the temperature, then remove the towels. When the animal is stable, radiographs should be taken to check for possible fractures, or any organ abnormalities (Ettinger and Feldman 1995; Plumb 1998).

When administering fluids to a patient in shock, we generally like to give half the dose quickly, monitor respiratory rate and effort of the animal, then continue to give the remainder of the fluids via a quick drip. Auscult the lungs regularly, and adjust the drip rate as needed. If the lungs have moist sounds on auscultation, then reduce the drip rate or discontinue fluids. Always consult a veterinarian to help determine the level of dehydration and formulate a fluid-treatment plan.

If the animal is not shocky and only mildly dehydrated, you can rehydrate it using lactated Ringer's solution subcutaneously or intravenously at a dose of 60 ml/kg/day (Murtaugh 1994). If administering the fluids SQ, you may divide the amount and give it in two to three doses over the course of the day.

Trauma and Fractures

Animals with trauma or fractures should be treated by a veterinarian.

Emaciation or Thin Animals

Emaciation is a condition that may be caused by poor nutrition, death/abandonment by the dam, or parasites (both endo and ecto). Blood and fecal samples should be taken and submitted to determine if any underlying problems exist, and a diet appropriate for the animal's age and level of emaciation should be initiated (Convy 2001; Ettinger and Feldman 1995). Diet changes may need to be made once laboratory results are finalized (e.g., low blood glucose may be corrected by giving SQ or IV dextrose (see Hypoglycemia above); calcium abnormalities should be corrected under the direction of a veterinarian (Morgan 1992). In rehabilitation situations, animals that present emaciated or thin may be treated with initial supportive care (fluids SQ or IV, +/− dextrose), and an appropriately balanced diet for the animal.

An emaciated animal should be given a bland diet once stabilized, warmed to normal body temperature, and rehydrated. The diet should be given as small frequent meals and not large meals all at once. The diet can be gradually modified for the kit's specific age and weight group over a period of a couple of days in order to give the animal's system an opportunity to digest and metabolize the food.

Ocular Lesions

Eye problems include corneal ulcers, foreign bodies, proptosed globes, and lens luxations (all due to trauma) and should be evaluated by a veterinarian and possibly a veterinary ophthalmologist (Slatter 1990).

Vomiting

Vomiting in young animals may be the result of ingesting foreign objects, from inappropriate dietary formulation or spoiled diet, medications, infectious agents, ulcers, heat stroke, or metabolic abnormalities (Ettinger and Feldman 1995).

Vomitus should be inspected for blood or a coffee ground consistency. The presence of blood or coffee ground material would indicate a severe problem and treatment plans should be conducted under the direction of a veterinarian (Ettinger and Feldman 1995).

Generally, one simple episode of vomiting can be treated by withholding food for a short period of time, giving SQ fluids to the kit, correcting the diet (provide a bland diet that is fresh), and monitoring for continuing signs (Ettinger and Feldman 1995). If the animal continues to vomit, a veterinarian should evaluate the animal and provide an additional treatment plan. Exploratory surgery may be necessary to correct the problem, especially if a foreign body is causing the vomiting.

Anemia

Anemia is not a disease, it is a symptom. It is decreased red blood cells in the blood as reflected by measuring packed cell volume (PCV) and red blood cells (RBC). Anemia is a complicated symptom to interpret and not as straightforward as simply reading a decreased PCV (Cotter 1993; Ettinger and Feldman 1995).

Clinical signs: Pale mucous membranes, dyspnea, tachycardia, and weakness may be further complicated by epistaxis, hematuria, continued hemorrhage, melena, and hematoemesis. Many of these signs are directly related to the decrease in oxygen delivery to the tissues by the resulting decrease in RBC (Cotter 1993; Ettinger and Feldman 1995).

Causes: It is important to assess the underlying condition, which causes blood loss or a decrease in RBC and leads to anemia. Obvious factors are hemorrhage due to trauma (punctures, lacerations, wounds, splenic fractures). Less-obvious causes are blood loss due to parasites (GI, urinary, pulmonary, cardiac, nasal heme), toxicities (rodenticide, copper, lead), infectious diseases (distemper virus, clostridial, leptospirosis), metabolic abnormalities (renal, hepatic, endocrine), vitamin deficiencies (some can be induced by drugs such as sulfas or poisons), and sepsis (Cotter 1993; Ettinger and Feldman 1995).

With an anemic animal, treatment is targeted at the underlying cause. Most of the animals that present as orphans, have anemias resulting from trauma, infections, parasites, toxicities, or debilitation (inappropriate nutrition). These problems all require different therapeutic plans. The goal of the therapy is to stabilize the patient, provide circulatory assistance, and enhance delivery of oxygen to the tissues until the underlying cause for the anemia can be corrected (Cotter 1993; Ettinger and Feldman 1995). Seek immediate veterinary assistance for a treatment plan.

RELEASE

Release fox kits at dusk or later in the evening as close as possible to the original pick-up site. Release at about six months of age. The foxes must be able to quickly catch and kill live prey. They should have been tested and proven this ability while they were being rehabilitated. They must also be able to run and jump well, and be fearful of humans.

SOURCES OF PRODUCTS MENTIONED

Bayer Corp., Shawnee Mission, KS

Boehringer Ingelheim Animal Health, Inc., St. Joseph, MO 64506; 1-800-821-7467

Goodwinol Products Corp., Pierce, CO; 1-970-834-1229

Jorgenson Laboratories, Inc., Loveland, CO; 1-800-525-5614

Kendall Company, Mansfield, MA 02048; 1-800-962-9888

PetAg Inc., 261 Keyes Ave., Hampshire, IL 60140; 1-800-323-0877, 1-800-323-6878; www.petag.com.

Pfizer Animal Health, Exton, PA

Ross Products Division, Abbott Laboratories, Columbus, OH 43215-1724; 1-800-986-8510; www.abbott.com, www.ross.com

REFERENCES

Bowman, D. D. 1999. *Georgis' parasitology for veterinarians*. Philadelphia, PA: Saunders.

Convy, J. 2001. *PAWS wildlife rehabilitation manual*. Spring. Lynnwood, WA: PAWS Wildlife Center.

Cotter, S. M. 1993. Pathophysiology of the hemiclymphatic system, course syllabus. Fall. North Grafton, MA: Tufts University School of Veterinary Medicine.

Ettinger, S. J., and E. C. Feldman. 1995. *Textbook of veterinary internal medicine*. 4th ed. Philadelphia, PA: Saunders.

Greene, C. E., ed. 1998. *Infectious diseases of the dog and cat*. 2d ed. Philadelphia, PA: Saunders.

Hanes, P. C. 1991. Red fox(*Vulpes vulpes fulva*) and gray fox *(Urocyon cinereoargenteus)*. *Wildlife Journal* 14(2): 9–16.

Macdonald, D., ed. 1995. *The encyclopedia of mammals*. New York: Facts on File.

Morgan, R. V., ed. 1992. *Handbook of small animal medicine*. 2d ed.. Philadelphia, PA: Saunders.

Murtaugh, R. 1994. Principles of medicine, course syllabus. Spring. North Grafton, MA: Tufts University School of Veterinary Medicine; Section on Small Animal Fluid Therapy.

Nowak, R. M. 1991. *Walker's mammals of the world*, vol. 2. 5th ed. Baltimore: The Johns Hopkins University Press.

Plumb, Donald C., 1998. *Veterinary drug handbook*. 3d ed. Ames: Iowa State University Press.

Slatter, D. 1990. *Fundamentals of veterinary ophthalmology*. 2d ed. Philadelphia, PA: Saunders.

White. J. 1983. Use of modified-live virus canine distemper vaccines in gray foxes. *Wildlife Journal* 6(1):16.

23
Black Bear Cubs

Sophia Papageorgiou, Darlene DeGhetto, and Jennifer Convy

NATURAL HISTORY

The black bear is of the order Carnivora, family Ursidae, genus *Ursus,* and species *americanus.*

Distribution

The American black bear (*Ursus americanus*) has a distribution from northern Mexico and California across northern America from Washington State to the Great Lakes, throughout Canada, and north into Alaska. There are populations also found in Newfoundland, Appalachia, and some areas of Florida in the northern Gulf Coast. They inhabit forests and woodlands (Macdonald 1995; Nowak 1991).

Description/ID

American black bears have light blondish-brown to black furcoat both dorsal and ventral (back and abdomen). They may occur with a white "blaze" on their chest. The snout is slightly lighter in color than body. They have a heavy body with relatively short legs and large curved claws on all four feet.

Reproduction

Females reach sexual maturity at four to five years, males at five to six years. Breeding season is generally June to mid-July. Gestation is 220 days but they have delayed implantation. Litters average one to three cubs and sows give birth every other year in January or February. The cubs remain denned with the sow until April to May when the family emerges from hibernation. The cubs are generally three to five months old at this time. Cubs are born in the den weighing approximately 8–10 oz. The cubs remain with the mother for 1 1/2 to 2 1/2 years (Macdonald 1995; Nowak 1991).

Habitat and Activity Period

Bears are crepuscular and nocturnal and range in forests and forested mountains. During fall and early winter they gain weight, which is stored as fat reserves. Eventually they stop eating in very cold weather, locate a den, and hibernate. They may not hibernate if they live in warmer climates of the southeastern United States (Macdonald 1995; Nowak 1991).

Natural Diet and Foraging Techniques

Black bears are omnivores but generally have a herbivorous diet (roots, berries, nuts), supplemented with insect protein and whatever they can find if scavenging. Seventy-five percent of their diet consists of natural vegetation: twigs, buds, leaves, nuts, acorns, grass, roots, tubers, fruit, skunk cabbage, salmonberries, and huckleberries. They also eat insects, small/medium-sized mammals, fish, honeycomb, and bee larvae (Macdonald 1995; Nowak 1991).

Denning

Black bears use a hollow log or burrow to sleep from late fall until early spring. The duration of hibernation inactivity varies in different parts of the United States and may also vary with the severity of the winter weather. Bears may not hibernate if they live in warmer climates of the southeastern United States. During winter sleep the bear's body temperature drops from 38°C to 31–34°C, the respiration slows, and metabolic rate is depressed. Black bears do not truly hibernate as they will get up every so often during warm-weather spells for water and then resume their winter sleep (Macdonald 1995; Nowak 1991; Wildlife Rehabilitation).

Additional Information

These animals are solitary as adults. They have a lumbering walk but are excellent climbers and swimmers and can move very fast if the need arises. They have strong claws used to tear apart logs in search of insects (Nowak 1991).

Behavior Considerations

Both wild and captive animals have a poor sense of sight, but their olfactory and auditory senses are very keen. The bear is plantigrade—it walks with heels touching the ground. Bears should flee from humans as soon as they see a person (even when they are in a captive rearing/rehabilitation situation). If the bear is unafraid of humans then a behavior problem may be involved and the bear should be reassessed before release back into the wild (Nowak 1991; PAWS 2001).

RECORD KEEPING

Detailed records must be maintained as in all captive animal situations. Accurate daily recording of attitude, weight, temperature, heart and respiratory rate (if possible), food fed (measured), and amount eaten (measured). All procedures, physical examinations, medications provided, or other information must be written in the animal's individual record file. Case number/tag numbers should be placed on all sheets of the animal's permanent record for identification purposes.

Age Determination

The following guidelines can be used to determine age (PAWS 2001):

Newborn: 225–330 g, mostly naked with some fine sparse, stiff hairs, blind, 6–8 in long
25 days: eyes open, short fuzzy brownish hair, begins playing with siblings soon
3 months: emerges from den
6 to 8 months: weaned but usually remains with mother until two years of age (Nowak 1991)
1 year old: 40–75 kg

Check teeth and body size to determine age, as well as the time of year the cub presents. Deciduous dentition is replaced between five and eight months. Bear cubs are generally born in January and February and leave the den in April to May depending on the winter weather that year (Macdonald 1995).

INITIAL CARE AND STABILIZATION

Perform a complete physical examination either by manual restraint or with sedation (depending on the size of the bear). The animal should be immobilized only if it is deemed in stable condition or poses a threat to the professionals assessing the animal. The level of restraint and sedation should be appropriate for the situation and procedure necessary at that time (Fig. 23.1).

The animal's individual situation will vary depending on its history, problems, and circumstances of

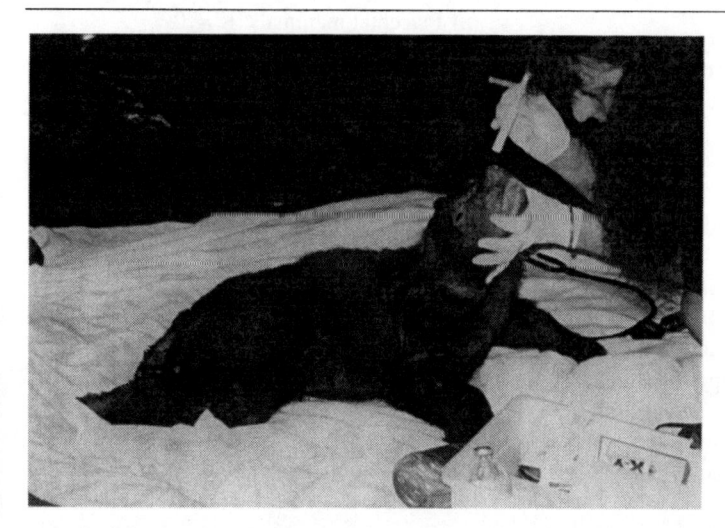

Figure 23.1. Physical examination of sedated black bear cub.

capture. A young cub may be debilitated with a low blood glucose level, or if it was suckling off of a dead sow it may be septic. All new bear cub patients should have the following workup.

Blood (CBC and chemistry panel) and a fecal sample should be submitted for analysis. The veterinarian should be present or called in if necessary. Check the packed cell volume (PCV), total protein, and blood glucose (BG) in order to initiate treatment for an immediate problem. If the BG is low, less than 80 g/dl, give subcutaneous or intravenous fluids (lactated Ringer's solution [LRS] or Normosol-R with a 2–1/2% dextrose solution SQ or higher percentage dextrose if given IV). Prepare blood slide smears for review by the veterinarian. Prepare equipment for IV catheter placement, fluid therapy, skin scraping, and possibly X rays. Be sure to provide the animal with heat, fluids, and appropriate medications based on physical examination findings.

FORMULAS: REHABILITATION DIET

We have had good results with the following rehabilitation diet.

Infant Formula: Use dilute Esbilac (PetAg) or any canine puppy formula, which may be purchased from feed stores, high-end pet food stores, many veterinary hospitals, or emergency clinics.

Mix one part powdered Esbilac (by volume) with two parts water. Gradually increase the strength of the formula by thirds from rehydrating solution to formula and then feed the formula until they are three to four weeks old.

Start with oral rehydrating solution (lactated Ringer's solution or Pedialyte)

Day 1: full rehydrating solution
Day 2: 2/3 rehydrating solution, 1/3 formula
Day 3: 1/3 rehydrating solution, 2/3 formula
Day 4: 100% formula (one part Esbilac powder to two parts water)

FORMULAS: WEANING DIET

The following bear mush recipe is good for weaning.

Bear mush recipe: Mix together 1/2 cup ground puppy chow, 1/2 cup baby cereal, 1 tablespoon powdered Esbilac or other puppy formula. Be consistent with the brand and type of puppy formula to decrease problems with diarrhea and indigestion. Add 1 cup warm water to make it oatmeal consistency. Finally add 3 tablespoons cottage cheese and mix together.

NURSING TECHNIQUE

If cubs' eyes are still closed, feed formula via a baby bottle with a premature-sized human nipple. If the cubs eyes are open, dish feed the formula. You may need to direct them to the dish and sometimes hold them still while they are very young until they focus on eating from the dish.

Once they catch on to feeding from a dish, then leave the enclosure while they eat to minimize human contact. Once they eat directly from the dish, give them their diet without the cubs visualizing you. To do this, separate them into an adjacent enclosure, clean the enclosure, place the food, leave, then allow the bears back into the original enclosure. If you have two cages/enclosures to use, place the food into the clean cage, move bears into the clean space, allow them to eat, then go in and clean the other exhibit once they have eaten. It is very important to minimize the association of humans and food to the bears, especially if there are plans to release the bear back into the wild (PAWS 2001).

AMOUNTS TO FEED

In order to figure out how much a bear cub should eat per day, it is first necessary to figure out how many kilocalories the cub requires per day and adjust that to the cub's stomach capacity. These calculations will determine the number of feeds and amounts per feeding required.

Daily caloric needs may be calculated as well as the exact volume the animal needs per day (PAWS 2001).

A. Mammals need 2–3 × Basal Metabolic Rate (BMR).
   1. BMR = (K) × (body weight in kg)$^{0.75}$
      (a) Placental mammals: K =70
      (b) Use a calculator with a y^x function
B. Beware of overfeeding.
   1. A guideline is to feed 10% of the bear's Body Weight (BW) per day divided into two to six feedings per day depending on age.
      (a) 1.5 oz/lb BW
      (b) 100 ml/kg BW
C. Observe the stomach and don't overfill.

Weigh the cub(s) daily while you're getting them started on their new formula/diet. Use recorded daily weights to calculate new formula amounts.

Feeding Guide

The following feeding guide has been successful for us (PAWS 2001):

Newborn to 4 weeks: Feed infant formula every four hours around the clock (six times a day).

4 to 8 weeks: Feed infant formula five times a day. When cub has been lapping formula from dish well for three to four days, then add baby cereal (Gerber baby cereal) to formula.

8 to 10 weeks: Gradually add bear mush to formula. Continue to feed five times daily.

10 to 12 weeks: Feed formula and bear mush mixed together. Feed four times per day. Dish feed, gradually increase ground puppy chow, and decrease the formula. Add no more than 10% fruit to mush.

12 to 14 weeks: Eliminate infant formula; should be on 100% bear mush/soaked puppy chow. Feed three times per day.

14 to 18 weeks: Require two to three feedings per day if the cub is weaning onto the bear mush/soaked puppy chow well. Include some fruits and natural vegetation. Dry puppy chow should be introduced and they ought to be eating it well at this point.

18 to 20 weeks: Should be completely weaned and eating dry puppy chow, fruit, and vegetables. Once they are consistently eating this diet they may be fed once a day until release.

HOUSING

A concrete enclosure/run enclosed on all six sides (preferably a combination of concrete with chain-link fence, with a concrete floor) with airline kennels and plenty of towels and blankets to provide warmth and a "denlike" environment is necessary. This space should be free from direct drafts and inclement weather conditions until the cubs are much older (eight months). Provide an external heat source if the animal is young, weak, or not thermoregulating well (Fowler 1978).

If a lone cub presents to a facility, attempts should be made to raise it with conspecifics (members of the same species) of similar size, age, and development once the animal is stable. If animals vary a bit by age and weight, they may be introduced slowly to one another, but if the larger animal is too aggressive and rough the situation may not work out (Fowler 1978). Appropriate pairing of animals may require sending the animal elsewhere (to an approved facility) in order that it may be raised in a more natural situation. Under no circumstances should the animal be exposed to or raised with any species other than black bears. Dogs, deer, small ruminants, or any other species is not acceptable.

The bear(s) should not be exposed to excessive human contact and care, especially if they are to be released back into a natural habitat.

As the cubs grow and age the airline kennels may be removed, logs can be added for climbing (be sure they can't hurt themselves if they fall off) along with small pools of water for swimming and playing. Culverts (large steel cylinders, both ends open that can fit a growing bear) may be used to simulate den structures. Indestructible toys, which can be properly sterilized, such as boomer balls or bowling balls, can be added to the enclosure as the cubs mature. Whole watermelons and apples tossed into pools make fabulous playthings. As the animals age it is also good to hide mealworms, grubs, raisins, and berries in crevices in the logs (feel free to be creative in this area). This stimulates foraging behavior and self-sufficiency, and decreases boredom for the animals.

It is necessary to have two enclosures assigned to the bears so that they can be moved to facilitate cleaning and food placement without visualizing humans. Access to the bear area should be limited to essential staff only for essential tasks. No talking in the area should be permitted at any time. Panic buttons or buzzers should be accessible to caretakers for emergency situations.

Be sure to have padlocks and secondary security clips on the doors of the enclosure. Enclosures should also have perimeter fencing around them in case bears escape the primary enclosure.

RESTRAINT AND HANDLING

Always wear gloves when handling any carnivores as a precaution against *Baylisascaris* sp. parasite worm, ringworm, and other diseases.

Young cubs under 16 lb (7.2 kg) may be handled by wearing work gloves over latex gloves. If cubs are very young, ill, or nonaggressive, latex gloves worn without the protective work gloves will be sufficient. Use a thick towel or blanket to trap and catch the cubs. Wrap them so they appear to be a burrito with their heads visible. Depending on the procedure/plan for the animals, you may not need to anesthetize them. If you are planning a long procedure, or the animal is extremely difficult to restrain, use Isoflurane inhalant anesthesia with oxygen (O_2) via a facemask. These animals are very young and should be given fluids (LRS or Normosol-R with 2 1/2% dextrose SQ) if sedated. Give 10 ml/kg IV for each hour of anesthesia or procedure time. The dextrose is recommended because of the glucose requirement of young animals. For longer procedures, an intravenous catheter should be placed in a cephalic (arm) vein to facilitate fluid therapy support.

Once cubs are approximately 16 lb (7.3 kg), they may be caught via manual restraint and bundled in a large towel. Wear thick work gloves over protective latex gloves when handling cubs this size. At this point sedate the cub using either Isoflurane inhalant gas anesthesia using a facemask, with or without endotracheal intubation, or injectable Telazol at approximately 2–4 mg/kg delivered intramuscularly. Use a lower dose for thin or young animals and a higher dose for more well-muscled older bear cubs. These animals should be restrained/handled with a veterinarian present performing the immobilizing, or supervising a trained staff member during the procedure. Immobilizing the cub without a veterinarian present should only be undertaken in an emergency situation by trained technicians, and preferably with a veterinarian on the way to assist in the situation.

With smaller bear cubs, 16–25 lb (7.3–11.4 kg), the sedatives may be delivered via a hand injection. For larger cubs, the drugs are delivered by cornering and restraining the animal with a rabies catch pole and injecting it, trapping it in a crate and injecting through the grates of a kennel, or via pole syringe or dart gun. Once immobilized, the animal should be supported with oxygen or a gas inhalant agent combined with oxygen via facemask or an endotracheal tube. Intubation and anesthetic support will depend on the procedure(s) being performed, length of time necessary for the animal to be immobilized, and trained staff available to intubate the animal. If the animal has been immobilized with a remote dart, give it an injection of broad-spectrum antibiotics (penicillin or cephalosporin at 10 mg/kg SQ).

IMMUNE STATUS AND SPECIAL NEEDS

In the wild, most cubs are three to five months old when they emerge from the den. They will have had colostrum from the dam and have been suckling for a few months until the time they are out of the den. Wild cubs that require hand rearing have generally lost their mom either from an accident or separation. They should have a complete physical examination, a treatment plan, and appropriate food and shelter. (For further information, see Chapter 24, Polar Bears, regarding raising younger bear cubs.)

COMMON MEDICAL PROBLEMS

Endoparasites

Fecal analysis will determine therapy. A fecal float to determine roundworm or coccidia infestation is part of a normal workup as well as a lugol (iodine) stain for identifying giardia. Roundworms are treated with fenbendazole (Panacur Suspension, 10% [Hoechst]) 50 mg/kg SID × 3–5 days, repeat in 10–14 days. Coccidia are treated with sulfadimethoxine oral suspension (Albon, 50 mg/ml [Roche]) 50 mg/kg SID × one dose, then 25 mg/kg SID × 7–10 days. Giardia is treated with Flagyl at a dose of 15 mg/kg once a day for 5–7 days (Bowman 1999; Plumb 1998).

Ectoparasites: Ringworm (dermatophytes), Mange

Ringworm is contagious to humans. It is a fungal disease and the lesions are characterized by a reddish ringed worm appearance on the skin in an area of alopecia (hair loss). Diagnosis is by clinical signs and doing a DTM/fungal culture. Treatment is with oral griseofulvin (Fulvicin [Schering]) microsize, 10 mg/kg PO BID for 4–6 weeks or for a minimum of 21 days with treatment of one to two weeks after resolution of clinical signs, and dips (spot or full bath) with lyme sulfur solutions. Griseofulvin may cause low white blood cell counts and other side effects, so a CBC should be done every two to three weeks on animals taking this medication or if any adverse clinical signs are seen. Again, this type of treatment should be done under veterinary guidance (Bowman 1999; Plumb 1998) (Fig. 23.2).

Sarcoptic mange is caused by sarcoptes mites, which are small arthropods visible by microscope. Clinical signs are diffuse alopecia +/– patchiness of the fur. Diagnosis is done by skin scraping. The mites are visible under 4× or 10× power on the microscope. Treatment is with ivermectin injections. Discuss treatment plan and doses with the veterinarian. Generally, one subcutaneous injection of ivermectin at 0.300 mg/kg can be given with a follow-up dose given three weeks later (Bowman 1999; Plumb 1998).

Demodectic mange is caused by a mite in primarily immunodeficient animals. Clinical presentation may be focal or diffuse and is seen as areas of alopecia with crusty scabs. Diagnosis is by skin scraping and viewing under the microscope. The mites look

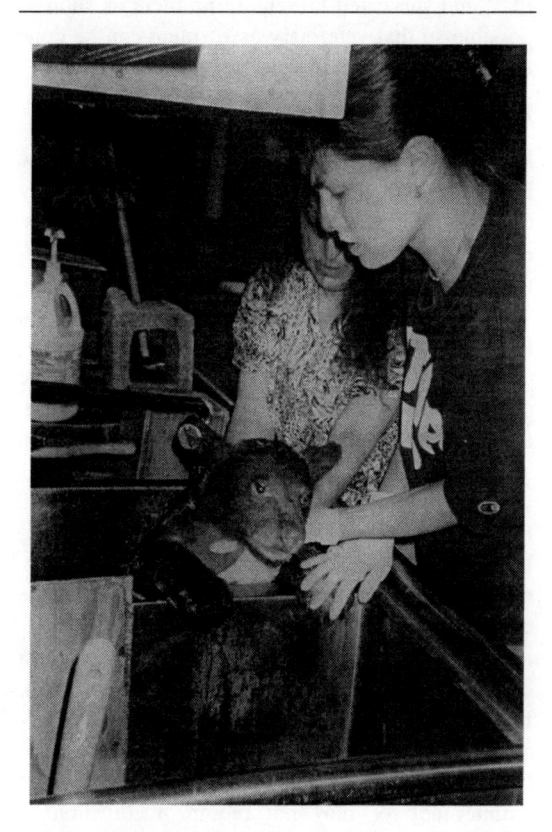

Figure 23.2. Lyme sulfur dip for bear cub with ringworm.

like small cigar-shaped creatures with eight waving arms. Treatment is with Goodwinol applied to small focal lesions, or dips with amitraz for generalized lesions. Ivermectin injections may also be used in the treatment as outlined for sarcoptic mange above. Diffuse demodecosis is difficult to treat and if incurable may lead to euthanizing the animal (Bowman 1999; Plumb 1998).

Ticks can be found in debilitated animals and should be removed using a hemostat clamp while the animal is sedated. Generally a very small number of ticks may live on the animal but they should not be present in overwhelming numbers. If that is the case, they are a result of the animal being debilitated. The animal may need to be dipped to eliminate all ticks (Bowman 1999).

Fleas may be present and if they are in large enough numbers a light flea bath may be used to treat them. Using a Vet-Kem flea powder, lightly distribute the powder on a towel, and rub the towel over the bear, staying away from face/eyes.

Trauma

Trauma in young bears is caused primarily by cars, gunshot, or attack by other animals. Head trauma can lead to neurological signs, including seizures, tremors, inability to thermoregulate, or other problems, such as trauma to the eyes, epistaxis (bleeding from the nose), aural (ear) bleeding, fractured jaw/ribs, and broken teeth (Ettinger and Feldman 1995). Treatment for trauma includes a thorough physical examination (if animal is stable), or therapy for shock as outlined below (fluids, steroids, heat, +/– antibiotics). If a fracture is detected or suspected, radiographs should be taken, only if the animal is stable. Stabilization of the fracture should be performed by a trained individual until further veterinary care is available.

Check the mouth for any tooth or jaw fractures. Also palpate the ribs and other bones for any abnormalities. If any fractures are evident or suspected, radiographs should be taken and reviewed by a veterinarian for appropriate treatment plan.

Anemia

Anemia is not a disease, it is a symptom. It is decreased red blood cells in the blood as reflected by measuring packed cell volume (PCV) and red blood cells (RBC). Anemia is a complicated symptom to interpret and not as straightforward as simply reading a decreased PCV (Cotter 1993; Ettinger and Feldman 1995).

Clinical signs include: pale mucous membranes, dyspnea, tachycardia, and weakness, and may be further complicated by epistaxis, hematuria, continued hemorrhage, melena, and hematoemesis. Many of these signs are directly related to the decrease in oxygen delivery to the tissues by the resulting decrease in RBC (Cotter 1993; Ettinger and Feldman 1995).

It is important to assess the underlying condition that causes blood loss or a decrease in RBC and leads to anemia. Obvious factors are hemorrhage due to trauma (punctures, lacerations, wounds, splenic fractures). Less-obvious causes are blood loss due to parasites (GI, urinary, pulmonary, cardiac, nasal heme), toxicities (rodenticide, copper, lead), infectious diseases (clostridial, leptospirosis), metabolic abnormalities (renal, hepatic, endocrine), vitamin deficiencies (some can be induced by drugs such as sulfas or poisons), and sepsis (Cotter 1993; Ettinger and Feldman 1995).

With an anemic animal, treatment is targeted at the underlying cause. Most of the animals that present as orphans have anemias resulting from trauma, infections, parasites, toxicities, or debilitation (inappropriate nutrition). These problems all require different therapeutic plans. Trauma, debilitation, and infections can be initially treated with fluid therapy—generally consider the animal shocky or 7% dehydrated (based on level of dehydration or assess for shock and consider replacing maintenance fluid levels as well) and replace fluid accordingly and start on broad spectrum antibiotics (ampicillin, Clavamox, trimethoprim sulfa). Monitor the animal's vital signs (temperature, heart rate, respiratory rate, CRT, and color). Additional treatment may include oxygen therapy (via facemask or endotracheal tube) or transfusion with whole blood, red cells, or Oxyglobin, under veterinary direction. Whole blood and RBC transfusions should be given IV at a rate of 1–3 ml over the first five minutes to monitor for a transfusion reaction. If a reaction occurs, give diphenhydramine (injectable Benadryl) at a dose of 2 mg/kg IM (Morgan 1992; Plumb 1998).

If Oxyglobin is administered it should be done under veterinary care at a dose of 10–30 ml/kg at a rate of 10 ml/kg/hr. The author recommends to start with the lower end of the dosage scale for Oxyglobin (Plumb 1998).

Broad-spectrum antibiotics (Clavamox 13.75 mg/kg PO, ampicillin 10 mg/kg SQ, Cefazolin 10–20 mg/kg SQ, or trimethoprim sulfas 15–20 mg/kg PO, SQ) should be given at appropriate doses. Steroids (an initial dose of 2–4 mg/kg SQ, IM, IV) may be administered once and continued based on the animal's continued assessment, physical reevaluation, and underlying problem causing the anemia (Plumb 1998).

The goal of the therapy is to stabilize the patient, provide circulatory assistance, and enhance delivery of oxygen to the tissues until the underlying cause for the anemia can be corrected.

Anemia from parasitism can be treated based on fecal/blood analysis along with supportive care outlined above (fluids and broad-spectrum antibiotics). Toxicities are trickier because the inciting toxin must be diagnosed and appropriate therapy initiated. If a toxin is suspected, consult with a veterinarian. Veterinarians should be made aware of an animal's PCV and suspected presenting problem as soon as possible so that veterinary assessment can be done and appropriate therapy instituted.

Foreign Bodies

Foreign bodies can be found in all orifices in the body and can enter the body via all orifices (body openings). Foreign bodies can be found in the eyes, ears, oral cavities, skin, and all sections of the gastrointestinal tract.

Ocular foreign bodies can be hidden deep behind the nictitans (third eyelid), entering via the eyelids, or seen penetrating the globe. Clinical signs include ocular discharge, usually unilateral, hemorrhage, and blepharospasm (Slatter 1990). A veterinarian should examine cubs with ocular foreign bodies.

Aural foreign bodies can be deep seated within the ear canal and may penetrate the tympanic membrane. Clinical signs include head shaking, head tilt, discharge from the ear, and pawing/scratching at the ear. The ear canal may be red, inflamed, and stenotic. You will probably have to use general anesthesia or heavy sedation in order to explore the ear canal. Have the veterinarian examine the ears with the animal under anesthesia. The animal must have the tympanic membranes evaluated for integrity. The animal may or may not require medication in the ear. Generally, Panalog ointment or Otomax ointment are used (Plumb 1998). If a veterinarian will be evaluating the animal within 12 hours, do not place any ointment in the ear canals so that the canals are clear of meds for easier visualization and evaluation of the tympanic membrane.

Oral foreign bodies may include grass awns, grass blades, fishhooks, bones, bullets, and string/line. Clinical signs include signs of increased ptyalism/drooling, sneezing, hemorrhage, head jerking, and excessive swallowing. Some foreign objects can be trapped behind a particular crevice in the soft palate or may be lodged in between teeth.

Nasal foreign bodies are generally caused by the inhalation of grass awns. Animals may have polyps that may cause similar clinical signs, but that is generally not the case in wild species. Clinical signs include excessive sneezing, discharge, epistaxis, or rubbing/pawing at the nose (Ettinger and Feldman 1995).

Foreign bodies of the skin may include bullets, fishhooks, nails, tape, fishing line, arrows/arrowheads, grass awns, or thorns. Check the skin for trauma or wounds. Check the interdigital spaces for penetrating foreign bodies. Clinical signs include hemorrhage, lacerations, punctures, limping, or gait abnormalities.

Treatment for all foreign bodies usually requires general anesthesia to remove them. If you suspect a foreign body is present, have a veterinarian examine the animal and treat it appropriately. Follow-up care may include any combination of the following: systemic antibiotics (Clavamox 13.75 mg/kg twice a day for 10–14 days—do not place on Baytril initially), wound dressings, wound flushes with sterile saline and dilute Nolvasan solution, or puncture/laceration repair with sutures by a veterinarian, and monitoring for wound dehiscence, abscess formation, or hemorrhage.

Gastrointestinal (GI) foreign bodies may include fishhooks, fish sinkers, or anything an animal can swallow that is not a normal food item. Clinical signs include vomiting, regurgitating, inappetence, fever, dark tarry stool, diarrhea, painful abdominal palpation (splinting), hunching over, pacing/not resting (Ettinger and Feldman 1995).

Diagnostics: If a GI foreign body is suspected, radiographs must be done, both v/d and lateral. The veterinarian should do a physical examination and review the radiographs and then determine a treatment plan. The treatment depends on the location of the foreign object. If possible, an attempt should be made to remove the object. It may be necessary to anesthetize the animal to accomplish removal.

Diarrhea

Diarrhea is defined as an increase in the frequency, fluidity, or volume of feces resulting from excessive fecal water content. Diarrhea can be characterized as acute or chronic and must be differentiated as occurring in the small versus the large bowel (Ettinger and Feldman 1995). Most of our patients present as acute cases of diarrhea and are either small or large bowel. Initial treatment of diarrhea, until it can be further characterized is fluid therapy, diet change and possibly broad spectrum antibiotics.

Acute diarrheas are generally caused by parasites, dietary indiscretion, drugs/medications, and toxins. Chronic diarrheas may be caused by uncorrected acute diarrhea problems and rectal anatomical abnormalities (strictures, masses), and can be seen in younger patients, infections (Salmonella, clostridial infection), ulcers, inflammatory bowel disease (both can be sequela of stress), toxins, or metabolic diseases (hepatic, kidney) (Ettinger and Feldman 1995).

Clinical signs include dehydration, bloat, loose/runny stool, fever, painful abdominal palpation with gaseous bowel loops, weight loss, tenesmus, and constipation.

Diagnostics include fecal examinations, fecal occult blood tests, CBC, radiographs, and fecal cytology. Fecal cultures may be necessary to determine the cause and characterize the type of diarrhea (Ettinger and Feldman 1995).

Treatment should be targeted at the underlying cause of the diarrhea. Young/baby animals should have diets reviewed and corrected. They should be given SQ fluids—crystalloids at appropriate dehydration/shock/maintenance doses—until they can be placed on the appropriate diet and clinical signs resolve. They may require systemic antibiotics (Clavamox [13.75 mg/kg twice a day for 10–14 days] or trimethoprim sulfas [15–20 mg/kg PO, SQ]) if they are compromised and appear debilitated (Plumb 1998). Fecal examinations should be done on all patients with diarrhea and appropriate anthelmintic therapy should be instituted (see Endoparasites above). Fluid therapy and dietary correction are the primary mechanisms to correct most of the acute diarrheas we see at the wildlife center.

Chronic diarrheas are more difficult to treat. Abdominal radiographs should be done. If parasites and dietary indiscretion have been ruled out and the diarrhea is persistent, the veterinarians should reassess the patient and decide on the next course of diagnostics and therapy. Maintaining fluid balance and correcting for dehydration and ongoing losses should continue in the patient (Ettinger and Feldman 1995; Plumb 1998).

Hypoglycemia

Young animals have higher glucose requirements than most adults of their species. The increased requirement is important as a source of energy for maturing metabolic functions, growth, and maintenance of normal blood glucose (BG) levels. They utilize all nutrients faster because of accelerated growth rates at young ages. It is important to restore and continue to meet their BG needs.

Clinical signs of hypoglycemia may be noted if the BG is less than 60 g/dl. Animals may appear hungry, shows signs of ataxia, or may have small seizures that may escalate and lead to loss of consciousness (Morgan 1992). Initially one can quickly apply Karo syrup to the gums and then give dextrose via gavage (stomach tube) or SQ. If giving dextrose SQ, give only a concentration of 2.5% dextrose. In most wildlife neonatal patients, it is difficult to place an IV catheter. An intraosseous (IO) catheter can be placed by the veterinarian, if the animal is severely dehydrated or hypoglycemic. Once a catheter is placed administer 5–10 ml/kg of a 20% dextrose solution (diluted from a 50% solution 2-ml sterile saline to 1.5 ml 50% dextrose) (Morgan 1992). Give this amount IV at a steady pace (not too fast and not too slow). Begin an IV drip of LRS or Normosol with an appropriate amount of dextrose added to the fluid bag to make a 2.5–10 or even up to 20% solution of dextrose (remember you can only give up to a 2.5% dextrose SQ but it is acceptable to give higher concentrations of dextrose intravenously or orally). Initially recheck the BG level (using a different vein than the one with the catheter) and modify the amount of dextrose in the fluids to accommodate the change in BG levels. If the dextrose drip is not maintaining or increasing/normalizing the BG level, give another bolus of the 20% dextrose solution. Once the BG has been corrected and the animal is stable, proper management with environmental control, nutrition, and additional SQ fluid therapy can normalize the patient.

Septicemia

Septicemia is defined as a systemic infection generally carried throughout the body via the bloodstream. The animals may or may not be febrile. Generally they are lethargic, weak, inappetent, have difficulty breathing, and have pale mucous membranes +/– small pinpoint red dots, which may also be on the skin. This can be caused by conditions of overcrowding, inappropriate nutrition or antibiotics, or wounds that are not treated.

Treatment includes immediate supportive care with fluids, warmth, and broad-spectrum antibiotics (trimethoprim sulfa or Clavamox)(Plumb 1998). Animals generally need aggressive care and veterinary evaluation.

Shock

Shock is usually a result of being hit by cars or attacked by dogs. The animals present with severe hypovolemia and hypoglycemia (see Hypoglycemia above). Animals have pale mucous membranes and glazed/glassy-appearing eyes, are recumbent, and may have an elevated temperature and a prolonged capillary refill time. If animals present with head trauma, they may have seizures, slip into a coma, have problems thermoregulating, or be hypoglycemic.

Initiate treatment with shock dose fluids (60–90 ml/kg) delivered via IV catheter if possible. After shock dose fluids have been administered, fluids with 5–10% IV dextrose may be required (unless the animal is having seizures and IV dextrose may need to be given in lieu of shock dose fluids until the animal stops seizing, then shock dose fluids may be resumed). Intravenous antibiotics and IV short acting steroids (Solu-Delta Cortef 0.2–1 mg/kg IV or 1–4 mg/kg IV). If the temperature is greater than 106°F(41°C) apply cold soaked towels to the animal. It is best to have traumatized or shocky animals evaluated by a veterinarian at the time of presentation (Ettinger and Feldman 1995; Morgan 1992; Plumb 1998).

Ocular Lesions

Eye problems include corneal ulcers, foreign bodies, lens luxations (all due to trauma). They should be evaluated by a veterinarian and possibly a veterinary ophthalmologist.

Vomiting

It is unusual to see vomiting in bear cubs. Vomiting in young animals may be the result of ingesting foreign objects, of inappropriate dietary formulation or spoiled diet, of medications, infectious agents, ulcers, heat stroke, or metabolic abnormalities (Ettinger and Feldman 1995).

Vomitus should be inspected for blood or a coffee ground consistency. The presence of blood or coffee ground material would indicate a severe problem and treatment plans should be conducted under the direction of a veterinarian (Ettinger and Feldman 1995).

Generally, one simple episode of vomiting can be treated by withholding food for a short period of time, giving SQ fluids, correcting the diet (provide a bland diet that is fresh), and monitoring for continuing signs (Ettinger and Feldman 1995). If the animal continues to vomit, a veterinarian should evaluate the animal and provide an additional treatment plan. Exploratory surgery may be necessary to correct the problem, especially if a foreign body is causing the vomiting.

Epistaxis

Epistaxis (bleeding from the nose) can be caused by a foreign body, trauma, fractures in the skull, pneumonia, or lung parasites (less likely). A rarer problem can be a coagulopathy (inappropriate clot formation/blood problem). An attempt to stop the bleeding and provide fluid therapy via an IV catheter should be instituted immediately. A physical examination should be done to search for obvious foreign objects, and radiographs should be taken to rule out any fractures or abnormal lung patterns. An activated clotting time test can be done to determine if prolonged clotting is present indicating an inherent blood factor complication or problem (Cotter 1993; Ettinger and Feldman 1995).

TAGGING

Metal ear tags should be placed in the ears upon initial physical examination to facilitate animal identification if a litter of cubs is being raised or if you anticipate receiving additional animals of similar age. Tagging also facilitates animal identification in the event an animal inadvertently escapes from an enclosure.

RELEASE

Bears that are unafraid of people should never be released. If possible, a cub can be put into a den with a hibernating female bear that has similar-sized cubs already. This would be arranged with state or federal wildlife departments, and knowledgeable local biologists. The release site should consist of water source, natural food types, and remote forested areas, preferably with minimal or no hunting of bear. It is best not to release close to the opening of bear-hunting season if the area allows bear hunting. Check the local hunting season guides. Any releases should be coordinated with the appropriate state or federal agencies for site selection, time of release, tracking, or other release considerations. Juvenile bears are often returned to the area of the original pickup location if appropriate and tracked with radio-tracking devices via an abdominal implant or radio collar. Each bear release is evaluated on a case-by-case basis with respect to postrelease research or complications.

Timing and Release Site

Behavior assessment should be monitored continually and proper steps should be taken to keep bears wild and afraid of humans. Bears that are unafraid of people should never be released. We try to release most bears in winter dens. The exceptions are:

1. Cubs that are received late in summer or fall and have not yet reached at least 65 pounds (30 kg) by the time a winter release is optimal (typically December, but some could be released as late as February). This is an average fall or pre-hibernation weight for wild bears. If they are not releasable by December, we can still do a winter release (into an artificial den) until February. Otherwise, the bear would not be released until the spring thaw when there is adequate food supply.
2. Any cub with a medical problem that necessitates holding the animal longer in captivity.
3. California bears, which are released in the fall season.
4. If a bear is released in the winter, we usually release it into a man-made den of straw bales. See Wildlife Rehabilitation for detailed guidelines on making a winter bear den. Before doing this, the bear needs to be in a dormant state, which is accomplished by decreasing food intake and encouraging hibernation behavior (Wildlife Rehabilitation). The bear will then be tranquilized, placed in a bear box, and transported to a release site (Wildlife Rehabilitation). Ensure all releases are coordinated with the state or federal departments of fish and wildlife (PAWS 2001).

Conditioning Schedule for Winter Den Release

The following schedule is appropriate for winter den release (Wildlife Rehabilitation):

- Begin reducing food no later than six weeks prior to release date, place a bear box with straw into the enclosure, and shut out all light sources.
- Twenty days prior to release, stop all food intake but offer fresh water. The bear should have access to two enclosures during food reduction stage. On day 21, confine the bear to one enclosure with the den box filled with straw and the water bucket secured to the door. Noise near the bear enclosure should be prohibited, and lights should remain off when checking the water source. Use a flashlight and insert a hose through the chain-link fencing on the door to replenish water quietly if need be every two days. At day 21 food ceases and you will no longer need to clean the cage. Food reduction takes three weeks and the bear should be in a dormant state for three more weeks before transport to the release site. This process can take longer but should never be shorter than six weeks (Table 23.1).

ACKNOWLEDGMENTS

We would like to thank Dr. John Huckabee for his contribution and training the authors to care for orphan bear cubs. We are especially thankful for his

Table 23.1. Black Bear Winter Den Prerelease Conditioning Food Guide

Day	What to Feed
1	15 cups dog food, 2 apples, 1 carrot, 1 cup mealworms, 1 cup berries
2	14 cups dog food, 2 apples, 1 carrot, 1 cup mealworms, 1/2 cup berries
3	14 cups dog food, 2 apples, 1 carrot, 1 cup mealworms, 1/2 cup berries
4	13 cups of food, 1 1/2 apples, 1 carrot, 1 cup mealworms, 1/2 cup berries
5	12 cups of dog food, 1 1/2 apples, 1 carrot, 1 cup mealworms, 1/2 cup berries
6	12 cups dog food, 1 1/2 apples, 1/2 carrot, 1 cup mealworms, 1/2 cup berries
7	11 cups dog food, 1 1/2 apples, 1/2 carrot, 1 cup mealworms, 1/2 cup berries
8	10 cups dog food, 1 apple, 1/2 carrot, 1 cup mealworms, 1/2 cup berries
9	10 cups dog food, 1 apple, 1/2 carrot, 1 cup mealworms, 1/2 cup berries
10	9 cups dog food, 1 apple, 1/2 carrot, 1/2 cup mealworms, 1/2 cup berries
11	8 cups dog food, 1 apple, 1/2 carrot, 1/2 cup mealworms, 1/2 cup berries
12	8 cups dog food, 1 apple, 1/2 carrot, 1/2 cup mealworms, 1/4 cup berries
13	7 cups dog food, 1 apple, 1/2 carrot, 1/2 cup mealworms, 1/4 cup berries
14	6 cups dog food, 1 apple, 1/2 carrot, 1/2 cup mealworms
15	5 cups dog food, 1 apple, 1/2 carrot
16	4 cups dog food, 1 apple
17	3 cups dog food, 1/2 apple
18	2 cups dog food
19	1 cup dog food
20	1/2 cup dog food
21	No food—stop cleaning cage, only check water
42	Tentative release time

expertise with the medical problems. We would also like to thank the staff, volunteers, and veterinary externs at PAWS Wildlife Center who assisted in all the medical, nursing, and orphan care responsibilities, which made it possible to treat and raise numerous bears and write this chapter during 1999–2000.

SOURCES OF PRODUCTS MENTIONED

Goodwinol Products Corp., Pierce, CO; 1-970-834-1229

PetAg Inc., 261 Keyes Ave., Hampshire, IL 60140; 1-800-323-0877, 1-800-323-6878; www.petag.com

REFERENCES

Bowman, D. D. 1999. *Georgis' parasitology for veterinarians.* Philadelphia, PA: Saunders.
Cotter, S. M. 1993. Pathophysiology of the hemiclymphatic system, course syllabus. Fall. North Grafton, MA: Tufts University School of Veterinary Medicine.
Ettinger, S. J., and E. C. Feldman. 1995. *Textbook of veterinary internal medicine.* 4th ed. Philadelphia, PA: Saunders.
Fowler, M. E. 1978. Carnivores. In *Zoo and wildlife medicine.* Philadelphia, PA: Saunders.
Macdonald, D., ed. 1995. *The encyclopedia of mammals.* New York: Facts on File.
Morgan, R. V., ed. 1992. *Handbook of small animal medicine.* 2d ed. Philadelphia, PA: Saunders.
Murtaugh, R. 1994. Principles of medicine, course syllabus. Spring. North Grafton, MA: Tufts University School of Veterinary Medicine; Section on Small Animal Fluid Therapy.
Nowak, R. M. 1991. *Walker's mammals of the world,* vol. 2. 5th ed. Baltimore: The Johns Hopkins University Press.
PAWS wildlife rehabilitation manual. 2001. Lynnwood, WA: PAWS Wildlife Center.
Plumb, Donald C. 1998. *Veterinary drug handbook.* 3d ed. Ames: Iowa State University Press.
Slatter, D. 1990. *Fundamentals of veterinary ophthalmology.* 2d ed. Philadelphia, PA: Saunders.
Wildlife Rehabilitation, Volume 13

24
Polar Bears

Gail Hedberg

INTRODUCTION

Polar bears (*Ursus maritimus*) are maintained in over 85 different captive settings throughout the world. International Species Inventory Systems (ISIS) records state that the number of captive births in the last 25 years is greater than one thousand. Table 24.1 summarizes ISIS data showing that the mortality rate for captive polar bear cubs in the first three months of life was approximately 56%.

The following information presents the most current data available. Detailed experiences from a successful hand-rearing polar bear project are provided. All products mentioned are listed in the "Sources of Products Mentioned" section at the end of the chapter. Collaborating with and compiling data from other zoological institutions may provide you with a foundation to further ensure survival for the polar bear, a noted difficult, sensitive, and delicate neonatal carnivore.

NATURAL HISTORY

Female polar bears become sexually mature at five to six years of age, while males become mature at eight. Breeding normally occurs between March and July.

The total gestation period is approximately eight months. Gestation includes a period of delayed implantation, in which the fertilized ovum stops maturing as it floats free within the uterus. Approximately six months later, the embryo attaches itself to the uterine wall and resumes development. The actual embryonic development is estimated to be four months.

The pregnant bear then "dens up" until the birth. Pregnant polar bears in captivity continue eating during this phase. A female in the den has a reduced heart rate and metabolism. Delayed implantation ensures survival for the pregnant female. In the event that the female has not put on enough fat reserves before denning, the embryo will not implant and is reabsorbed by her body. The captive female will need to gain an additional 200 kg between the time of conception and the time of denning so that she can have the fat reserves to allow the embryo(s) to reach full term, and begin lactating for rearing cubs (Hanning 1992).

Loud noises may bother many captive polar bears. Environmental noise, such as construction projects within close proximity to the bear habitat, must be eliminated for the entire two- to three-month denning period. Providing access to secure off-exhibit cubbing dens is the key to successful captive births of polar bear cubs. I have had experience with successful monitoring of the birth process in which an infrared camera was set up to record the female in the den. Daily review of the 24-hour videotape provided a record of the female's movements. The complete birth cycle was recorded and reviewed. This visual husbandry management tool has had extreme importance in monitoring the neonate and the maternal capacity of the female postpartum.

Average birth weight is 454–680 g. Average litter size is two, with litter size ranging from one to four. Litters greater than two are rare.

Preparation (Three Months Prior to Birth)

Birth patterns for captive polar bears are very predictable. Captive births begin in October and continue through January. It is important to prepare for any circumstances that may present a cub for hand rearing. A video monitoring system is extremely helpful if maternal neglect is a concern. Cubs are

Table 24.1. Historical Data for Captive Polar Bear Births (No. of Births = 1115)

		Age	Deaths	Per day	Per week	Per month
Month 1	Week 1	0 days	213	19.10%	45.50%	53.40%
		1 day	98	8.80%		
		2 days	85	7.60%		
		3 days	51	4.60%		
		4 days	24	2.20%		
		5 days	19	1.70%		
		6 days	17	1.50%		
	Week 2		57		5.10%	
	Week 3		22		2.00%	
	Week 4		9		0.80%	
Month 2			21			1.90%
Month 3			16			1.40%
			632			

Note: Based on all ISIS data on captive-born animals: 31-Dec-00 (raw data as received from participating zoos). The following data are for captive-born animals (Polar bear, *Ursus maritimus*), births by region: European, 471; North American, 588; Asian, 23; African, 17; Australian/New Zealand, 14.

often presented in a hypothermic, weakened state. The primary cause of mortality in newborns is maternal neglect and trauma.

The following are some important steps that may be taken to assist care providers in hand rearing polar bear cubs:

- Research and discuss milk formula diet options with other institutions. (See Table 24.3 for complete historical listing of hand-rearing projects by institution.)
- Maintain a minimum of two incubators (isolettes) in ready state for use with multiple cubs (thermostat controlled internal temperature capacity of 90°F [32.5°C] with humidity option).
- Acquire assorted presterilized bottles, nipples, gowns, and surgical gloves designated for this project.
- Keep a supply of frozen polar bear serum for alternate source of immunoglobulins.
- Have a written plan ahead of time and review it with all care providers.

RECORD KEEPING

Table 24.2 is a sample form for keeping track of essential data.

CRITERIA FOR INTERVENTION

Newborn cubs are rarely presented in plain view for the animal care staff to hear or see. A well-cared-for cub will be content to sleep between feedings. A natural posture for the sow is to lie on her back and allow the cub to nurse. Excessive grooming may cause trauma to a cub. The most noteworthy signal for initially distressed cubs is loud, excessive bawling or crying. The dam should surround the cubs with her body. If cubs are left unattended, then hypothermia and/or hypoglycemia will occur. A weak or compromised cub cannot vocalize.

INITIAL CARE AND STABILIZATION

A cub should be transported in a heated, towel-lined Styrofoam box. Use latex exam gloves filled with warm water to maintain a constant heat source until the cub is transferred to a more sophisticated incubator. Human infant-care isolettes provide the optimum space and needed temperature gradient control for the duration of this controlled environment (Fig. 24.1).

An immediate action to warm the cub's core body temperature is critical. Normal newborn cub body temperature ranges from 96.8°F (36.0°C) in the first days to 97–99°F (36.2–37.2°C). After one to two

Table 24.2. Sample Record

Date _____ Age (days) _____ Weight _____ (+/−) _____ % _____

Location _____ Littermates _____

	FOOD OFFERED			CONSUMED				EVALUATION				
Time	Type/Amount	Solids	Liquids	CC	Grams	How Long	Response	Feces	Urine	B-Temp	Attitude	Medical
Totals												

Common name _____

Zoo ID _____

FECES
0 - None
F - Firm
SF - Semifirm
SL - Semiloose

URINE
0 - None
N - Normal
A - Abnormal

RESPONSE
0 - No Response
1 - Poor/Slow
2 - Moderate
3 - Enthusiastic

ATTITUDE
D - Depressed
S - Sedate/Resting
A - Active/Alert
HT - Hypertense/Stressed

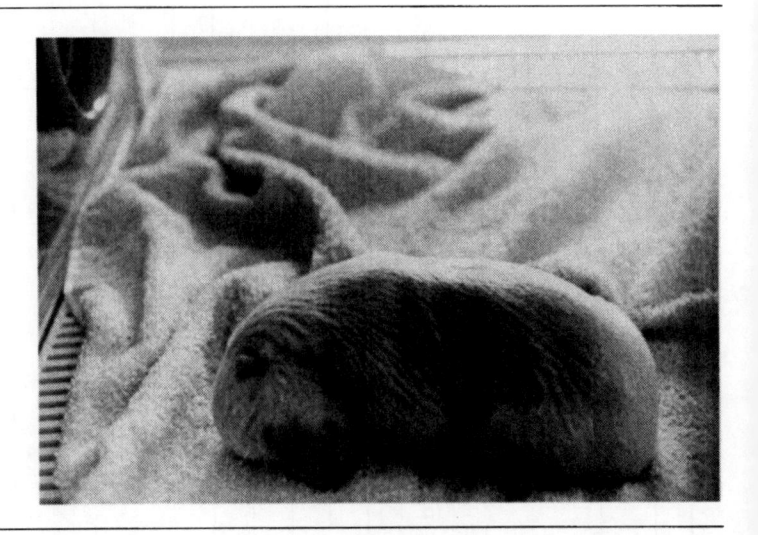

Figure 24.1. Polar bear cub sleeping in incubator.

weeks of age, the temperature range is near 100°F (37.8°C). Temperature monitoring is best accomplished with a pediatric digital rectal thermometer. Once the cub is placed in an incubator at 86–88°F (30–32°C), surround the compromised cub with fresh latex gloves filled with warm water or small 250-ml saline IV bags warmed in a microwave oven. Replace these bags as they become cool.

Multiple incubators facilitate quick transfer to a clean, warm environment.

Generally, multiple conspecifics can remain together but it may be necessary to separate cubs because nursing on a littermates genitals is a potential problem.

Maintaining clean incubators is mandatory and cubs cannot be exposed to changes in ambient temperatures, even for just routine cleaning. Padding the incubator minimizes irritation to the muzzle from excessive "rooting around." A 6-in stockingette filled with rolled cotton or Styrofoam beads from a beanbag chair works extremely well. Line the perimeter of the incubator. These bumpers are reusable if care is taken when washing and drying. Always have extra sets ready for replacement. "Bumper guards" also give a solitary cub an artificial surrogate with which to bond. Polyester fleece (see Sources of Products Mentioned) is another suitable bedding source. This product is very durable and seems to hold up the best even when left with unsupervised animals. Extreme caution should be used, however when selecting synthetic fleece. Animals that suckle on these fabrics may ingest fibers and cause constipation. Many artificial fabrics ("fake furs") are available and can be sewn in shapes that resemble fabric-covered bolsters. This replicates the shape of a maternal sow's abdomen or appendage, and all cubs feel more secure when draped over their mother.

Initial care of the umbilicus is of utmost importance as this is a primary source for entry of bacterial pathogens. One method for the care of the umbilicus includes the application of chlorhexidine (0.5%) (Nolvasan 2% solution diluted 1:2 with sterile water) every 6 hours for a minimum of 72 hours and watch the site for heat or swelling. This is more effective than 2% iodine or Betadine. Seven percent iodine is caustic, burns the end of the umbilicus, and traps bacteria within the stump. Dilute Betadine has been substituted with the theory that it is less caustic, but the potential for bacterial entrapment still exists. Now chlorhexidine is used because it is less caustic and has a wider bacterial spectrum (Madigan 1997). The umbilicus "tag" will dry and dissappear approximately 48 hours after birth.

Literature indicates that serum from an adult polar bear should be given to a neonate whenever possible (Kenny, Irlbeck, and Eller 1999; Torgerson 1990; Michalowski 1971). I followed that recommendation and gave serum orally and subcutaneously to a one-day-old cub. The eighteen cc of banked frozen serum was obtained from a nonrelated captive polar bear housed at another institution. The initial dose was 9.0 ml subcutaneously followed by 9.0 ml orally, divided equally into the next three feedings. The cub's weight was 645 g.

New research for serum as a source for antibody protection in dogs states that both oral administration and subcutaneous injection are used, but intestinal absorption is minimal after 12 hours. The dose is 22.0 ml/kg as a single dose. Higher IgM concentrations were achieved with the S/C route (Bouchard et al. 1992; Poffenbarger et al. 1991; Glickman et al. 1988). Utilizing this new research information, the recommended amounts of frozen stored serum (at −70°C) is 10–15 cc per cub, depending on the animal's presenting weight.

A review of available literature for maternal polar bear milk analysis shows that the overall composition changes throughout the lactation cycle (Cook et al. 1970; Roken and Roken 1981). A milk sample from day 13 of lactation showed the fat level to be 14.9% in a captive sow (Roken and Roken 1981). Other samples from wild-caught sows approximately at 16 months of lactation are 33.1–69.5% fat. Changes in milk composition may also act to conserve maternal energy stores to ensure survival of the sow (Derocher, Andriashek, and Arnould 1993). This once again validates the need for captive sows to be in optimum nutritional status for adequate lactation.

The fat component of maternal polar bear (*Ursus maritimus*) milk has a wide range of reported concentrations. The range is 14.9% to 69.5%. This information shows the importance of a gradual increase in the fat component for hand-rearing milk formulas.

The use of commercial feline and canine milk replacers for hand rearing exotic carnivores has been well documented by published accounts in the *International Zoo Yearbook* and AZA's *Infant Diet Notebook*. A complete resource guide is listed at the end of this chapter (see Sources).

In 1993 a reformulation occurred with Esbilac. Butterfat was added to improve mixability. Some exotic species exhibited digestive problems with this new formulation. Lactobezoar was reported in tiger and leopards. In conjunction with the above change came the development of Zoologic, a line of products made by PetAg, Inc. This system of seven milk replacers is mixed and matched to meet the appropriate maternal milk analysis. The Zoologic products appropriate in ursid hand rearing are Milk Matrix 33/40 and Milk Matrix 42/50. The product numbers represent the minimum crude protein and fat percentages. Note that these two formulations are original pre-1993 powdered Esbilac and KMR product without *butterfat*. These PetAg products are accessible for the international market.

Nurturall milk replacers by Veterinary Products Laboratories and Just Born milk replacers by

Table 24.3. Historical List of Polar Bear Cub Hand-Rearing Projects and Base Diet

Date	Institution	Formula
Jan 2000	Adventure World, Japan	Esbilac Powder
Oct 1999	Brookfield Zoo, Illinois	Esbilac Powder/MultiMilk
Mar 1998	Alaska Zoo, Anchorage	Esbilac Powder, cream
Nov 1994	Denver Zoo, Colorado	Esbilac Powder, half/half cream
1989	Rostock Zoo, Germany	Soyaval
Dec 1988	Rostov-on-Don Zoo, Russia	Goat's milk
1985	Leningrad Zoo, Russia	10% cream
Nov 1985*	San Diego Zoo, California	Esbilac Liquid, cream
Jan 1984	Knoxville Zoo, Tennessee	Esbilac Powder
Dec 1982	Zoo Atlanta, Georgia	Cream/water
Nov 1982	San Francisco Zoo, California	Esbilac Powder
Jan 1980	Toronto Zoo, Canada	Esbilac Powder
1980	Leningrad Zoo, Russia	Soy powder, goats milk, cream
Nov 1976	Lincoln Park Zoo, Illinois	Esbilac Liquid, cream
Nov 1972	Kolmarden Zoo, Sweden	Sobee, milk powder, egg yolk powder
Nov 1971*	Topeka Zoo, Kansas	Esbilac Powder, cream
Dec 1969*	St. Paul Zoo, Minnesota	Esbilac Powder
Dec 1969	Rochester Zoo, New York	Esbilac Powder

*Did not survive.

Farnam Pet Products are basically the same products. It is a marketing clarification only. Nurturall is only available through a licensed veterinarian. Just Born is available through a retail outlet. Both of the above products are labeled for use in puppies or kittens, as is Lactol milk replacer manufactured by Sherley's Limited available in the United Kingdom. All of these are available to the international market. Artificial milk diets have limitations when compared to maternal milk. The formulations cannot fully duplicate maternal milk composition.

Esbilac Powder or Milk Matrix 33/40 is the recommended product for hand rearing polar bears. Esbilac Powder is a canine (puppy milk replacer). See table 24.3 for a complete international summary of polar bear hand-rearing projects. Esbilac has been used successfully with and without the addition of whole milk products. Table 24.4 outlines in detail the ratio of Esbilac Powder to sterile water. I prefer using sterile water when making formula because of the potential risk of contaminants in tap or bottled water. This precaution can be relaxed when the neonate is stable. Note the concentration increases as the cub matures. If Esbilac Powder is unavailable, then review the European accounts for alternative milk products.

DAILY NURSERY CARE ROUTINES

Weigh the cub daily at the same time. Expect a weight gain of 30–90 g/day after initial stabilization.

An initial feeding schedule is every 2.5 hrs × 24 hrs for the first seven days. Dietary adjustments and manipulations are introduced gradually and only one item adjusted at a time. This species does not tolerate rapid changes in diet. I followed a strong recommendation to limit the amount of formula fed at each feeding (see Table 24.4; also Michalowski 1982, Phone conversation with author).

The Playtex nurser system with plastic liners is suggested because of the expanded surface area of the latex nipple as it attaches to the bottle (see Fig. 24.2). The nose of the cub hits the plastic rim of the standard baby bottle. Polar bear cubs have a very strong suckle response. The orthodontic NUK nipple should be used to replace the standard Playtex nipple after the initial artificial rearing protocol has been established. The Playtex disposable plastic liners help keep the formula sterile.

Constipation is the most commonly reported medical problem. The addition of corn syrup in the milk formula has been beneficial as an aid in reducing the tendency for constipation. The osmotic property of glucose in corn syrup acts as a natural laxative in the gastrointestinal tract. Use 1.0 ml corn syrup per 25 ml prepared formula. Retention of water by osmosis promotes consistent defecation. ABDEC, a pediatric liquid oral vitamin source, is recommended at a dose of 0.5 ml per 100 ml of prepared formula.

A dose of cod liver oil initially at 5 ml/day supported the increased fat requirement. Vitamin A

Table 24.4. Polar Bear Cub Milk Replacer Feeding Schedule, San Francisco Zoo, 1984

Age	Weight	Esbilac Powder	Daily Intake (limit feedings)
1 day	645 g	1:3 powder/sterile water	9 feedings/day 28 ml feeding
9 days	1020 g	1:2 powder/sterile water	9 feedings/day 28 ml feeding
16–22 days	1.57 kg (17 days)	1:1.5 powder/sterile water	8 feedings/day 28 ml feeding
23–29 days	1.85 kg (23 days)	1:1.5 powder/sterile water	7 feedings/day 42 ml feeding
30–47 days	3.82 kg (45 days)	1:1 powder/sterile water	6 feedings/day 56 ml feeding
48–50 days		1:1 powder/sterile water	6 feedings/day 71 ml feeding
51–74 days	4.9 kg (52 days)	1:1 powder/sterile water.	
	6.3 kg (66 days)	Add 15 g (1 TBS) increments Hills Feline Science Diet CD every day = 120 g maximum	6 feedings/day 85 ml feeding
75 days	8.0 kg	Eating from bowl above formula 1:1 powder/sterile water + Hills Feline Science Diet CD 2:1	4 feedings/day 120 ml feeding

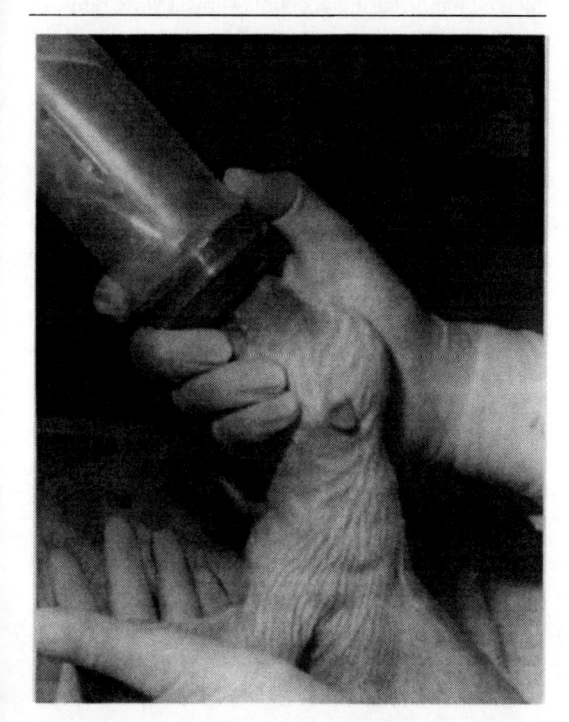

Fig. 24.2. Polar bear cub nursing on a bottle.

requirements have not been established for this species. It is uncertain if they are predisposed to an increased requirement for vitamin A or have a high tolerance. Use caution when feeding fish as part of the weaning diet. Certain fish like carp, herring, mackerel, smelt, and capelin, have the enzyme thiaminase. Thiaminase destroys thiamine (vitamin B_1). Supplement with 25 mg of thiamine per kilogram of fish fed (Allen, Oftedal, and Baer 1996).

TIPS FOR WEANING FROM FORMULA TO SOLID FOOD

My personal experience confirms that weaning a polar bear is challenging. Having gone through the mechanics of bottle-feeding for the preceding six weeks, the basic emotional and psychological needs of a cub will have been satisfied. Now the cub and caregivers must overcome two major developmental hurdles: teething and weaning.

Teething is a very difficult developmental process. The cub may have intense "bawling" or crying episodes. The cub can exhibit signs of colic and refuse scheduled feedings. This begins at six to eight weeks of age. It seems to last for one week. Massaging the gums and using frozen teething rings are helpful. Pediatric Anbesol Gel may be used topically on the affected area for short-term relief for cub and caregiver.

Early weaning may be necessary due to aggressive biting and chewing of the nipple. The normal dentition of a neonate begins at approx 45 days of age. Begin offering one tablespoon per day (15 g/day) of solids in the formula at 50 days of age. This can be a commercial canned carnivore diet.

Begin offering a bowl of formula/gruel in the morning after the first bottle. This can begin at age 70 days. One suggested source for solids is Science Diet Feline Maintenance prescription diet. Gradually introduce and make transitions to soaked omnivore biscuit at age 80 days.

OTHER PRACTICAL INFORMATION

This species normally exhibits slow physical development when compared to exotic felids and canids.

Day 28: ears open, eyes beginning to open
Day 33: eyes completely open
Day 40: tries to walk
Day 45: out of incubator
Day 56: molars erupt; prefers cooler environment (65°F)
Day 63: Offer shallow pan of water due to cub's tendency to immerse entire head into bowl when learning to drink water.

The period from bottle nursing to independence from caregivers is approximately eight months. This species requires detailed attention 24 hours a day. The intense monitoring of a cub is what increases survivability during the first 30 days.

Be aware of a cub's sensitivity to increased levels of environmental stimulation. All external ambient noise should be minimized. Room lighting should be dim and the incubator should be covered for the first three weeks.

During this time the normal development of the cub requires it to be maintained in a constant temperature-controlled environment until fully furred. The importance of hygiene and sterile handling of all equipment and utensils cannot be emphasized enough. The caretaker's initial direct contact with the animal should occur with sterile gloves and surgical gown in a nursery environment. This will minimize exposure to potential pathogens. Change gloves each time the cub is fed. A change of gloves is required between multiple cubs, although this added precaution might be lifted after the first week of age. No other animals should be housed in the immediate vicinity.

Proper elimination of urine and feces from the animal should occur outside of the incubator. The use of absorbent disposable pads is helpful. Stimulate the cub to urinate and defecate by gently patting the perineal area with warm-water-soaked gauze or cotton pad. This is done each time the cub is handled for a scheduled feeding. Wear latex gloves when stimulating the cub to urinate and defecate.

The cub should never be exposed to a fecal-contaminated environment. This is why multiple incubators are useful. The cub may be placed directly into the second unit while the first unit is cleaned. Also in the event of equipment failure, a back-up unit is always available. Once the cub is fully furred, it will be more content to spend time out of the incubator. This is evident at about three to four weeks of age. This is when you can begin to lower the temperature of the incubator a few degrees a day until it reaches room temperature. There will be a time when the cub needs an ambient temperature much cooler than is comfortable for its human surrogates. This occurs about seven to eight weeks of age.

The emotional needs of polar bear cubs require the caregiver(s) to fill the role as a surrogate for an extended period. Behaviors such as swimming can be gradually introduced when cubs are 18 weeks of age. A small wading pool can be filled with just enough water to wet the cub's feet. This process can be repeated as often as two to three times a week until it is time to find a deeper pool.

The most important factor is the slow introduction of water. A shallow pan of drinking water was introduced at 63 days of age. Polar bear cubs have a tendency to immerse their entire head into a bowl of water. They need to learn how to drink. The same holds true when introducing a large body of water for swimming. Caretaker and cub should walk in the shallow end before the cub faces a water level that is over its head. The caregiver should constantly give reassurance as the cub follows. The caregiver should wear waders or a wet suit to facilitate constant supervision. A dog harness with a long lunge line keeps the bear within reach. This process should be slow and controlled as the cub learns to handle water. Later, crushed ice may be introduced for enrichment.

CONCLUSIONS

The key to a successful outcome is commitment and extreme dedication from the caregiver(s). This species presents unique challenges. Limited documented hand-rearing accounts show a wide range of formula trials. It is important to continually make adjustments and modifications. With careful planning and skilled implementation of hand-rearing protocols, a well-adjusted cub can reach adulthood.

ACKNOWLEDGMENTS

I would like to thank Laurie Gage, Daniel Michalowski, Andrew Derocher, Ann Malley, Debra Hoffman, Diana Weinhardt, Forrest Townsend, Laurie Bingaman Lackey, Lydia Kolter, Karin Linke, Malcom Ramsay, Pat Lampi, Koji Imazu, Andrew Malov, Nataly Popova, Tatiana Voltchenko, Marina Poltavskaja, Rita McManamon, Ellen Dierenfeld, Kerri Slifka, Carrie Cramer, Lisa Cline, Quinton Rogers, Rosemarie Hughey, and Svetlana Pyke for information. For editorial support, a special thank you to Freeland Dunker and Ellen Williams. Digital imaging assistance was provided by Sherrie Ransom.

SOURCES OF PRODUCTS MENTIONED

ABDEC: Parke-Davis & Co., Detroit, MI 43232

Anbesol: Whitehall-Robbins Healthcare, Madison, NJ 07940; 1-888-797-5638; www.anbesol.com/index.asp

Beaphar, Inc., 6200 Falls of Neuse Rd., Suite 102, Raleigh, NC 27609; 1-919-855-9990, FAX 1-919-855-9991

C/D Hills Prescription Diet: PO Box 148, Topeka, KS 66601; 1-800-445-5777; www.hillspet.com

Esbilac: PetAg, Inc., 261 Keyes Ave, Hampshire, IL 60140; 1-800-323-6878; www.petag.com

Isolette: Used Air Shields Incubator, Rankin Biomedical Corporation, 9580 Dolores Dr., Clarkston, MI 48348; 1-248-625-4104, FAX 1-248-625-1070; E-mail: rankin@tir.com

Just Born: Farnam Pet Products, A division of Farnam Companies, Inc., Phoenix, AZ 85013; 1-800-234-2269; www.farnam.com

Lactol: Sherley's Limited, Homefield Rd., Haverhill, Suffolk CB9 8QP U.K.; Phone 01440 715700, FAX 01440 713940; E-mail: sherleys@dial.pipex.com

Mead Johnson Nutritionals: 1-812-429-6339, FAX 1-812-429-7189; 24-hour toll-free fax on demand 1-888-606-7737; E-mail: www.mead-johnson.com

NeoCalglucon: Geneva Pharmaceuticals, Division of Sandoz, Inc.; 2655 W. Midway Blvd., PO Box 446, Broomfield, CO 80038-0446; 1-800-525-8747, FAX 1-303-469-6467; www.novartis.com

Nurturall: Veterinary Products Laboratories, PO Box 34820, Phoenix, AZ 85067-4820; 1-888-241-9545; www.vpl.com

Playtex Products, Inc.; PO Box 7016, Dover, DE 19903-1516; 1-800-222-0453, 1-302-678-6000, FAX 1-302-678-6200; www.playtexbaby.com

Polar Bear Diet-Dry: Animal Spectrum, Inc., PO Box 721, North Platte, NE 69103-0721; 1-800-228-4005, FAX 1-308-534-7015

Polyester Fleece: Body Gear for Pets, PO Box 5924, Petaluma, CA 94955; 1-800-699-4050, FAX 1-707-792-2262; E-mail: bodygear@pacbell.net

Stockingette: Balfour Health Care, Div. Of Kayser-Roth Hosiery, Inc., 425 N. Gateway Ave., Rockwood, TN 37854

Wireless Thermometer: Oregon Scientific International, Ltd., 19861 SW 95th Place, Tualatin, OR 97062; 1-888-274-7980, FAX 1-541-465-9406; E-mail: www.oregonscientific.com

Zoologic Milk Matrix: PetAg Inc., 261 Keyes Ave., Hampshire, IL 60140; 1-800-323-0877, 1-800-323-6878; www.petag.com

REFERENCES

Allen, M., O. T. Oftedal, and D. J. Baer. 1996. Feeding and nutrition of carnivores. In *Wild mammals in captivity: Principles and techniques*. Chicago: University of Chicago Press.

AZA. 1999. *Infant diet notebook*. Silver Spring, MD: American Zoo and Aquarium Association.

Bouchard, G., et al. 1992. Absorption of an alternate source of immunoglobulin in pups. *American Journal of Veterinary Research* 53(2): 230.

Cook, H. W., J. W. Lentfer, A. M. Pearson, and B. E. Baker. 1970. Polar bear milk. IV. Gross composition, fatty acid, and mineral constitution. *Canadian Journal of Zoology* 48: 217–19.

Derocher, A. E., D. Andriashek, J. P. Y. Arnould. 1993. Aspects of milk composition and lactation in polar bears. *Canadian Journal of Zoology* 71 561–67.

Hanning, J. 1992. Keeping and breeding polar bears at Edinborough Zoo. In *Management guidelines for bears and raccoons*. Bristol, U.K.: ABWAK.

Glickman, L. T., F. S. Shofer, A. J. Payton, L. L. Laster, and P. J. Felsburg. 1988. Survey of serum IgG and IgM concentrations in a large Beagle population in which IgG deficiency has been identified. *American Journal of Veterinary Research* 49(8): 1240–45.

Kenny, D. E., N. A. Irlbeck, and J. L. Eller. 1999. Rickets in two hand-reared polar bear (*Ursus maritimus*) cubs. *J Zoo Wild Med.* 30(1): 132–40.

Madigan, J. E. 1997. Medical care. In *Manual of equine neonatal medicine*. Woodland, CA: Live Oak Publishing.

Michalowski, D. R. 1971. Hand rearing a polar bear cub at Rochester Zoo. *International Zoo Yearbook*. London: Zoological Society.

Poffenbarger, E. M., P. N. Olson, M. L. Chandler, H. B. Seim, and M. Varman. 1991. Use of adult dog serum as a substitute for colostrum in the neonatal dog. *American Journal of Veterinary Research* 52(8):1221.

Raby, K., G. Hedberg, K. Hobson, F. H. Dunker, and R. A. Bennett. 1996. Clinical aspects of a neonatal care program. *Proceedings of the American Association of Zoo Veterinarians*. Lawrence, KS.

Roken, B. O., and B. Roken. 1981. Successful rearing of young male polar bear *Thalarctos maritimus* in Kolmardens Zoo (Kunstliche Aufzucht Eines Neugeborenen Mannlichen Eisbaren [Thalarctos Maritimus Phipps 1774] in Kolmardens Djurpark). *Zool. Gart.* 51(2):119–22.

Torgerson, W. R. 1990. Polar bear biology and medicine. In *Handbook of marine mammal medicine*, edited by Leslie A. Dierauf. Boca Raton: CRC Press.

SUGGESTED READING

Arnould, J. P. Y., and M. A. Ramsay. 1994. Milk production and milk consumption in polar bears during the ice-free period in western Hudson Bay. *Canadian Journal of Zoology* 72: 1365–70.

Baker, B. E., C. R. Harington, and A. L. Symes. 1963. Polar bear milk: Gross composition and fat constitution. *Canadian Journal of Zoology* 41: 1035–39.

Baker, B. E., F. Y. Y. Huang, and C. R. Harington. 1963. The carbohydrate content of polar bear milk casein. *Biochemical and Biophysical Research Communications* 13: 227–30.

Baker, B. E., V. B. Hatcher, and C. R. Harington. 1967. Polar bear milk. III. Gel electrophoresis studies of protein fractions isolated from polar bear milk and human milk. *Canadian Journal of Zoology* 45: 1205–10.

Bannikov, A. G., ed. 1969. *The polar bear and its conservation in the Soviet Arctic*. Leningrad: Hydrometeorological Publishing House.

Colby, R. H., C. A. Mattacks, and C. M. Pond. 1993. The gross anatomy, cellular structure, and fatty acid composition of adipose tissue in captive polar bears (*Ursus maritimus*). *Zoo Biol.* 12(3):267–75.

Forthman, D. L., S. D. Elder, R. Bakeman, T. W. Kurkowski, C. C. Noble, and S. W. Winslow. 1992. Effects of feeding enrichment on behavior of three species of captive bears. *Zoo Biol.* 11(3):187–95.

Foster, W. J. 1981. Dermatitis in polar bears—A nutritional approach to therapy. *Proceedings of the American Association of Zoo Veterinarians.* Seattle, WA.

Grams, K., and G. Ziegler. 1998. Enrichment options: Large carnivores-bears (*U. maritimus, U. americanus, U. arctos*) *Animal Keepers' Forum* 25(7): 282–83.

Hedberg, G. E., R. A. Bennett, and F. H. Dunker. 1995. Preliminary studies on the use of milbemycin oxime for treatment of polar bears (*Ursus maritimus*) with chronic balisascaris transfuga infection. *Proceedings of the American Association of Zoo Veterinarians.* East Lansing, MI.

Hess, J. K. 1971. Hand rearing polar bear cubs at the Saint Paul Zoo. *International Zoo Yearbook: Zoological Society of London* 11: 102.

Jenness, R., A. W. Erickson, and J. J. Craighead. 1972. Some comparative aspects of milk from four species of bears. *Journal of Mammalogy* 53: 34–47.

Joseph, B. E., E. D. Asper, and J. E. Antrim. 1990. Marine mammal transport. In *Handbook of marine mammal medicine: Health, disease, and rehabilitation*, edited by Leslie A. Dierauf. Boca Raton: CRC Press.

Kenny, D. E., et al. 1998. Determination of vitamins D, A, and E in sera and vitamin D in milk from captive and free-ranging polar bears (*Ursus maritimus*), and 7-dehydrocholestrol levels in skin from captive polar bears. *Zoo Biology* 17: 285–93.

Kohm, A. 1991. Vitamin A, D, and E supplement revitalized breeding of polar bears in Karlsruhe. *Zool. Gart.* 61(1):21–23.

Latinen, K. 1987. Longevity and fertility of the polar bear, *Ursus Maritimus Phipps*, in captivity. *Zool. Gart.* 57(2–3):197–99.

———. 1984. Polar bear management at the Detroit zoo. *Am. Assoc. Zool. Parks Aquariums Regional Conf. Proc.*119–26.

Law, G, H. Boyle, and J. Johnston. 1986. Notes on polar bear management at Glasgow Zoo. *Ratel* 13(2):56–58.

Leatherland, J. F., and K. Ronald. 1981. Plasma concentrations of thyroid hormones in a captive and feral polar bear (*Ursus Maritimus*). *Comp. Biochem. Physiol. A Comp. Physiol* 70(4):575–77.

Linke, K. 1989. Hand raising an Ice Bear (*Thalarctos maritimus*) at the Garten Rostock Zoo. *Jahresbericht 1990*, 36–44.

Miller, G. D. 1983. Responses of captive grizzly and polar bears to potential repellents. *Int. Conf. Bear Res. Manage.* 5:275–79.

Nunley, L. 1977. Successful rearing of polar bears / Thalarctos Maritimus/ at Tulsa zoo. *International Zoo Yearbook* 17:161–64.

Papini, R., P. Cavicchio, and L. Casarosa. 1991. *Baylisascaris transfuga* found in captive polar bears (THALARCTOS MARITIMUS) in Italy. *Ann. Fac. Med. Vet. Pisa* 43: 151–55.

Poulsen, E. M., V. Honeyman, P. A. Valentine, and G. Teskey. 1996. Use of fluoxetine for the treatment of stereotypical pacing behavior in a captive polar bear [see comments]. *Journal of American Veterinary Medical Association* 209(8):1470–4.

Teskey, G. C., P. A. Valentine, E. M. B. Poulsen., V. Honeyman, and R. M. Cooper. 1996. Treatment of stereotypic behavior in the polar bear (*Ursus maritimus*) (Tratamiento de la conducta esterotipada en el oso polar [*Ursus maritimus*]). *Am. Assoc. Zoo Vet. Annu. Proc.*, 334–36. (Proceedings of the American Association of Zoo Veterinarians Annual Conference, November 3–8, 1996, Puerto Vallarta, Mexico, abstracts only.)

Thomas, W. D. 1968. Mixed exhibit for polar bears and arctic foxes, Thalarctos Maritimus and Alopex Lagopus, at the Omaha Zoo. *International Zoo Yearbook* 8:18–19

Wortman, J. D., M. D. Larue. 1974. Hand rearing polar bear cubs at the Topeka Zoo. *International Zoo Yearbook: Zoological Society of London* 14: 215.

25
Raccoons

Darlene DeGhetto, Sophia Papageorgiou, and Jennifer Convy

NATURAL HISTORY

The raccoon is of the order Carnivora, family Procyonidae, genus *Procyon*, and species *lotor*.

Description

Raccoons are brownish-gray with interspersed black hair above and a grayish coat below. They have a bushy tail with four to six alternating black and brownish-gray rings. A black mask is evident on their face, which is outlined in white. The adult head to rump length is 24–27 in. with a 7.5–16-in. long tail (Macdonald 1995; Nowak 1991).

Reproduction

Mating season is from December to August, and the gestation period is approximately 63 days. Peak mating occurs in February and March. Females usually have one litter per year with one to seven kits per litter born in April and May. Weaning of wild kits takes place between two and four months of age (Macdonald 1995; Nowak 1991).

Habitat and Activity

Raccoons are nocturnal and successfully occupy diverse habitats. They prefer forested bottomlands near streams, but also thrive in cities and suburbs. Dens are usually made of leaf litter in hollow trees or any protected area including attics and crawl spaces. They do not hibernate, even in very cold climates (Macdonald 1995; Nowak 1991). They are excellent swimmers and climbers. Their forepaws articulate and are capable of opening latches on cage doors, making them great escape artists. Raccoons tend to become desensitized to humans easily so it is very important to keep the kits fearful of humans.

Natural Diet

Raccoons will consume a variety of foods including fruits, nuts, insects, small mammals, birds, eggs, crayfish, frogs, worms, fish, clams, turtles, and acorns (Macdonald 1995; Nowak 1991).

Behavior Considerations

Captive and wild raccoons are primarily nocturnal. If they are out and about during daylight hours this can be a clue to a significant medical problem. Raccoons are very territorial but social animals. In captivity they are aggressive and easily bored. Juveniles require a behaviorally enriched environment such as climbing structures/tools, water access, natural foliage, and live-prey training. Raccoons become easily accustomed to humans. We cannot stress enough that human contact should be minimal (as is necessary for feeding/cleaning/medical care). This is especially important because in many communities raccoons are considered nuisance animals (Macdonald 1995; Nowak 1991; PAWS 2001).

Physiological Parameters

Adult raccoons weigh 5.4–21.6 kg. Their body temperature ranges from 100 to 102°F (37.8 to 38.9°C). Their heart rate ranges from 128 to 180 beats per minute (Macdonald 1995; Nowak 1991)

RESTRAINT AND HANDLING

Raccoons are definitive hosts for the roundworm *Baylisascaris*, which can be transmitted to humans and other animals via unprotected physical contact, primarily with raccoon feces. This roundworm may cause severe central nervous system damage that could be fatal in humans and other animal species.

Therefore, IT IS MANDATORY THAT PROTECTIVE GLOVES ALWAYS BE WORN WHEN HANDLING THESE ANIMALS. In addition to latex protective gloves, workman's leather gloves may be worn, and may actually be necessary when handling older animals (Bowman 1999; PAWS 2001). *Baylisascaris procyonis* ova are virtually indestructible and may last in the environment for years. Other animals in a facility should also be protected from contact with raccoon feces; for example, the runoff from cleaning a raccoon pen should not pass through another animal enclosure.

Infant and juvenile raccoons can be held by the scruff of the neck or by the forelegs. They tend to scream, grasp, or bite at the gloves, and may often urinate with handling. For an older, aggressive juvenile, restrain by the "foreleg method." With the animal's back toward your abdomen, pin the raccoon down with a gloved hand or towel. Grasp the raccoon by the shoulder region of the forelegs. You should have one leg in each hand. Make sure you are holding the forelegs as close as you can to the shoulders (armpit area). The raccoon should not be able to bite you and the animal can be restrained for miscellaneous procedures using this technique (PAWS 2001).

While working with the animals, do not speak to the animals or encourage behavior that will condition the animals to humans (PAWS 2001).

ASSESSMENT OF THE NEONATE: AGE DETERMINATION

Age can be determined with the following guidelines (Huckabee 1999–2000):

Newborn: weighs 60–75 g; their back is sparsely furred and the eyes and ears are closed.
2 weeks: face mask is fully haired as well as the back.
2 1/2 to 3 weeks: ears and eyes are open.
3 weeks: tail rings are fully furred.
3 to 4 weeks: kits squirm actively and chitter, but cannot support their weight on their legs at this time.
4 weeks: deciduous (milk teeth) first, second, and third incisors erupt.
4 to 6 weeks: animals begin walking.
6 weeks: deciduous second, third, and fourth premolars erupt.
8 weeks: deciduous first premolars and permanent first incisors erupt.
10 weeks: permanent second incisors and first molars erupt.
12 weeks: permanent third incisors erupt.
14 weeks: permanent canines erupt.
16 weeks: most of the animals in the wild are weaned at this time.

INITIAL CARE AND STABILIZATION

Perform a complete physical examination either by manual restraint or with sedation. The animal should only be immobilized if it is in stable condition and only if necessary to perform a physical examination or do a diagnostic workup (blood panel, radiographs, etc.). Be sure to wear examination gloves when handling raccoons. The physical exam should include palpating the hard palate to check for lesions. If the animal has a cleft palate it could affect its ability to suckle and cause complications such as aspiration pneumonia.

If the kit appears injured or ill, obtain a blood sample to run a CBC and a chemistry panel if enough blood is available; a fecal sample should be submitted for analysis. The veterinarian should be present or called if necessary depending on the condition of the animal. Check the packed cell volume (PCV), total solids (TS), and blood glucose (BG) in order to initiate treatment for immediate problems. If the BG is low, less than 60, give subcutaneous or intravenous fluids (lactated Ringer's solution or Normosol-R with a 2 1/2% dextrose solution SQ or higher percentage dextrose if given IV). Prepare two to three blood slide smears for review by the veterinarian. Prepare equipment for skin scrape, and possibly IV catheter placement, fluid therapy, and X rays. Be sure to provide the animal with an external heat source, fluids, and appropriate medications based on physical examination findings (Morgan 1992; PAWS 2001).

Once the initial exam has been performed, formulate a treatment plan for any problems the animal may have. Remember these animals are not domesticated, but many of their medical problems can be treated similarly to those of domestic cat and dog species. If you do not have access to a veterinarian with wildlife experience, a small-animal practitioner should be quite helpful in caring for these species. Keep in mind these are still wild animals and must function in a harsh, unforgiving environment in nature. Fractures and other medical problems must heal well enough to enable the animal to catch prey items for food, climb, escape from predators, and protect itself (PAWS 2001). Isolate and quarantine the raccoon (or litter) from other raccoons and other mammals upon arrival.

FORMULAS, SUPPLEMENTS, AND CALORIC REQUIREMENTS

Rehydrating solutions used for raccoons include Pedialyte (Ross) or an electrolyte solution such as lactated Ringer's solution (LRS) (PAWS 2001).

KMR (Kitten Milk Replacer, available at most veterinary hospitals, pet food and feed stores) and Zoologic 42/25 (available through local feed stores) are both made by PetAg, Inc., and have been used successfully with baby raccoons. For either product, mix one part powder with two parts water by volume.

Start by feeding 100% rehydrating solution. Follow the feeding guide for amounts to feed. Once the infant is rehydrated, begin to add in the formula gradually. Start with 75% rehydrating solution and 25% formula. At the next feed give 50:50 rehydrating solution to formula; the next feed 75:25, and finally give 100% formula as described below.

Weaning Diet

Raccoon Mush is composed of soaked puppy chow, Gerber high-protein baby cereal, and KMR powder, with enough water added to achieve an oatmeal-like consistency (PAWS 2001). Gerber high-protein baby cereal is available from Gerber Products Company.

Juvenile Diet

During and following weaning, offer a diversity of food items including dry dog food, fish, mice, fruits, and nuts (PAWS 2001).

TUBE FEEDING

To tube feed a raccoon, you will need (PAWS 2001):

Red rubber catheter (Kendall Sovereign Feeding Tube and Urethral Catheter, sizes 8, 10, and 12 French)
Lubricant (KY Jelly, for instance)
Light source (flashlight or ophthalmoscope)
Syringe (3, 6, or 12-ml)
Joint to attach the syringe to the red rubber catheter (Christmas Tree Connector or Barbed Connector—Jorgenson)
Formula (see above)

Infants are fed via gavage tube if their eyes are still closed or they are too weak to eat out of a dish. Before placing the tube into the esophagus, measure the length of the tube to be passed from the nose to the last rib of the animal. Mark the length with a permanent marker. Apply a small amount of lubricant to the tip of the red rubber catheter but avoid lubricating the holes toward the end of the tube. One should be trained in this technique to avoid accidentally placing the tube into the trachea. The gavage tube is passed into the esophagus to the stomach, while the animal is held ventral-side down in a normal position. If the head is pulled upward or the neck bent downward forming a right angle to the body, the tube may be accidentally placed into the trachea and the food delivered into the lungs. If the food enters the lungs the animal will quickly asphyxiate and die. This can be avoided by keeping the head and neck normally positioned. If the animal is overfed or regurgitates during feeding, it may lead to aspiration pneumonia (Huckabee 1999–2000; PAWS 2001).

FEEDING AND HUSBANDRY TIPS

The animals may be dish fed if they are strong enough to eat and their eyes are open. The raccoon mush is a good choice for dish feeding because the animals are able to eat it easily.

After each feeding be sure to stimulate the neonates to urinate and defecate. This is done by gently rubbing their genital and rectal areas using a moist soft cloth. This should stimulate them to defecate and urinate. It is important to perform this with young animals until they begin to urinate and defecate on their own, at approximately three to four weeks of age (Huckabee 1999–2000; PAWS 2001).

In addition to formula feedings, the raccoons are given solid food items when they are 400 g in weight. Tables 25.1 and 25.2 provide details on formula feeding, housing, and adding solid food to the diet.

HOUSING

Raccoons housed alone become very lonely and should be given a stuffed animal and extra towels to help them feel secure until the single animal can be introduced to a conspecific (same species) (PAWS 2001). Raccoons also like to sleep above the ground; therefore, providing hammocks hanging in all of their enclosures is important to simulate their natural environment. They may occasionally use kitty litter boxes, which can be placed in the kennels and enclosures for the animals that choose to use them. The best setup is to hang a hammock toward the rear of the crate with a litter box beneath the hammock. The food and a secured water dish can be placed in the front of the crate near the door.

Table 25.1 Raccoon Feeding Formula and Housing Guide

Housing	Weight	Amount per Feeding	No. Feedings/day
Incubator			
	100 g	5.0 ml	6
	150 g	6.5 ml	6
	200 g	10 ml	5
	250 g	12 ml	5
	300 g	13 ml	5
	350 g	15 ml	5
	400 g	17 ml	5
	450 g	18 ml	5
Place in aquarium with heating pad half way under the aquarium in a warm room			
	500 g	25 ml	4
100/200 size crates/kennels with hammocks in a warm room			
	550 g	27 ml	4
	600 g	28.5 ml	4
200/300 size crates with hammocks in a warm room			
	650 g	30.5 ml	4
	700 g	32 ml	4
	750 g	34 ml	4
	800 g	36 ml	4
200/500 sized crates with a hammock in an area free of drafts, but still indoors			
	850 g	37 ml	3
	900 g	39 ml	3
	950 g	40.5 ml	3
	1000 g	42 ml	2
	1050 g	43 ml	2
	1100 g	44 ml	1
Secure enclosure, indoors; crates and hammocks should be available for the animals to use freely			
	1200 g	Should be fully weaned	
	1300 g	Weaned	

Source: PAWS (2001).

Raccoon enclosures must be cleaned at least once a day, but they generally require more frequent cleaning throughout the day because these animals can be very messy.

VACCINATION AND DEWORMING PROTOCOLS

Upon their arrival at the rehabilitation center, we determine the age and stabilize the patients. Once the animals are stable (this may be the next day or so), we initiate vaccinations and deworming according to the following schedule (PAWS 2001; Plumb 1998).

Deworming

Use Nemex-2, concentration 4.54 mg/ml, with dosage of 10 ml/kg orally. Give on arrival if the animal is two weeks of age (over 200 g) and repeat every 14 days for a total of four treatments. [Note: Do not deworm with Panacur (fenbendazole)—see Toxicity below.]

Table 25.2 Raccoon Solid Food Addition Guidelines

Body weight	Solid food added to diet
400–800 g	Provide raccoon mush
850–1500 g	Provide soaked puppy chow with small amounts of cut fruit
1525–2000 g	1/2 soaked puppy chow with 1/2 hard puppy chow, small pieces of cut fruit, fish, and vegetables
2000+ g	Provide hard puppy chow, live prey items (mice, fish), fish, fruits, and vegetables. Fruits and vegetables should only comprise 10% of the diet at this point

Vaccines

The following vaccines are recommended (Huckabee 1999–2000; PAWS 2001):

1. Fervac vaccine (a distemper vaccine manufactured for ferrets by United Vaccines). Dosage: 1.0 ml administered subcutaneously. Frequency: give on arrival if the animal is six weeks of age (over 850 g) and repeat every 21 days for a total of four injections.
2. Biovac Mink Enteritis Virus vaccine (KV) by United Vaccines. Check administration instructions on vial for dosage and frequency.
3. Feline Panleukopenia Vaccine. Feline panleukopenia vaccine is generally purchased as part of a combination vaccine with other viral diseases. Only administer the panleukopenia, the liquid portion, and dispose of the vial containing the dry material that is the other vaccine portion. Dosage: 1.0 ml administered subcutaneously. Frequency: give on arrival if the animal is six weeks of age (over 850 g) and repeat in 30 days for a total of two injections.

COMMON MEDICAL PROBLEMS

Parasites

[Note: Always wear gloves when handling raccoons because of the potential zoonotic and detrimental effects of *Baylisascaris*.]

Gastrointestinal Parasites (Endoparasites)

Baylisascaris procyonis is a roundworm (nematode), the eggs of which are shed in the feces and can be transmitted to all mammal species via the fecal-oral route. Raccoons are definitive hosts for this parasite, which means that the worm can progress through a normal life cycle and reproduce in this species only. Raccoons live normal lives with this parasite, but other mammals cannot. If the eggs find their way into an aberrant host they will not complete a normal life cycle and begin abnormal migrations through the host's organs. They can migrate anywhere, including into the brain, thereby causing abnormal neurological signs, which can be fatal. In a fecal float, the eggs of this worm species resemble most other roundworm eggs and can be definitely diagnosed by histopathology. Treat roundworm infections with Nemex (see instructions under Deworming, above) (Bowman 1999; Plumb 1998).

As with any endoparasites, fecal analysis will determine therapy. A fecal examination by direct smear and a float to determine worm infestation is part of a normal workup. The direct smear may be stained with lugol (iodine) stain for identifying giardia. If giardia is suspected and not seen on direct float, a fecal sample may need to be submitted to a veterinary diagnostic laboratory for analysis. Coccidia, a protozoal endoparasite, is treated with Albon at an initial dose of 55 mg/kg once, then at a dose of 27 mg/kg once a day for ten days. Giardia is treated with metronidazole (Flagyl) at a dose of 15 mg/kg once a day for five to seven days. If tapeworms are found, give a dose of praziquantel (Droncit) based on current weight and recommended dose on the bottle of the drug (Bowman 1999; Plumb 1998).

In young raccoons coccidia and nematodes will be the most common endoparasites seen.

Ectoparasites

Ringworm

Ringworm is contagious to humans. Always wear gloves when handling/treating an animal suspected of having ringworm. It is a fungal disease and the lesions are characterized by a reddish ringed worm appearance on the skin in an area of alopecia. Diagnosis is by clinical signs and doing a DTM (dermatophyte type medium) culture, which can be obtained from a local veterinary diagnostic laboratory. Consult a veterinarian for treatment. Griseofulvin ultramicrosize has been used successfully at an oral daily dose of 5–10 mg/kg for a minimum of three weeks (Bowman 1999; Plumb 1998). It is not as commonly diagnosed in raccoons as it is in foxes and bears (Bowman 1999).

Mange

If the animal presents with alopecia (fur loss) always perform a skin scraping to rule out sarcoptic or demodectic mange. Sarcoptic mange is caused by sarcoptes mites, small arthropods visible by microscope. Clinical signs are diffuse alopecia +/– patchiness of the fur. Diagnosis is accomplished by having your veterinarian do a skin scraping. Treatment is with ivermectin injections (0.300 mg/kg SQ) repeated every 14 days. It may take up to five treatments to resolve. Discuss dosages with a veterinarian if you have any questions (Bowman 1999; Plumb 1998).

Demodectic mange is caused by a mite in primarily immunodeficient animals. Clinical presentation may be focal or diffuse and is seen as areas of alopecia with crusty scabs. Diagnosis is by skin scraping and viewing under the microscope. The mites appear like small cigar-shaped creatures with eight waving arms. Treatment is with Goodwinol topical ointment or dips with amitraz (Mitaban, Pharmacia & Upjohn, Kalamazoo, MI). Ivermectin injections may also be used in the treatment (see dose mentioned above). Diffuse demodecosis is difficult to treat, and if incurable may lead to euthanizing the animal (Bowman 1999; Plumb 1998). It is not as commonly diagnosed in raccoons as it is in foxes and bears (Bowman 1999).

Fleas and Ticks

Ticks can be found in debilitated animals and should be removed using a hemostat clamp. Generally a very small number of ticks may live on the animal but they should not be present in overwhelming numbers. If that is the case, they are a result of the animal being debilitated. The animal may need to be dipped with a veterinary-approved tick dip to eliminate all ticks. Be sure to use a product safe for young animals (Bowman 1999).

Fleas occasionally may be present and if they are in large enough numbers, a light flea bath or dusting with flea powder, preferably a pyrethrin-based product may be used to treat them. Diluted Permectrin II (Boehringer Ingelheim) works well. Dilute it by using 3.5 cc Permectrin II to 1500 ml water.

One of the safest ways to treat is to place a small amount of dust on a towel, remove the excess powder, and use the towel to rub the animal's torso, legs, and feet, avoiding the head and face. With the babies use only a minimal amount. If the animal has an adverse reaction (respiratory distress, bluish gums), immediately bathe the animal and remove the flea product. With animals that react to the powder, use a flea comb to remove fleas and lightly dust the underside of the kit's bedding. Be sure to monitor the kits for adverse reactions before leaving them overnight with the powdered towel.

Toxicity

A fenbendazole toxicity has been suspected in some rehabilitated raccoons. It causes intestinal lesions that are similar histopathologically to parvoviral lesions as seen in canids. Fenbendazole may be used judiciously for individual cases under veterinary care. Raccoon kits receiving this drug should be monitored for adverse side effects (severe diarrhea, vomiting, lethargy) (PAWS 2001).

Preputial Sucking

Management problems include preputial suckling on themselves or by conspecifics. The urge to suckle is strong in many of the young neonates and if they are not with their mothers, they mistake the preputial structures as nipples and suckle on them. This results in inflammation, irritation, and possibly infection of the prepuce (Huckabee 1999–2000). If this is noted keep the preputial area clean with dilute chlorhexidine (Nolvasan) solution and apply topical agents such as Panalog cream, Desitin, or silver sulfadiazene to the area affected two to four times a day. The animals may need to be housed individually until the skin is normal because of the common problem of other individuals licking off the topical medication. However, this creates a vicious cycle of the problem because the little kits may stress if housed alone and continue to suck on this area. A number of wraps have been attempted to avert the kits from suckling but raccoons are very adept at removing most wraps from their bodies, even at a very young age (Huckabee 1999–2000; PAWS 2001).

If the problem is treated early on, there is a better chance of healing. Rarely a kit cannot be treated successfully, becomes septic, is unresponsive to treatment, and may need to be humanely euthanized.

Metabolic Bone Disease

Metabolic bone disease (MBD, rickets, osteomalacia, and a number of other names) is the result of a number of abnormalities and imbalances involving many complex endocrine pathways, improper nutrition, and husbandry mismanagement (Ettinger and Feldman 1995). Basically, it is an imbalance of calcium, vitamin D, and phosphorus causing bones to become flexible and bendable, and can lead to folding fractures of the long bones. Clinical signs include lameness, fractures, bone deformities, reluctance to move or walk, painful joints/bones on palpation, and anorexia (Ettinger and Feldman 1995). Diagnosis in young animals is generally achieved with a thorough physical exam and radiographs.

Treatment depends on the age of the animal, duration of the metabolic problem, and the clinical signs. Calcium injections, vitamin D (orally), and proper diet are primary treatment regimens. Therapy with medication should be under the direction of a veterinarian. If corrected early, the animal may recover and the bones remodel to normal configuration. If the disease has progressed, it may not be reversible and the animals must be euthanized (Ettinger and Feldman 1995; Huckabee 1999–2000; PAWS 2001).

Bloat and Indigestion

Young raised on formula may develop bloat and/or indigestion Ettinger and Feldman 1995; PAWS 2001). Episodes of gastritis can be caused due to diet (spoiled formula, inappropriate formula, allergies), infectious etiologies (bacterial, viral, parasites), or toxins. In babies it is generally due to dietary or infectious agents. Initial signs include bloated or distended abdomen, abnormal fecal output or abnormal feces, restlessness, and decreased interest in suckling or eating. It is critical to assess the animal early in the disorder to correct the problem and avoid secondary complications (dehydration, weight loss, bacterial infections, shock, death), which can ensue quickly in a neonate.

Diagnosis is by exclusion of other potential problems. Fecal exams as outlined above under Parasites should be done, along with a thorough physical examination and radiographs to assess for abnormal organ pattern.

Treatment is straightforward for simple indigestion. Provide fluid support via subcutaneous fluids (see Shock and Dehydration below) and withhold feeding for one or two feeds. Fluids should be continued for the duration of time that formula feeding is withheld. Be sure to stimulate the kit periodically to encourage passing of stool and urine. If the kit is stable, modify the formula and feed the less-concentrated formula that the kit was fed prior to presenting with bloat for a number of feeds. Then slowly increase the concentration of formula to the appropriate formula for the animal's weight level. Therapy may include pink bismuth (Pepto-Bismol), at a dose of 1 ml/10 lb (1 ml/4.5 kg) orally twice daily (Plumb 1998). We also use simethecon drops.

If the kit does not improve within a few hours and the bloat is not subsiding, or it rebloats, a veterinarian should assess the animal for further diagnostics and treatment.

Trauma

Generally, most young raccoons do not present with significant trauma; however, the possibility of attack by other animals or being hit by a vehicle exists. When a young raccoon presents to your facility, perform a thorough exam and check for fractures of the skull, spine, long bones, jaws, and teeth. Often a predisposing cause to trauma is canine distemper virus (see below), which may occur even in young raccoons.

Check the skin for evidence of wounds (lacerations, bite wounds, or bruises). Bite wounds and lacerations can be treated by cleansing the wounds with dilute Nolvasan solution and rinsing with physiologic saline solution (0.9% saline). Bite wounds should be left open and draining, while lacerations may require drain placement and/or sutures. A veterinarian can assist with these procedures. Subcutaneous fluid therapy and broad-spectrum antibiotics (amoxicillin or cephalosporins at 10 mg/lb) may be required depending on the extent of trauma (PAWS 2001; Plumb 1998).

For more severe trauma (blood in the ear, epistaxis), a veterinarian should be consulted for evaluation and a treatment plan. If the animal is having seizures, the underlying cause needs to be determined and corrected or treated. Causes include head trauma, hypoglycemia, sepsis, or infectious diseases (see all below). Initial treatment for seizures is diazepam 0.5–1.0 mg/kg (Plumb 1998). It may be given intravenously or per rectum. Delivery of the drug rectally may be quicker to administer to a seizing patient. Until a veterinarian can examine the animal, keep it warm and well hydrated (SQ or IV fluids) and monitor attitude and neurologic signs.

The animal may not be aware enough to eat and swallow, so do not offer food for a few hours until it can be stabilized and further evaluated (Ettinger and Feldman 1995; Morgan 1992; PAWS 2001).

Fractures

During an initial physical exam, check the skull and mouth for any cranium, tooth, or jaw fractures. Cranial fractures may not be repairable, but jaw and tooth fractures can be repaired. Proper alignment of the jaw is fairly important so that the animal is capable of killing and eating well. Palpate the ribs and other bones for any abnormalities in bone integrity. If any fractures are evident or suspected, radiographs should be taken, once the animal has been stabilized. Long-bone fractures may require stabilization (e.g., Robert-Jones bandage) by an appropriately trained individual until further veterinary care is available.

Most fractures in young animals will heal well with proper treatment. Radiographs should be reviewed by a veterinarian who can then formulate an appropriate treatment plan.

Diarrhea

Diarrhea is defined as "an increase in the frequency, fluidity, or volume of feces" (Ettinger and Feldman 1995). Diarrhea can be characterized as acute or chronic and must be differentiated as originating in the small versus the large bowel. Most of our patients with diarrhea have the acute form, which is caused by problems in either the small or large bowel. Initial treatment of diarrhea, until it can be further characterized, is fluid therapy, diet change, and gastrointestinal protectants (see treatment section below). It is best to hold off on antibiotic therapy initially, and attempt supportive care and diet change to correct the diarrhea. Most therapies suitable for young domestic dogs would be appropriate in young raccoon kits as well (i.e., Pepto-Bismol at 1 ml/10 lb [4.5 kg] orally two to three times a day, and cimetidine 7–10 mg/kg PO, SQ, IV two to three times daily) (Ettinger and Feldman 1995; Plumb 1998).

Causes: Acute diarrheas in young animals generally are caused by parasites, inappropriate formula or feeding methods, medications, and toxins. Chronic diarrheas may be caused by uncorrected acute diarrhea problems and rectal anatomical abnormalities (strictures, masses) and can be seen in our younger patients with infections (salmonella, clostridial), ulcers (due to stress or trauma), or toxins. Clinical signs include dehydration, bloated abdomen, loose/runny stool, fever, pain on abdominal palpation with gaseous bowel loops, weight loss, and tenesmus (Ettinger and Feldman 1995; Morgan 1992).

Diagnostics: Fecal analysis (direct and float), hemaoccult fecal tests, CBC, radiographs, fecal cytology, and fecal cultures may be necessary to determine the cause and characterize the type of diarrhea (Ettinger and Feldman 1995).

Treatment: Treatment should be targeted at the underlying cause of the diarrhea. Young and baby animals should have diets reviewed and corrected and be given SQ fluids—crystalloids at appropriate dehydration/shock/maintenance rate until they can be placed on the appropriate diet and clinical signs resolve. A veterinarian should calculate the amount of fluids necessary to treat the raccoon, but approximately 60–90 ml/kg/day of crystalloids (Normosol-R or lactated Ringer's solution) delivered via IV catheter is reasonable. The young raccoons may require broad-spectrum systemic antibiotics (Clavamox, 13.75 mg/kg PO BID for seven to ten days or metronidazole at 15 mg/kg PO SID for five to seven days) if they are compromised and appear debilitated (Plumb 1998). Fecal examinations should be done on all patients with diarrhea and appropriate anthelminth therapy instituted (see Endoparasites above). Fluid therapy and correction of formula are the primary mechanisms to correct most of the acute diarrheas we see in babies and juveniles at the wildlife center.

Chronic diarrheas are more difficult to treat. Abdominal radiographs should be done. If parasites and dietary problems/indiscretion have been ruled out and the diarrhea is persistent, the veterinarians should reassess the patient and decide on the next course of diagnostics and therapy. Maintaining fluid balance and correcting for dehydration and ongoing losses should continue in the patient (e.g., ongoing fluid therapy IV, PO, SQ at appropriate fluid rates) (Ettinger and Feldman 1995).

Hypoglycemia

Young animals have higher glucose requirements than most adults of their species (Ettinger and Feldman 1995; Morgan 1992). The increased requirement is important as a source of energy for maturing metabolic functions, growth, and maintenance of normal blood glucose (BG) levels. They utilize all nutrients faster because of accelerated growth rates at young ages. It is important to restore and continue to meet their BG needs.

Clinical signs of hypoglycemia may be noted if the blood glucose (BG) is less than 60 g/dl. Animals may appear hungry, show signs of ataxia, or have small seizures that may escalate and lead to loss of consciousness. Initial therapy is to quickly apply Karo syrup to the gums and then give dextrose via gavage tube (orogastric tube), subcutaneously, or intravenously. If giving dextrose SQ, remember to give only a concentration of 2.5% dextrose. In most wildlife neonatal patients, it can be difficult to place an IV. An intraosseous catheter may be placed by a veterinarian, if the animal is severely dehydrated or hypoglycemic, in order to deliver fluid therapy. Once a catheter is placed, administer 5–10 ml/kg of a 20% dextrose solution, which may be diluted from a 50% solution using a ration of 2-ml sterile saline to 1.5 ml 50% dextrose. Give this amount IV at a steady pace. Begin an IV drip of LRS or Normosol-R with an appropriate amount of dextrose added to the fluid bag to make a 2.5–10% or even up to a 20% solution of dextrose. Remember you can only give up to a 2.5% dextrose SQ but it is acceptable to give higher concentrations of dextrose intravenously if warranted. Initially recheck the BG level within the first two hours of therapy (using a different vein than the one with the catheter) and modify the amount of dextrose in the fluids to accommodate the change in BG levels. If the dextrose drip is not maintaining and/or increasing, or normalizing the BG level, give another bolus of the 20% dextrose solution as outlined above. Once the BG has been corrected and the animal is stable, proper management with environmental control, nutrition, and additional SQ fluid therapy can normalize the patient. Young raccoons will generally normalize with a minimal therapy/intervention and maintain their BG level once placed on a well-balanced diet. If simple intervention does not bring them to a normoglycemic state, then a veterinarian should be involved in establishing a treatment plan (Ettinger and Feldman 1995; Morgan 1992).

Septicemia

Septicemia is a problem manifested as a systemic infection generally carried throughout the body via the bloodstream (Ettinger and Feldman 1995; Morgan 1992). The animal may or may not be febrile. Generally they are lethargic, weak, inappetent, may have difficulty breathing, and have pale mucous membranes. This can be caused by conditions of overcrowding, infections, inappropriate nutrition or antibiotics, or wounds that are not properly treated. Diagnosis is via clinical signs, a complete blood count, and a blood glucose level. The CBC will generally indicate a severely elevated or decreased white blood cell count. The blood glucose level will usually be low (below 60 g/dl).

Immediate supportive care should be initiated with fluids (see Anemia below), warmth, and broad-spectrum antibiotics (trimethoprim sulfa or Clavamox, see doses in Anemia below) (Ettinger and Feldman 1995; Morgan 1992; Murtaugh 1994; Plumb 1998). The animal may need aggressive care and veterinary evaluation. We have not seen this as a common problem in raccoon kits, but if you suspect this problem, have a veterinarian evaluate the animal immediately and formulate a treatment plan for the individual animal.

Shock and Dehydration

Shock is usually a result of trauma, disease, hypoglycemia, or severe malnutrition in wildlife patients. An affected animal may present with severe hypovolemia and possibly hypoglycemia (see Hypoglycemia above). Animals may have pale mucous membranes and glazed/glassy-appearing eyes, may be recumbent, and may have an elevated temperature and a prolonged capillary refill time. If animals present with head trauma, they may have seizures, slip into a coma, or have problems thermoregulating (Morgan 1992; Murtaugh 1994; PAWS 2001). For more information, see Shock/Dehydration in Chapter 22.

Infectious Diseases

Canine distemper virus (CDV), parvovirus, and rabies virus have been seen in raccoons.

Canine Distemper Virus

Canine distemper virus is a paramyxovirus. It is transmitted via aerosolization (respiratory secretions) and invades epithelial cells, entering via the respiratory tract. This is a very serious disease, generally with a grave prognosis. Young, unvaccinated animals between three to six months old are most susceptible and affected. The "virus can be excreted for 60–90 days." It is susceptible to most veterinary disinfectants (Ettinger and Feldman 1995; Greene 1998).

CDV causes a variety of clinical signs including weakness, lethargy, inappetence, diarrhea, respiratory signs, mucopurulent oculonasal discharge, hyperkeratosis of the foot pads, and, as the disease progresses, neurological signs with characteristic retinal abnormalities in the eye. Initial nonspecific clinical signs begin two to four days postinfection with more severe signs occurring within a week. If you suspect the kit has distemper, it should be isolated and evaluated by a veterinarian for diagnosis and treatment. Treatment is often unrewarding and recovered animals may shed the virus, thereby infecting other animals. Usually, animals diagnosed with canine distemper are humanely euthanized (Convy 2001; Ettinger and Feldman 1995; Greene 1998; Morgan 1992).

Towels, blankets, kennels, food bowls, enclosures, toys, or other items should be completely disinfected before being used for any other animal. Allow the enclosure/kennel space to air out for 48–72 hours before putting another animal into the enclosure (Greene 1998).

Prevention is vaccination. See schedule under Vaccination Protocols in Chapter 22.

Parvovirus (Canine Viral Enteritis)

Parvovirus is a DNA virus that "requires rapidly dividing cells for replications" (Greene 1998). The virus is quite resistant in the environment and is spread from contact with feces or oronasal secretions of infected animals. The virus will also attack lymphoid tissue causing decrease of white blood cells. Clinical signs include severe lethargy, foul smelling hemorrhagic diarrhea, and vomiting. The clinical signs have a rapid onset and the animals can fail quickly. The myocardium of the heart may also be affected causing cardiac disease. Depending on the level of cardiac involvement, the kit may die suddenly from this virus. Kits exhibiting any of these signs should be treated by a veterinarian (Ettinger and Feldman 1995; Greene 1998; Morgan 1992).

Diagnosis is via a canine parvovirus CITE snap test using a fecal sample. The test is specific and sensitive for this virus. The test is available through most veterinary drug distributors. If an animal is positive on the CITE test, isolate the animal from other carnivores in a warm temperature-controlled room and consult with a small-animal veterinarian to establish a treatment plan and assess the animal periodically (Ettinger and Feldman 1995).

Animals can be treated successfully if therapy is started early in the disease process or as soon as the diagnosis is confirmed. If the animal improves and recovers, it should be isolated from other raccoons as well as carnivores for at least two weeks. The kit will continue to shed the virus for that amount of time and can transmit the virus to other vulnerable animals (Ettinger and Feldman 1995).

All towels, blankets, kennels, food bowls, enclosures, toys, or other items should be completely disinfected before being used for any other animal. Allow the enclosure/kennel space to air out for 48–72 hours before putting another animal into the enclosure.

Prevention is vaccination. See schedule under Vaccination Protocols in Chapter 22.

Rabies Virus

Rabies is an RNA virus that is easily killed by a variety of disinfectants used in animal and veterinary facilities (Ettinger and Feldman 1995; Greene 1998). This virus is transmitted via saliva from bite wounds of infected animals. The virus affects the central nervous system (CNS) and causes aberrant neurological behavior usually exhibited as severe aggression.

If rabies is suspected, the animal is euthanized and the head submitted to a special lab for rabies testing. If rabies is suspected and the animal bites someone, it should be immediately humanely euthanized and the head submitted for special lab testing (Ettinger and Feldman 1995; Greene 1998). If someone was bitten or in contact with the animal's saliva, the person should see a physician immediately and begin prophylactic shots for exposure. This is a fatal disease if not treated immediately once someone has been exposed. Your local public health office should be informed immediately if you suspect an animal is rabid and you plan to euthanize it.

All staff members at a facility that accepts mammals to raise and/or release should have prophylactic rabies vaccinations done with the guidance of your local public health officer.

Rabies virus lives in wild mammal populations throughout the United States (except in Hawaii). There are different wildlife reservoirs of the virus in different areas of the United States. Raccoons, skunks, foxes, dogs, and bats (migratory) are the primary wild and domestic animals that carry rabies in this country. A level of enzootic infection is maintained in various wild animal populations. Problems arise in an area when an epizootic or epidemic occurs in an area. When this occurs, it's possible to see an increase in the carnivores presenting to wildlife centers (Greene 1998).

While most of the young neonates that you may see will not have rabies, there is a chance a juvenile raccoon that is positive for rabies may present to your facility and may have signs of a rabid animal. There are two forms of rabies: the furious form, with which most people are familiar, and the dumb/paralytic form that seems to allude many individuals, including many practitioners. Clinical signs of the furious form are change in demeanor/personality, excessive licking of the bite wound site, and anxiety, which lasts for approximately a week. Animals exhibit a fear of water because they cannot swallow and therefore cannot drink. They drool excessively for the same reason. The paralytic form is seen as a lower motor neuron paralysis from the site of the bite and progresses along the nerve until it reaches the CNS and lasts about two to four days. Animals occasionally exhibit choking during this phase, but it is actually a paralysis of the laryngeal nerves. Do not place your hand in the animal's mouth without protective gloves if you attempt to relieve a choking situation (Greene 1998).

For safety purposes, any towels, blankets, toys, or other items should be disinfected and thrown away. Kennels, water bowls, and food bowls should be completely disinfected before being used for any other animal. Allow the enclosure/kennel space to air out for at least 48 hours before putting another animal into the enclosure.

Ocular Lesions

Eye problems include corneal ulcers, cataracts, foreign bodies, proptosed globes, and lens luxations (all due to trauma) and should be evaluated by a veterinarian and possibly a veterinary ophthalmologist (Huckabee 1999–2000; PAWS 2001; Slatter 1990).

Vomiting

Vomiting in young animals may be the result of ingesting foreign objects, from inappropriate dietary formulation or spoiled diet, medications, infectious agents, ulcers, heat stroke, or metabolic abnormalities (Ettinger and Feldman 1995).

Vomitus should be inspected for blood or a coffee ground consistency. The presence of blood or coffee ground material would indicate a severe problem and treatment plans should be conducted under the direction of a veterinarian (Ettinger and Feldman 1995).

Generally, one simple episode of vomiting can be treated by withholding food for a short period of time, giving SQ fluids to the kit, correcting the diet (provide a bland diet that is fresh), and monitoring for continuing signs (Ettinger and Feldman 1995). If the animal continues to vomit, a veterinarian should evaluate the animal and provide an additional treatment plan. Exploratory surgery may be necessary to correct the problem, especially if a foreign body is causing the vomiting.

Anemia

Anemia is not a disease, it is a symptom. It is a decreased number of red blood cells in the blood, as reflected by measuring packed cell volume (PCV) and red blood cells (RBC) (Cotter 1993). Clinical signs include pale mucous membranes, dyspnea, tachycardia, and weakness, and may be further complicated by epistaxis, hematuria, continued hemorrhage, melena, and hematoemesis. Many of these signs are directly related to the decrease in oxygen delivery to the tissues by the resulting decrease in RBC (Cotter 1993; Morgan 1992). A veterinarian should examine the anemic patient, determine a cause and establish a treatment plan complete with parameters for monitoring the animal's progress. For more information, see Anemia in Chapter 22.

RELEASE CRITERIA

Behavior should be assessed continually during the development and growth of the raccoons while undergoing rehabilitation. Proper steps must be taken to keep the raccoons wild and afraid of humans (no talking when working in raccoon areas, minimal and necessary handling only, no playing or hand feeding the animals, etc.). Experienced staff or personnel should evaluate the animals regularly for health and human fear.

For optimal chances of survival, the animals should weigh a minimum of 3500 g prior to release. The juveniles must be fearful of humans and be able to forage and hunt live prey successfully. The raccoons should be released with conspecifics into an unused shed or barn with natural foods available in the immediate surroundings. Water access is vital in a release site, and water should be easily accessible (creeks are favored). If the animals are soft released, supplemental feedings will be necessary. If the animals are hard released, leave puppy chow at the release site. Release the animals at the original site they were found whenever possible. It is preferable to release animals at dusk or in the evening (PAWS 2001).

ACKNOWLEDGMENTS

We would like to thank Dr. John Huckabee for his contribution and for training the authors to care for orphan raccoons. We are especially thankful for his expertise with the medical problems. We would also like to thank the staff, volunteers, and veterinary externs at PAWS Wildlife Center who assisted in all the medical, nursing, and orphan care responsibilities, which made it possible to treat and raise numerous raccoons and write this chapter during 1999–2000.

SOURCES FOR PRODUCTS MENTIONED

Boehringer Ingelheim Animal Health, Inc., St. Joseph, MO 64506; 1-800-821-7467

Gerber Products Company, c/o Consumer Affairs, 445 State Street, Fremont, MI 49413-0001; www.gerber.com; 1-800-443-7237

Jorgenson Laboratories, Inc., Loveland, CO; 1-800-525-5614

Kendall Company, Mansfield, MA 02048; 1-800-962-9888

PetAg, 30 W. 432 Rt. 20, Elgen, IL 60120; 1-800-332-0877, 1-800-323-6878; www.petag.com

Ross Products Division, Abbott Laboratories, Columbus, OH 43215-1724; 1-800-986-8510; www.abbott.com, www.ross.com

United Vaccines, Madison, WI 53713; 1-800-283-6465

REFERENCES

Bowman, D. D. 1999. *Georgis' parasitology for veterinarians*. Philadelphia, PA: Saunders.

Convy, J. 2001. PAWS wildlife rehabilitation manual. Spring. Lynnwood, WA: PAWS Wildlife Center.

Cotter, S. M. 1993. Pathophysiology of the hemiclymphatic system, course syllabus. Fall. North Grafton, MA: Tufts University School of Veterinary Medicine.

Ettinger, S. J., and E. C. Feldman. 1995. *Textbook of veterinary internal medicine*. 4th ed. Philadelphia, PA: Saunders.

Greene, C. E., ed. 1998. *Infectious diseases of the dog and cat*. 2d ed. Philadelphia, PA: Saunders.

Huckabee, J., ed. 1999-2000. Wildlife medicine. A manual for the NWRA wildlife medicine course. Lynnwood, WA: National Wildlife Rehabilitators Association

Macdonald, D., ed. 1995. *The encyclopedia of mammals*. New York: Facts on File.

Morgan, R. V., ed. 1992. *Handbook of small animal medicine*. 2d ed. Philadelphia, PA: Saunders.

Murtaugh, R. 1994. Principles of medicine, course syllabus. Spring. North Grafton, MA: Tufts University School of Veterinary Medicine; Section on Small Animal Fluid Therapy.

Nowak, R. M. 1991. *Walker's mammals of the world*, vol. 2. 5th ed. Baltimore: The Johns Hopkins University Press.

PAWS wildlife rehabilitation manual. 2001. Lynnwood, WA: PAWS Wildlife Center.

Plumb, Donald C. 1998. *Veterinary drug handbook*. 3d ed. Ames: Iowa State University Press.

Slatter, D. 1990. *Fundamentals of veterinary ophthalmology*. 2d ed. Philadelphia, PA: Saunders.

26
Ferret Kits

Vickie McKimmey

INTRODUCTION

It is extremely difficult to hand rear ferret kits from birth without a good supply of ferret milk and 24-hour-a-day attention. If the jill is unable to care for her offspring, they should be fostered to another lactating jill if possible. This is highly recommended and it is also recommended that you work closely with other breeders in order to know who has a lactating jill if the need would ever arise. Most jills accept kits of any size or age at any stage of lactation. It's best if the kits are no more than one week different in age, since the larger kits will tend to push the smaller, younger ones away. Jills can successfully rear more kits than she has nipples for by rotating the kits as they nurse and sleep.

HOUSING AND FEEDING TIPS FOR JILLS AND METHODS TO MAXIMIZE GOOD PARENTING

Experienced jills rarely reject their kits, but first-time jills often do. They may not mother their litter for several days, which is too late for many kits that are not aggressive enough to follow the jill and nurse. The more privacy these jills have, the more likely they are to bond with their litter. Handling of the kits does not cause the jills to reject their litter, but unusual noise and confusion nearby do. Ferrets get very excited and may bury the kits in the bedding or put them in a pile in a corner of the enclosure or in food or water containers. Some jills cannibalize the first few or all of their kits as they are born.

If a first-time jill rejects but does not cannibalize her kits, place her and the litter inside a very small, full plastic bottomed cage only large enough for her litter box and a dishpan with bedding for the next box. Offer moist food frequently and attach a water bottle. Do not let her have too much room and keep her in close quarters with the kits. This sometimes helps her to concentrate, allowing her to more readily accept her litter. Once she accepts the kits, the jill can be allowed to move around more freely; however, some young jills get out to play and seem to forget their young.

If the room temperature is too warm, over 70°F (21°C), the jill may be reluctant to stay in the nest. To avoid accidental chilling of the kits, place a heat lamp near but not directly over the nest so that the jill can move away from it when she becomes too warm.

Jills that fail to produce enough milk to feed their kits may be genetically incapable of doing so. Before this conclusion is made, at least four variables should be examined: management, nutrition, systemic diseases of the jill, and chronic mastitis.

First-time jills or older jills that are poorly managed at whelping time may never settle down with their newborn kits and quickly dry up when the stimulus from nursing is inadequate. Make sure the jill is housed away from unaccustomed noisy activity, and until the litter is more than five days old, discourage visits by people unfamiliar to the jill. A good mother rarely leaves the nest for the first few days after whelping. Inadequate access to food and water limits the jill's ability to make milk. Low-sided dishes of food and water should be placed close enough to the nest so that the jill can reach them without leaving her kits.

Nutrition determines the difference between adequate and outstanding milk production. Jills fed a maintenance diet raise slow-growing kits with poor coats that are more susceptible to infectious diseases than well-nourished kits. Three-week-old kits that are doing poorly benefit from milk and moist food supplements, but nothing ensures that kits will be healthy and robust as much as a steady and plentiful supply of ferret milk. Offer the best quality diet available to lactating jills; the dietary fat level should be 25–30% at two to three weeks after birth. High protein (min 34–36%) and high fat (min 20%) is about the best you can get with any dry diet. Supplementing with a milkshake using Ensure Plus, whipping cream, a whole egg, or Nutrical (Tomlyn Co.), or even offering Hill's AD or Nutrical from the tube is good to start two to three weeks before birth and continue afterward. Also, jills need access to water at all times.

Nursing jills with serious systemic diseases stop producing milk. Their kits look thin and are noticed crying and moving around instead of nursing or lying quietly next to the jill. The common reasons for a sudden reduction in milk production are mastitis and metritis. Other diseases that may appear during nursing include bladder infections, urolithiasis, and lymphosarcoma.

If acute infections are promptly treated, the jill usually continues lactating; however, if she is very ill for a few days early in lactation, she will probably dry up. Feed the litter of a sick jill at least four times a day when their mother has little milk, but leave them with her so that as soon as she is able to produce milk the stimulus of nursing will induce lactation. Later in lactation, the jill has a lesser tendency to dry up immediately when sick or dehydrated. Whenever a lactating jill is ill, encourage her to take as much nourishment as possible by frequently offering high-calorie treats such as Nutrical or Ensure Plus (Ross) as well as her regular food, dry or mixed with warm water, or even offer Hill's AD diet.

NATURAL HISTORY

Ferret kits are helpless, naked, and blind and have little ability to maintain their body temperature for the first two weeks of life. Normal kits weigh about 8–10 g at birth, 30 g at one week, 60–70 grams at two weeks, and over 100 g at three weeks of age. Their eyes usually open at 30–35 days of age, although in some they open as early as 27 days of age.

Healthy, normal litters lie quietly and close to the jill and nurse or sleep except when the jill leaves the nest. By three weeks of age, even though their eyes are still closed, kits begin to explore and nibble on soft food, such as the regular diet moistened with water. Ferrets are weaned at six to eight weeks of age.

WHAT TO FEED

Supplementing milk for the kits is often the best alternative when the jill's milk production is reduced after birth. Leave the kits with her so that the stimulus of nursing induces some lactation and she can stimulate and clean them between feedings. Supplement newborn kits with puppy or kitten milk replacer enriched with cream until the fat content is 20%. One formula that works well is three parts dog milk replacer, such as Esbilac (PetAg) to one part whipping cream.

NURSING TECHNIQUES AND AMOUNTS TO FEED

You might have to teach the kit for the first feed or two. Wrap its body in a towel, with its head protruding. Do not have the kit on its back; hold it at the angle it would naturally assume if suckling from a jill. Handle it gently and talk softly. With a drop of milk on it, coax the tip of the cannula (BD Interlink Cannula)/nipple very gently into the kit's mouth, slightly off center. Be prepared to take plenty of time over the first feeding. Do not force the kit if it really does not take to the nipple, the more you struggle, the worse you will make it. If the bottle and nipple are not working, use a 1–3-cc syringe with a feeding tip (or cannula). Dribble the liquid in very, very gradually and be extremely careful not to choke the infant.

Kits drink much more if the milk is warm. Feed them as much as they will take at least four times a day from a dropper or plastic pipette. Start by feeding about 0.5 cc per feed and increase to 1 cc per feed by the end of the first week, but as a rule of thumb let the kit determine the amount.

A 3-cc feeding syringe or a syringe fitted with a cannula works best until the kit is large enough to handle nursing from a small pet nursing bottle. The aim is to feed until the kit shows signs of refusing, then stop. Do not overfeed, if anything, underfeed. Feed amounts equal to approximately 10% of body weight. If you see signs of diarrhea, you are overfeeding either in strength of mixture or in quantity of total liquid intake. Check for a steady weight gain to ensure you are feeding enough, but expect a loss of weight for the first day or two until the kit's system gets used to the milk substitute and the shock of being separated from its mother. The amount fed will of course increase as the kit grows. Be aware that kits grow very fast. Be careful to never give so much milk that the kit's stomach bloats. By three weeks of age, the kit should be nursing approximately 6–8 cc of formula from the bottle. At that point start feeding milk or mush from a small bowl.

For the first week, feed every two hours, including nights. Then gradually reduce the number of nighttime feedings over the next couple of weeks. By three weeks of age, the feedings should be adjusted to every three or four hours and you can start offering the softened adult diet at this time.

Kits that have reached three weeks of age can survive on supplemental feedings of milk, with no milk from the jill, until they are old enough to subsist on solid food. Use the same formula as that for newborn kits, and offer as much as they will take at least three times daily. Feed three-week-old kits individually with a plastic pipette, dropper, or small animal nursing bottle because at this age they crawl into milk in a dish and get wet and cold. Older kits drink well from a dish after a few lessons. A low flat dish is preferable to a saucer because ferrets put their feet on the dish when they eat or drink. Kits cannot live on solid food without milk until they are over four weeks old, and they do poorly on an adult diet before five weeks of age.

HUSBANDRY

Every time you feed, or shortly afterward, you must stimulate the kit's bowels and bladder because its muscles are not yet developed. Stroke the stomach and back legs. Use a cotton ball or wash cloth moistened in warm water to wipe its anogenital area very gently until something happens—and it will probably urinate and defecate almost simultaneously. It may not defecate after every feed, but you must make sure that it urinates each time. Kits will start defecating and urinating on their own at about three weeks of age. This is about the same time they start eating mush and moving out of the nest box.

TIPS FOR WEANING FROM FORMULA TO SOLID FOOD

Feed the mother's dry kibble softened with water. Mix in a little AD Diet (Hills) to make it into a "gravy." Make it soupy at first and work up to just softened. Do not feed fruit or vegetables. Ferrets are strict carnivores and have a very difficult time digesting carbohydrates. Examples of good diets are:

High-quality dry ferret feed: Totally Ferret, Zupreem, Mazuri Ferret, 8-in-1 Ultimate (Performance Foods, Inc.)

High-quality dry kitten feed: Purina Pro Plan, Iams, Eukenuba
Canned diets: Science Diet Feline Growth, Hill's AD

COMMON MEDICAL PROBLEMS

Hypothermia

If the jill is sick or a poor mother and the nest area is not sufficiently warm, the kits may become chilled. They chill quickly and do not attempt to nurse when they are cold. Hold chilled kits in warm water or place them on a heating pad until they are active. If they have been extremely cold, give a few drops of glucose solution orally. Dehydrated newborn kits rapidly absorb 0.5–1.0 ml of SC fluids warmed to body temperature.

When antibiotic therapy is necessary for newborn kits, the dose is only one or two drops of most antibiotics. Amoxicillin must be diluted 4:1 with water so that a dose sufficiently low for a baby kit is obtained. Chloramphenicol formulated for IV use is effective orally in newborn kits.

Diarrhea

Diarrhea in newborn kits may be caused by rotavirus, secondary bacterial agents, or bacteria. Ferret rotavirus is not identical to rotaviruses of human infants, pups, calves, and pigs. It is carried by adult ferrets and may affect even unstressed litters that have no passive immunity. Rotavirus diarrhea is life threatening in kits one to seven days of age. Older kits may not require treatment.

Kits with rotavirus diarrhea look wet and the hair on the heads and necks is slicked down. Because the jill licks away all evidence of diarrhea, you many not recognize the problem. Newborn kits with severe enteritis dehydrate rapidly. Most survive if treated with subcutaneous electrolyte solutions (0.5–1.0 ml per kit several times a day) and oral antibiotics for four to five days for the prevention of secondary bacterial enteritis. Useful antibiotics include amoxicillin, tylan, and chloramphenicol.

SOURCES FOR PRODUCTS MENTIONED

BD Company, 1 Becton Drive, Franklin Lakes, NJ 07417; 1-201-847-6800; www.BD.com

Eight In One Pet Products, 2100 Pacific Street, Hauppauge, NY 11788 or The Ferret Store: www.theferretstore.com; 1-888-833-7738

Hills Diets, 1-800-445-5777,
www.sciencediet.com

Performance Foods, Inc., 3001 Industrial Lane, #4, Broomfield, CO 80020; www.totallyferret.com

PetAg, 30 W. 432 Rt. 20, Elgen, IL 60120; 1-800-332-0877, 1-800-323-6878; www.petag.com

Ross Products Division, Abbott Laboratories, Columbus, OH 43215-1724; 1-800-986-8510; www.abbott.com, www.ross.com

Tomlyn Company, 711 S. Harding Hwy., Buena, NJ 08310; 1-800-866-5582; www.tomlyn.com

RESOURCES

American Ferret Association (AFA): www.ferret.org afa@ferret.org

Ferret Central: FAQ's at www.ferretcentral.org

Just a Business of Ferrets: www.mindspring.com/~jbferret jbferret@mindspring.com

For Ferrets Only, PO Box 1760, Dunnellon, Fl 34430-1760; 1-888-340-7671; www.craftycreatures.com/forferretsonly/contact.html

27
Exotic Felids

Gail Hedberg

INTRODUCTION

It is common for facilities with an exotic feline animal collection to suddenly have a need for hand-rearing protocols. Zoos, circuses, trainers for film work and corporate collectors/displayers—all have had a time when parental inability or mortality leaves them with one or more newborn cubs to raise. Rejection during the neonatal period (initial lactation) is frequently due to the mother's not being physiologically or behaviorally adapted to successfully rear her cubs. Hand rearing may also be a matter of choice rather than necessity if it is desirable to socialize the animal for tractability. Conversely, an injured or abandoned cub may require hand rearing with an eye toward release into the wild as the goal.

If orphaned cubs are to survive, strict husbandry guidelines must be observed. Stabilization includes a complete physical examination to determine the overall health status. Appropriate supportive therapy may be necessary to assist the animal's ability to thermoregulate and to correct dehydration. Well-formulated nutrition will promote proper development, and strict cleanliness standards will help ensure success (Fig. 27.1).

All factors contributing to a successful outcome are based on a proactive approach. Imagine the worst-case scenario, be prepared with a plan, and have the necessary items commonly used in hand rearing on hand. These include nipples, bottles, assorted milk replacers, an accurate scale, incubator or source of heat, blender, methods for warming the formula, assorted fleece bedding, and methods for sterilizing utensils, bottles, and nipples. Time and attention to detail are required for the 24-hour monitoring that is initially required to hand rear exotic felids. Hand rearing is as much of an art as it is a science. Utilizing these two concepts together will lead to a successful outcome.

CRITERIA FOR INTERVENTION

Sometimes cubs appear to be secure with the dam, but poor milk production causes weight loss and increased dehydration, combined with low rectal temperatures. Cubs may be observed to nurse but do not receive enough nutrition. Initial physical exam after 24 hours postpartum provides a baseline for monitoring the weight, temperature, and hydration for questionable situations. Continue to monitor these parameters at 48- and if necessary at 72-hour intervals.

FORMULAS AND FEEDING GUIDELINES

The criteria to determine which formula to use are based on comparing the analysis of maternal milk with product availability and individual species tolerance and acceptance. Nutritional requirements vary among individual members of the same species and members of the family Felidae. It is important to compare the maternal milk analysis with the selected milk substitute for each hand-rearing project (see Table 27.1).

There are significant differences among formulas in percentage of solids, fats, proteins, and carbohydrates. For example, puppy milk replacers are high in fat, and kitten milk replacers are high in carbohydrate and protein. Milks high in carbohydrates are often not tolerated well by *Panthera* sp. and this frequently leads to diarrhea. The inability to digest the carbohydrate lactose may be corrected by adding lactase enzyme such as Lactaid to the stock formula. Add 2 drops per 100 ml of prepared formula then refrigerate for 24 hours before feeding.

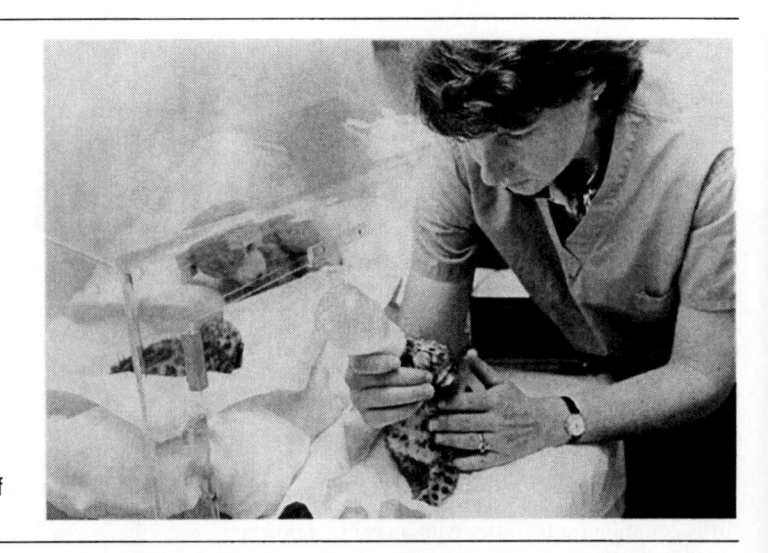

Figure 27.1 Feeding a snow leopard cub (photo courtesy of the San Francisco Zoo).

Table 27.1 Maternal Milk Analysis for Selected Nondomestic Felids

Species	Solids g/100g	Fats		Protein		Carbohydrate	
		g/100g	% g/g	g/100g	% g/g	g/100g	% g/g
Domestic cat, *Felis catus*[a]	17.7	5.0	28.0	7.2	40.5	4.9	27.8
Lynx, *Felis lynx*[e]	21.7	6.2	28.6	10.2	47.0	4.5	20.7
Puma, *Felis concolor*[b]	35.5	18.6	52.4	12.0	33.8	3.9	11.0
Leopard, *Panthera pardus*[e]	22.6	6.5	28.8	11.1	49.1	4.2	18.6
Jaguar, *Panthera onca*[c]	28.2	7.8	27.7	13.7	48.6	2.7	9.6
Lion, *Panthera leo*[d]	30.2	17.5	57.9	9.3	30.8	3.4	11.2
Tiger, *Panthera tigris*[c]	24.4	8.4	34.4	10.5	43.0	3.0	12.3
Cheetah, *Acinonyx jubatus*[b]	23.7	9.5	40.1	9.4	39.7	3.5	14.8

Source: Results were calculated from data obtained from [a]Abrams (1950); [b]Ben-Shaul (1962); [c]Jenness, Personal communication to author; [d]Jenness, Regehr, and Sloan (1970); [e]Anonymous undated. Also, M. Ewing, Personal communication to author.

Many *Panthera* species benefit from formulas that include a portion of strained-poultry-meat baby food added to the milk as early as one to two weeks of age. The added meat source provides extra calories without increasing the volume when the animal needs to begin the weaning phase (Table 27.2).

Chicken and turkey commercial baby foods are two well-accepted sources of easily digestible meat proteins. Maintaining the total percent solid content is helpful in preventing loose stools. Formulas that are low in protein may cause hair loss, which I observed when snow leopard cubs were fed straight Esbilac. When strained-chicken baby food was added, the hair coat improved. This technique is also beneficial in preparing for the weaning process. As a rule, it is best to introduce meat baby food gradually over the course of a week, not exceeding one jar (71.0 g) of baby food per 12.5 oz (370 ml) of prepared formula. This process can begin as early as twelve days of age if a predicable weight gain and acceptable stools are observed.

A complete list of nutritive composition of baby foods and common milk products is provided as a reference in this chapter. Creating formula may be necessary when commercial milk replacers are unavailable. There are other suitable options. Examples of successful homemade formulas are listed in Table 27.3.

Weaning/Enrichment Diet

A nutritious enrichment diet was developed by Liliana Abascal Johnson of the Guadalajara Zoo, Mexico. Use cooked (boiled) 1.5 kg whole chicken and remove skin, grind with 300 g dry commercial

Table 27.2 Tiger Cub Stock Formula

Age-Day		Ready to Feed Liquid
12	30 gms (2 TBS) Chicken Baby Food	370cc (12.5 oz can) Esbilac
13	45 gms (3 TBS) Chicken Baby Food	370cc (12.5 oz can) Esbilac
14	60 gms (4 TBS) Chicken Baby Food	370cc (12.5 oz can) Esbilac
15-20	70 gms (1 jar) Chicken Baby Food	370cc (12.5 oz can) Esbilac
21 **	140 gms Chicken Baby Food (2 jars), 8 gms ZuPreem Feline Diet (1.5 tsp)	740cc 2 (12.5 oz cans) Esbilac
22	140 gms Chicken Baby Food (2 jars), 15 gms ZuPreem Feline Diet (1 TBS)	740cc 2 (12.5 oz cans) Esbilac
23	140 gms Chicken Baby Food (2 jars), 22 gms ZuPreem Feline Diet (1.5 TBS)	740cc 2 (12.5 oz cans) Esbilac
24	105 gms Chicken Baby Food (1.5 jars), 30 gms ZuPreem Feline Diet (2.0 TBS)	740cc 2 (12.5 oz cans) Esbilac
25	70 gms Chicken Baby Food (1 jar), 37 gms ZuPreem Feline Diet (2.5 TBS)	740cc 2 (12.5 oz cans) Esbilac
26	70 gms Chicken Baby Food (1 jar), 45 gms ZuPreem Feline Diet (3 TBS)	740cc 2 (12.5 oz cans) Esbilac
27	70 gms Chicken Baby Food (1 jar), 60 gms ZuPreem Feline Diet (4 TBS)	740cc 2 (12.5 oz cans) Esbilac
28***	75 gms ZuPreem Feline Diet (5 TBS), Continue increasing ZuPreem Feline Diet in 15 gm increments daily	740cc 2 (12.5 oz cans) Esbilac
31	135 gms ZuPreem Feline Diet (9 TBS) or 1 can ZuPreem Feline Diet. This final concentration blends well and flows through an adjusted nipple.	740cc 2 (12.5 oz cans) 2220cc 6 (12.5oz cans) Esbilac

** Strain the formula through a cheesecloth, enlarge the nipple
*** Omit chicken baby food

cat food pellets. Prepare small meatballs and freeze. Also use an ice cube tray to form and freeze small quantities.

The use of commercial feline and canine milk replacers for hand rearing exotic felids has been well documented by published accounts in the *International Zoo Yearbook* and AZA's *Infant Diet Care Notebook*. A complete resource list is contained in Sources of Products Mentioned, below.

A recent survey shows an equally divided preference for Esbilac, KMR, and Zoologic Milk Matrix Formulation milk replacers. Goat's Milk Esbilac is a milk replacer for puppies with sensitive digestive systems. When using the powdered Esbilac or Milk Matrix 33/40 to make formula, the recommended ratio, by volume, of powder to water is 1:2 as the stock formula (see Table 27.4).

In 1993 a reformulation occurred with Esbilac and KMR. Butterfat was added to improve mixability. Some exotic species exhibited digestive problems with these new formulations. Lactobezoar was reported in tigers and leopards.

In conjunction with the above change came the development of Zoologic, a line of products made by PetAg, Inc. This system contains seven milk replacers to mix and match to meet the appropriate maternal milk analysis. The Zoologic products appropriate in felid hand rearing are Milk Matrix 33/40 and Milk Matrix 42/50. The product numbers represent the minimum crude protein and fat percentages. Note that these two formulations are original pre-1993 powdered Esbilac and KMR product without butterfat. These PetAg products are accessible for the international market.

Nurturall milk replacers by Veterinary Products Laboratories and Just Born milk replacers by Farnam Pet Products are basically the same products. It is a marketing clarification only. Nurturall is only available through a licensed veterinarian. Just Born is available through retail outlets. Both of these products are labeled for use in puppies or kittens, as is Lactol milk replacer manufactured by Sherley's Limited available in the United Kingdom. Wombaroo Food Products also markets specific

Table 27.3 Custom Recipes for Selected Species

Lion Cub Formula

As Fed	Maternal g/100g	Artificial g/100g	Ingredients	Amount
Solids	34.1	37.2	Cow's milk	160 ml
Fat	18.9	18.5	Cream	10 ml
Protein	12.5	13.6	1 Egg yolk	20 ml
Carbohydrate	2.7	3.2	Gelatin powder	30 ml
			Sunflower oil	30 ml

Leopard Cub Formula

As Fed	Maternal g/100g	Artificial g/100g	Ingredients	Amount
Solids	27.50	25.00	Cow's milk	180 ml
Fat	7.98	7.96	Glucose powder	3 ml
Protein	13.60	11.80	2 Egg yolk	40 ml
Carbohydrate	5.40	4.60	Gelatin powder	20 ml

Puma Cub Formula

As Fed	Maternal g/100g	Artificial g/100g	Ingredients	Amount
Solids	34.5	32.8	Cow's milk	168 ml
Fat	18.6	16.6	Cream	10 ml
Protein	12.0	12.0	1 Egg yolk	20 ml
Carbohydrate	3.9	4.1	Gelatin powder	25 ml
			Glucose powder	2 ml
			Sunflower oil	30 ml

Cheetah Cub Formula

As Fed	Maternal g/100g	Artificial g/100g	Ingredients	Amount
Solids	22.4	21.8	Cow's milk	185 ml
Fat	9.48	9.4	Water	20 ml
Protein	9.41	8.8	1 Egg yolk	20 ml
Carbohydrate	3.51	3.6	Gelatin powder	15 ml
			Sunflower oil	25 ml

5 g = 5 ml = 1 teaspoon; Gelatin and Glucose are in a granule form.

powdered milk replacer for the cheetah, lion, tiger, and puma. All of these are available to the international market. Artificial milk diets have limitations when compared to maternal milk. The formulations cannot fully duplicate maternal milk composition.

Taurine is an amino acid essential in the diet of felids. It is essential to other species but they synthesize taurine from cysteine. Mother-reared cubs receive taurine when nursing. Taurine deficiency has been reported to cause serious changes in heart function and retinopathy (Burton et al. 1988; Howard et al. 1987). It is an essential to supplement taurine when the artificial formula of choice is puppy milk replacer or cow's milk. A daily liquid taurine supplement, DYNATaurine, can be added to a bottle-feeding. Taurine is also available in a chewable tablet. Zoo infant felids should be supplemented with 250 mg of taurine per day. (McMannamon and Hedberg 1993). Commercial kitten milk replacer has been supplemented. Current preliminary

Table 27.4 FELID Taxonomy-Formula Guidelines and Birth Weights

	Species	Formula	Weight
Subfamily Acinonychinae			
Acinonyx jubatus	Cheetah	Milk Matrix 33/40, KMR, Custom	0.375–0.575 kg
Subfamily Felinae			
Caracal caracal (Felis or Lynx caracal)	Caracal	Milk Matrix 33/40 KMR	0.21–0.26 kg
Catopuma badia (Felis badia)	Bay cat	Milk Matrix 33/40 KMR	0.18 kg
Catopuma temminckii (Felis temminckii)	Temmincki's or Asian golden cat	Milk Matrix 33/40, 42/25, KMR, Esbilac	0.195–0.235 kg 0.18 kg
Felis bieti	Chinese desert cat	Milk Matrix 33/40, KMR	0.10 kg
Felis chaus	Jungle cat	Milk Matrix 33/40, KMR	0.19 kg
Felis margarita	Sand cat	Milk Matrix 33/40, KMR	0.09 kg
Felis margarita scheffeli	Pakistan sand cat	Milk Matrix 33/40, KMR	0.04–0.09 kg
Felis nigripes	Black-footed cat	Milk Matrix 33/40, KMR	0.085 kg
Felis sylvestris (includes Felis catus, ornata, lybica)	European, African, Indian wild cat	Milk Matrix 33/40, 42/25 KMR, Esbilac	0.113 kg
Herpailurus yaguarondi (Felis yagouarundi)	Jaguarundi	Milk Matrix 33/40, KMR	0.134 kg
Leopardus pardalis (Felis pardalis)	Ocelot	Milk Matrix 33/40, 42/25, KMR, Esbilac	0.215–0.250 kg 0.22 kg
Leopardus tigrinus (Felis tigrinus)	Tiger cat, tigrina or oncilla	Milk Matrix 33/40, KMR	0.08–0.13 kg
Leopardus wiedii (Felis wiedii)	Margay	Milk Matrix 33/40, 42/25, KMR, Esbilac, Lactol	0.17 kg
Leptailurus serval (Felis serval)	Serval	Milk Matrix 33/40, 42/25, KMR, Esbilac, Lactol	0.2–0.25 kg
Leptailurus serval (Felis serval)	Serval	Milk Matrix 33/40, 42/25, KMR, Esbilac	0.26 kg
Lynx canadensis (Felis canadensis), (Lynx lynx canadensis)	Canadian lynx	Milk Matrix 33/40, 42/25, KMR, Esbilac	0.155 kg
Lynx lynx (Felis lynx)	Eurasian lynx	Milk Matrix 33/40, 42/25, KMR, Esbilac	0.40 kg
Lynx pardina (Felis or Lynx lynx pardina)	Iberian lynx	Milk Matrix 33/40, 42/25, KMR, Esbilac	
Lynx rufus (Felis rufus)	Bobcat	Milk Matrix 33/40, 42/25, KMR, Esbilac	0.20 kg
L. r. escuinapae (F. r. escuinapae)	Mexican bobcat	Milk Matrix 33/40, 42/25, KMR, Esbilac	
Oncifelis colocolo (Felis colocolo)	Pampas cat	Milk Matrix 33/40, KMR	0.14 kg
Oncifelis geoffroyi (Felis geoffroyi)	Geoffroy's cat	Milk Matrix 33/40, KMR	0.07 kg
Oncifelis guigna (Felis guigna)	Kodkod	Milk Matrix 33/40, KMR	
Oreailurus jacobitus (Felis jacobita)	Mountain, Andean cat	Milk Matrix 33/40, KMR	

(continues)

Table 27.4 FELID Taxonomy-Formula Guidelines and Birth Weights (continued)

	Species	Formula	Weight
Subfamily Felinae			
Otocolobus manul (Felis manul)	Pallas's cat	Milk Matrix 33/40, KMR	0.08–0.15 kg
Prionailurus bengalensis (Felis bengalensis)	Leopard cat	Milk Matrix 33/40, KMR	0.08 kg
P. b. iriomotensis (Felis or Mayailurus iriomotensis)	Iriomote cat	Milk Matrix 33/40, KMR	
Prionailurus planiceps (Felis planiceps)	Flat-headed cat	Milk Matrix 33/40, KMR	
Prionailurus rubiginosus (Felis rubiginosus)	Rusty-spotted cat	Milk Matrix 33/40, KMR	0.07 kg
Prionailurus viverrinus (Felis viverrinus)	Fishing cat	Milk Matrix 33/40, 42/25, KMR, Esbilac	0.176 kg
Profelis aurata (Felis aurata)	African golden cat	Milk Matrix 33/40, KMR	
Puma concolor cougar (F. c. cougar)	Eastern cougar or puma	Milk Matrix 33/40, 42/25, KMR, Esbilac, Custom	0.22–0.68 kg
Subfamily Pantherinae			
Neofelis nebulosa	Clouded leopard	Milk Matrix 33/40	0.205 kg
Panthera leo	Lion	Milk Matrix 33/40, 42/25, KMR, Esbilac, Lactol, Custom	1.10 kg
P. l. persica	Asian or Indian Lion	Milk Matrix 33/40, 42/25, KMR, Esbilac, Custom	1.13–1.19 kg
Panthera onca	Jaguar	Milk Matrix 33/40, 42/25, KMR, Esbilac	0.59 kg
Panthera pardus	Leopard	Milk Matrix 33/40, 42/25, KMR, Esbilac, Custom	0.482–0.653 kg
Panthera tigris	Tiger	Milk Matrix 33/40, 42/25, KMR, Esbilac	0.68–1.40 kg
Pardofelis marmorata (Felis marmorata)	Marbled cat	Milk Matrix 42/25 Esbilac	0.095 kg
Uncia uncia (Panthera uncia)	Snow leopard	Milk Matrix 33/40, 42/25, KMR, Esbilac	0.510–0.594 kg

Note: Taxonomy data-Reprint with permission from Kristin Nowell (Nowell and Jackson, 1996). Average birth weights from AZA (1985).

research from this author indicates taurine levels in commercial chicken baby food to be a good dietary source. Once the animal is receiving a meat-base diet, the taurine supplement may be discontinued.

Formula preparation should follow certain critical guidelines. If multiple caregivers are involved, one individual should be designated as the advisor to set the feeding schedule and to provide instructions on how to mix the formula. Use only presterilized bottles and nipples. Prefill bottles for the total number of scheduled feedings needed for 24 hours. Make enough formula for an extra feeding in case of loss or spillage. Label bottles with the date, time prepared, and amount. If a bottle is designated for a particular feeding, label it accordingly. Any equipment used for formula preparation must not be used for other purposes. Clean all equipment well with hot soapy water and rinse thoroughly as some ingredients may leave a thin, greasy film on plastic. Rufect is an effective enzymatic detergent-degreaser with disinfectant properties. If feeding equipment is not thoroughly rinsed, soap residue may cause loose stool. A basic sterilization method of boiling feeding utensils, bottles, and nipples once a day is a good practice. The use of sterile, bottled, or boiled water until such time that an animal's stability is no longer at risk is extremely important. Do not use distilled water because it lacks essential minerals. An animal that has normal stool and has slowly been introduced to a normal adult environmental can be considered stable.

An animal's response to hand rearing is measured by satisfaction between feedings, acceptable stool, and adequate weight gain. Proper hygiene, strict handling and storage of ingredients, and utensil sterilization contribute to the overall health of the animal and cannot be emphasized enough.

BOTTLE-FEEDING GUIDELINES

A bottle should be offered only if an animal is stable, alert, and responsive. The first bottle-feeding should be done with an oral electrolyte solution and is to primarily strengthen the suckling response. If a strong suckle response is present, then a dilute milk formula can be offered. Introduce the stock formula gradually to newborns as well as older neonates. Initially offer a dilute formula that is 25% formula and 75% electrolyte solution. Gradually increase the strength of the formula over the next 24 to 36 hours. It is important to note that dehydration can still be present and subcutaneous fluids may need to be continued until the first bowel movement.

The suckling response may be stimulated and encouraged with proper nipple selection and is critical in successfully starting the hand-rearing process (Fig. 27.2). The emotional gratification of the neonate may be ensured when that time spent nursing from the bottle is slow and consistent. Frustration from the animal occurs when inappropriate nipples are used or when the flow of the formula is inappropriate. Too much formula too fast is not good either. Extensive experience shows that selection and use of specialty natural latex nipples have been valuable in bottle-feeding. See Sources of Products Mentioned, below, for available nipples.

The goal in nipple selection is to find the perfect nipple and make modifications in the flow rate to encourage a slow, passively controlled feeding.

The smaller felid species respond well to the Pet Nurser system as well as the elongated, conical shaped nipple by Four Paws. Two other uniquely shaped nipples (balloon-shaped and elongated) made by PetAg are other acceptable options to have available. *Panthera* species initially respond well to a shorter, softer version of a standard human infant nipple. There are two specialty nipples for premature human infants that work very well for

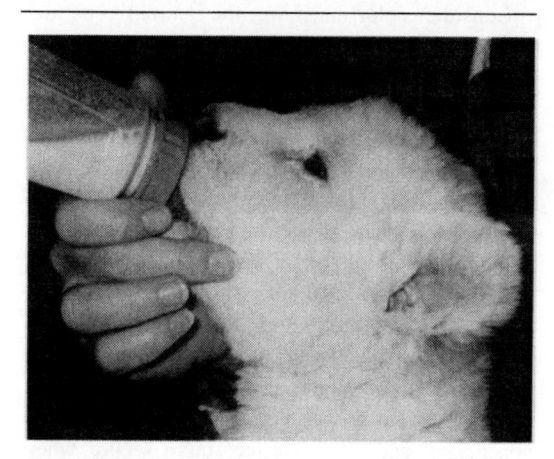

Figure 27.2 White lion nursing (photo by Kent Hedberg, courtesy of Siegfried and Roy Productions).

Panthera. Mead-Johnson manufactures two standard nipples and a "NUK"-shaped orthodontic preemie-size nipple. The next size that works well is the Evenflo Preemie Nipple. This is available at the larger human-infant retail outlets. It does collapse with a strong aggressively nursing cub so it is recommended that these be used only in the early development stages in cubs that are one to ten days of age. The flow rate is adjusted to maintain a slow flow to minimize aspiration from too much milk being suckled too fast. Venting the bottle by tightening or loosening cap rings will adjust the flow. An animal should never nurse so aggressively that it collapses and pulls the nipple out of the cap. This usually occurs when the nipple is too soft. Standard latex infant-formula nipples are ideal for older lion, tiger, and leopard cubs and will last until the animal is weaned because they are more durable. Cubs may be finicky and develop a preference for a certain nipple. Care should be taken to use that specific brand of nipple throughout the nursing period. Always have adequate nipple replacements in case a new nipple is needed. In this way negative behaviors, such as possessiveness, can be minimized. The cub will be less likely to get frustrated. Ultimately the goal is to wean a cub off the bottle and onto solid food with minimal stress and effort.

HOUSING

Incubators provide a controlled temperature environment for severely compromised newborns. See the product list at the end of this chapter for sources. It is extremely important to avoid overheating newborns.

Consider color-matching the animal's natural coat to the artificial bedding. Polyester fleece (see Sources) is available in assorted colors—white, cream, and gray. This product is very durable and seems to hold up the best even when left with unsupervised animals. Extreme caution should be used, however, when selecting synthetic fleece. Animals that suckle on these fabrics may ingest fibers, which could cause constipation. Many artificial fabrics ("fake furs") are available and can be sewn in shapes that resemble fabric-covered bolsters. If Velcro is used, laundering and restuffing with rolled terry-cloth towels is the most hygienic. This replicates the shape of a maternal felid's abdomen or appendage, and all felids feel more secure when draped over their mother.

With multiple cubs, use color-coded file-folder charts that match the available colors for baby bottle cap rings, nipple covers, and I.D. collars. Colored nail polish applied to one or more nails on one foot may also be incorporated during the early days for ease in identification.

To prevent the potential exposure to environmental contaminants, caregivers should avoid contact with other animals while hand rearing. If caring for other animals and crossover is to occur, strict hygiene measures should be practiced before returning to the hand-rearing facility. A change of clothing and washing hands and arms with an antibacterial soap is mandatory. Basic quarantine guidelines should be implemented. When entering the facility, shoes should be removed and replaced with alternate footwear that is designated for use only when working with the hand-reared animal.

History has shown that the number of participants involved in hand-rearing programs should be limited to two to three caregivers. The fewest number of caregivers ensures reduced stress on the animal, provides better consistency with record keeping, and provides continuity with all aspects of husbandry. Individuals not providing care must wait until the animals receive their first scheduled vaccination before they may handle them. Each hand-rearing project presents with a unique set of circumstances. If solid routines and guidelines are established, the potential risks can be minimized.

FEEDING STRATEGIES

Certain sensitive species like leopard species may be difficult for the caregiver to manage and acclimate to hand rearing. Using the appropriate nipple is helpful. Often it requires great patience while convincing a cub to relax and focus. Waiting until the cub is drifting off to sleep to insert the nipple into its mouth will allow the bonding process to proceed. Another method has also proven successful. While seated, scruff the cub and gently suspend and slowly swing it with one hand. This mimics the same motions as if the mother were carrying the cub in her mouth. Slowly lower the cat to your lap. When the cub is relaxed, insert the nipple/bottle. Repeat this process for short periods in a dark room.

The amount to feed is usually based on the total volume calculated for the day, based on a percentage of the animal's weight. For this reason it is imperative to have an accurate scale.

Cubs and kittens can consume as much as 15–20% of their body weight per day. The small felids seem to require the higher percentage. Using a conservative figure of 12–18% per day is a good starting point. After the first three days, the daily amount may be adjusted. The first feed should be promptly at 0800 (8 A.M.) and the cub should be fed every 2.5 to 3 hours; this would be six to eight feedings a day. Once the total daily amount has been determined, divide that by the total number of feedings in 24 hours to determine the amount to be offered at each feed. A weight gain trend of 100 to 200 grams a day in large felids and 50 to 100 grams a day in smaller species is acceptable. When the calculated amount of formula has been consumed, most felids do not require feedings past 2100 (9 P.M.).

For the first feeding of the day, it is easier to feed the amount calculated and prepared from the day before. Once the morning routine is under way, calculate the amount needed to meet the nutritional goals for that day. Weigh the animal after it has been stimulated to urinate and defecate. If inadequate weight or lower than desired weigh gain is recorded, formula percentages may be increased slowly with each bottle. Often animals require a second feeding within one to one and a half hours after the initial morning feed. Feedings after this "catch-up" period should allow the schedule to level out. The rest of the feedings will satisfy the cub and normal sleep periods will occur after feeding. Animals should not be overfed. Do not allow the animal to consume all that it wants. Diarrhea will often occur when an animal is fed more than 25% of its body weight per day. Animals may gain weight too quickly and have difficulty supporting their own body weight. It can also predispose them to bone developmental abnormalities. Supplementing with sterile water or oral electrolytes post-feeding often provides the cubs with an extra feeling of fullness without the risk of overfeeding.

Assessing the feeding response each time a bottle

is offered is a good indicator for evaluating overall attitude and demeanor. Kittens and cubs should always be eager to be fed. Each case requires modification and a certain customization to meet the individual needs of the animal.

The normal digestive process occurs while the cub sleeps undisturbed until sunrise. This is where the benefits of having a premeasured bottle for this first feeding prove helpful. Critical-care newborns may need intense monitoring for the first week if the nutritional goals cannot be met within the above time schedule. Daily total formula consumption records are important to see exactly what percentage of body weight the animal actually did consume. If the diet provides the proper level of satiation, the cub or kitten will be content to sleep between feedings. However, with the larger cubs, it is not recommended to exceed 8 oz (240 ml) of formula per feeding. Note that strained meat baby food may be slowly reduced and canned feline ZuPreem added and pureed in the formula starting at three to four weeks of age.

The weaning process may be instituted as soon as the incisors have erupted. Canned ZuPreem or other nutritionally balanced carnivore diets are introduced from a pan. This is as early as 4.5–5.5 weeks of age. I have experienced situations in which cubs had difficulty during the weaning phase. Vomiting, diarrhea, and refusal of the bottle for one to two feedings have occurred. The bottle becomes a tool for maintaining the established bond between the caregiver and cub. Weaning to an adult diet often depends on available products. The most important consideration is to provide a nutritionally balanced diet for continued growth and development.

Each animal experiences levels of frustration when the volume or numbers of bottle feedings are changed. Cubs may become possessive over the bottle or feed/water pan sometimes without provocation. Forced weaning occurs because attempts to bottle-feed may become dangerous to the surrogate. It is at this time that assorted adult food items should be gradually introduced to reduce potential problems with diarrhea. These products must be suitable nutritionally balanced adult zoo carnivore diets. Time and patience are required to carry the animal through this critical period. Daily weight checks need to be continued to evaluate the overall transition to an adult diet.

EXPECTED WEIGHT GAIN

Expect an initial gain of 100 grams per day for large species (lions, tigers, leopards) and 50 grams per day for smaller species (serval, bobcat, caracal). These figures will double when solids are introduced.

IMPORTANCE OF ADEQUATE TRANSFER OF IMMUNOGLOBULINS

Although the immune system of felid neonates is capable of responding at birth, environmental pathogens present a considerable risk to newborns. Some of these organisms are innocuous to an adult but when a neonate is exposed, an overwhelming infection may occur before the immune system can generate a primary immune response. Maternal antibodies help protect the neonate while they develop the ability to mount an immune response to the antigens in their environment. Kittens and cubs are vulnerable to systemic bacterial infections, particularly those causing bronchopneumonia during the first few weeks of life.

Recent studies have revealed that domestic kittens receive 95% of their maternal antibodies from the colostrum and milk of the queen (Levy and Crawford 2000; Casal, Jesyk, and Giger 1996).

Exotic felid species may be at risk for failure of passive transfer of these antibodies if the young are rejected before receiving colostrum. This is of greater concern in underweight and weak neonates or those that lack the strength to compete with siblings. Offspring in large litters may be at risk because they have dams with inadequate colostrum production for the entire litter. If a kitten or cub has a questionable history of nursing, it may have problems with infections during the first two months of life because its immune system may not be well developed. In such cases, animals will need to be managed with additional supportive care and/or antibiotic therapy.

New research studying failure of passive transfer in kittens indicates the (domestic) feline gut closes to transfer of IgG by 16 hours after birth. (Casal et al. 1996). The intestine is unable to absorb these large molecules at later times. There are several tests available to determine if a neonate has adequate IgG levels. The most definitive is serum radial immunodiffusion. This quantifies levels of immunoglobulins. Although one report found no difference in IgG concentrations between feline milk and colostrum, preliminary data from the University of Florida found colostral IgG concentration of to be 4000–8000 mg/dl (Levy and Crawford 2000). This falls rapidly until by approximately one-week postpartum the level in milk is closer to 250 mg/dl or lower. These findings are more typical of other species that have been studied.

Failure of passive transfer can be corrected in kittens by administration of adult cat serum either IP or SQ. The dose required to reach the normal IgG levels of nursing kittens is 150 ml/kg of serum to colostrum-deprived kittens less than 24 hours old (Levy and Crawford 2000). However, the minimum concentration of IgG required to protect neonates from infection is unknown. In foals, failure of passive transfer (FPT) treatment goals include raising serum IgG concentration to at least half of normal (Levy and Crawford 2000). If the same holds true for exotic felids, then a minimum of 75 ml/kg IP or SQ BID would be appropriate for a tiger cub that was at risk at 24 hours postpartum (Levy, Phone conversation with author).

Collection and long-term storage of serum and or plasma from all exotics that have breeding potential is recommended as a source for supplemental IgG. It is necessary to screen potential donors because of the risk of disease transmission with blood products. Continued research is ongoing to establish a more practical source of supplementation of IgG in domestic kittens (Levy, Phone conversation with author). Further research is needed on the problem of correction of failure of passive transfer in exotic felids.

COMMON MEDICAL PROBLEMS

Respiratory Infections

Managing a neonate requires that every effort be made to reduce the risk of exposure to potential pathogens. Necropsy results compiled from 116 kittens that died within the first 8 weeks of life indicated that bacterial bronchopneumonia was the most common finding (Casal et al. 1996). The bacterial isolates from the kittens included *E. coli*, hemolytic streptococci, *Pasteurella multocida*, *Staphylococcus aureus*, and gram-negative enteropathogens (Casal et al. 1996). Their isolates were similar to bacteria found in the respiratory and gastrointestinal tracts of healthy cats, indicating that fatal respiratory infections in preweaned kittens may arise from the normal flora of the queens (Casal et al. 1996).

Umbilical Stump Treatment

Newborns have a decreased resistance to bacterial infections, which makes them prone to sepsis when they are stressed. The most common route of entry is the umbilicus. Apply chlorhexidine (0.5%) (Nolvasan 2% solution diluted 1:3 with sterile water or saline) to the umbilical stump every 6 hours for 24 hours and examine for heat or swelling. This is more effective than 2% iodine or povidone-iodine. Seven percent iodine is caustic and burns the end of the umbilicus trapping bacteria within the stump. Dilute povidone-iodine also has the potential for bacterial entrapment. Chlorhexidine is used because it is less caustic and has a wider bacterial spectrum. It also has longer residual antimicrobial activity (Madigan 1997).

Hypothermia

The ability of neonatal felids to thermoregulate is limited. Normal rectal temperatures range from 96.8°F (36.0°C) in the first days to 97–99°F (36.2–37.2°C) in the first two to four weeks. If a newborn's body temperature drops below 94°F (34.5°C), its suckling response may be diminished or absent.

Hypothermia may be caused by a number of factors such as low ambient temperature, weak or immature cubs, insufficient maternal instinct causing neglect of care, or excessive grooming. Insufficient mammary development in the dam can also reduce a cub's ability to receive warmth when they nestle against the mammary glands for heat. A chilled cub should never be warmed rapidly as this results in tissue damage and hemorrhage. The use of heat lamps is not advisable as they may cause severe burns and dehydration if left unattended. Heating pads should be covered and set at the lowest setting. Heating pads that are used incorrectly may also cause severe burns, which may only be evident days later when the tissue begins to slough. Circulating warm-water heating pads and ICU water-lined warmers see Sources below) are the safest methods to heat the cubs. It is best to maintain a temperature gradient within a neonate's confined space. A range of 5–10°F (3–5°C) from the warmest to the coolest spot will allow the animal to either seek heat or to select the area most comfortable. It is important to monitor the temperature of the enclosure using either traditional or electronic environmental thermometers. Using a remote digital sensor (see Sources below) provides a method of precisely monitoring ambient temperature from a remote location. This device has the ability to monitor changes within a preset margin and to sound an alarm when the temperature changes suddenly or moves outside the set range. The caregiver may monitor the base station while the animal setup is in another room. This can be extremely valuable if a power or equipment failure occurs in the middle of the night when the cubs are not under immediate supervision.

Hypoglycemia and Dehydration

In cases of hypothermia, the suckling response may be virtually nonexistent. Often an underlying factor contributing to hypothermia is hypoglycemia. A combination of supplemental heat and subcutaneous fluid electrolytes with 2.5% dextrose will help to stimulate the suckle response.

A dehydrated newborn should not be given any formula, as this will dehydrate the animal more. The total normal oral and parenteral fluid maintenance requirement in neonates is 50 ml–75 ml/kg/day. This can be divided into two or three doses over a 24-hour period. These guidelines depend on how rapidly the fluids are absorbed and the animal's demeanor. Neonates seem to have a higher fluid maintenance requirement. Starting at the higher dose is appropriate for the first assessment. Then taper to the lower dose until the animal is stable.

Calcium Deficiency

Balanced calcium and phosphorus ratios should be maintained throughout the hand-rearing process. Commercial kitten and puppy milk replacers provide the appropriate ratio. Abnormal calcium and phosphorus ratios may result in metabolic bone disease, and may be a result of inadequate formula intake during the weaning process. Adequate calcium levels must be maintained until the felid reaches maturity. Weaning diets of chicken and organ meat are extremely high in phosphorus. Special attention to calcium supplementation to balance the phosphorus is required. If a cub presents with lameness, take radiographs to rule out inadequate cortical bone development.

Diarrhea

Note: If the reader follows the recommendations in this section exactly, problems with diarrhea may be avoided. Diarrhea is fairly common in hand-reared felids. Generally, it is caused by a dietary imbalance, which could be a result of a variety of factors. The formula may be inappropriate for the species, may be too concentrated or offered too much or too often. Diarrhea may occur if the ingredients of the formula are changed too quickly, for example, during the addition of meat. Most commonly, diarrhea is caused by powdered formula that is made up and offered too concentrated in the initial feeds to cubs that are less than four weeks of age. Occasionally cubs will develop diarrhea when a new batch of powdered product is introduced. Batches of powdered product may vary and if the consistency of the stock formula changes with the new batch, adjustments in the powder-to-water ratio will need to be made. Cultures of the feces should be taken to rule out bacterial causes. If there is no underlying medical problem, often giving the cubs straight Pedialyte (Ross) or an electrolyte solution for one feed, and then half-strength formula for several feeds after that, may help. Gradually increase the strength of the formula as the consistency of the feces improves. Sometimes this process takes several days to a week or more. The *gradual* addition of meat to the formula, such as chicken baby food (with no onion), or ZuPreem often results in improved fecal consistency. If the diarrhea persists and/or is severe, the cub should be evaluated by a veterinarian and may require fluid therapy.

SOCIALIZATION

As human surrogates for their mothers, we are responsible for addressing the emotional needs of each animal. Experienced individuals share the viewpoint that a human-animal bond is created with the intense nursery care. This can be measured in the animal's ability to adapt to a captive environment. The strength of an established relationship is often underestimated. The goals of any hand-rearing project should have been defined at the start. Is the animal going to be used as a contact animal for education or is it an exhibit animal? Sometimes it may take intense effort and time to see that an animal's full potential is not compromised or damaged as a result of our intervention. Improper training techniques at an early age are an example. A commitment and attention to the style of care can have a significant impact on potentially negative stereotypic behaviors often reported in accounts of hand-reared animals.

The following scenarios may be useful guidelines when considering hand-rearing options. If a single animal is presented for hand rearing, it may be beneficial to network with other neighboring institutions to locate similar situations. Consider consolidating the hand-rearing efforts at one facility and then shift to the other for the remainder of the weaning phase. This will allow both institutions to share the project. Rearing animals together provides benefits both to animals and institutions until a semipermanent status is reached. Because birth season for felid species in captivity is somewhat predictable, this is a practical approach.

Providing the cubs with a variety of safe and interesting "toys" will help to prevent boredom. Boredom may lead to undesirable behaviors. Plan on rotating the toys as interest declines. Simple toys made from socks as well as "puppy" toys are safe and interesting in the first phase of development. Toys should provide independent exploration of the environment. The surrogate should not try to play with the animal and its toys. This promotes aggressive play. Keep in mind what seems acceptable for a 5 kg animal may not be acceptable when it weighs 50 kg. Shaping a cub's behavior in nonconfrontational, positive ways reduces fear and distrust. The most important step in reducing undesirable behaviors is to try to understand the origin of the undesirable behavior and use redirection to correct it. Cubs kept busy several times per day with physical, challenging activities are much less likely to develop into animals that bite. A caregiver who has an ability to anticipate and predict certain moods and attitudes will have the most successful approach.

A lion as an adult is an aggressive, fearless cat that is typically silent when threatened. On the other hand, tigers are far more demonstrative in conveying their moods. When comparing tiger and lion cubs, two-month-old lion cubs are slower to develop emotionally. They require selective levels of security when compared to tiger cubs of the same age. This means periodic reassurance by the surrogate. Negative snarling and growling are symptoms of poor socialization, temperament defects, and a caregiver's failure to establish clear leadership.

When caretakers provide socialization and good leadership, they increase the animal's confidence and feeling of security, and reduce excessive inappropriate, dangerous behaviors. For weaned cubs, examples include feeding and taking cubs out at regularly scheduled times each day. Early acceptance of leash training will help facilitate this. Introduction of collar and leash can start at two to four weeks of age. This method of animal handling must be introduced with patience and caution. For those unfamiliar with this style of training, seek outside help and guidance.

Human surrogates that initiate play behavior are viewed by the cub as a "play toy." The cub's mouth is a tool for exploration, acquisition, social advancement, stress reduction, vocal expression, and survival. In social groups, cubs bite each other to test relative strength and establish rank without causing serious trauma. The human surrogates need to learn and understand play behaviors. This requires an ability to react effectively and redirect these aggressive instincts.

Possessiveness is a behavior resulting from a dominant animal establishing control over food, food dishes, toys, brooms, and territory. This defensive, self-protective trait is the cub's attempt to keep an impending threat away. Usually it is the inexperienced caregiver that promotes this behavior. Early signs may be apparent when bottle-feeding. If a feeding frenzy is allowed to proceed, this behavior will only accelerate as the cub matures. The bottle-feeding period can be gratifying and comforting for the adolescent cub well beyond the nutritional requirement for a milk diet. It must be decided if this is promoting the established bond or challenging it. This negative behavior cannot be changed, only minimized. It is in the early days of bottle-feeding that possessive behavior can be discouraged.

ACKNOWLEDGMENTS

I would like to express appreciation to Freeland Dunker, Karen Schuester, Ellen Williams, Avery Bennett, and Laurie Gage for reviewing and offering helpful criticism of an earlier draft. Ellen Dierenfeld, Quinton Rogers, Mary Ewing, Penny Andrews, Debra Hoffman, July Levy, and Scott Citino provided information.

SOURCES OF PRODUCTS MENTIONED

Animal Intensive Care Unit (AICU): 30 lb table top acrylic forced air incubator by Lyon Electric Company, Inc., 1690 Brandywine Ave., Chula Vista, CA 91911; 1-619-216-3400; FAX 1-619-216-3434; www.lyonelectric.com lyonelect@cts.com

Beaphar Inc. (USA), 6200 Falls of Neuse Rd., Suite 102, Raleigh, NC 27609; 1-919-855-9990; FAX 1-919-855-9991

Dyna-Taurine: Harlmen Corporation, PO Box 371073, Omaha, NE 68114; VOICE/FAX 1-800-393-0794; E-mail: info@harlmen.com

Esbilac: PetAg Inc., 261 Keyes Ave., Hampshire, IL 60140; 1-800-323-0877, 1-800-323-6878; www.petag.com

Evenflo latex nipples, rings, nipple covers, sealing disc: Evenflo Company, Inc., 1801 Commerce Dr., Piqua, OH 45356; 1-800-233-5921; www.evenflo.com

Four Paws Pet Nurser: Four Paws Products Limited, 50 Wireless Blvd., Hauppauge, NY 11788; 1-516-434-1100; www.fourpaws.com

Goat's Milk Esbilac: PetAg Inc., 261 Keyes Ave., Hampshire, IL 60140; 1-800-323-0877, 1-800-323-6878; www.petag.com

Intensive Care Systems: Portable water-lined warmers by Thermo Care, PO Box 6069, Incline Village, NV 89450; 1-800-262-4020; FAX 1-775-831-1230; E-mail: staff@thermocare.com

Isolette Infant Incubator: Used Air Shields Incubator, Rankin Biomedical Corporation, 9580 Dolores Dr., Clarkston, MI 48348; 1-248-625-4104; FAX 1-248-625-1070; E-mail: rankin@tir.com

Just Born: Farnam Pet Products, A division of Farnam Companies, Inc., Phoenix, AZ 85013; 1-800-234-2269; www.farnam.com

KMR: PetAg Inc., 261 Keyes Ave., Hampshire, IL 60140; 1-800-323-0877, 1-800-323-6878; www.petag.com

Lactol: Sherley's Limited, Homefield Rd., Haverhill, Suffolk CB9 8QP, U.K.; Phone: 01440 715700; FAX 01440 713940; E-mail: sherleys@dial.pipex.com

Mead Johnson Nutritionals: Nipples; 1-812-429-6339; FAX 1-812-429-7189; 24-hour toll-free fax-on demand 1-888-606-7737; www.mead-johnson.com

Nurturall: Veterinary Products Laboratories, PO Box 34820, Phoenix, AZ 85067-4820; 1-888-241-9545; www.vpl.com

Pedialyte: Ross Products Division, Abbott Laboratories, Columbus, OH 43215-1724; 1-800-986-8510; www.abbott.com, www.ross.com

Polyester Fleece: Body Gear for Pets, PO Box 5924, Petaluma, CA 94955; 1-800-699-4050; FAX 1-707-792-2262; E-mail: bodygear@pacbell.net

Rufect: Detergent/Disinfectant by the Ruhof Corporation, 808 West Merrick Road, Balley Stream, NY 11580; 1-800-537-8463; FAX 1-516-285-5888; www.ruhof.com

Wireless Thermometer with remote sensor: Oregon Scientific International, Ltd. 19861 SW 95th Place, Tualatin, OR 97062; 1-888-274-7980; FAX 1-541-465-9406; info@oscientific.com; www.oregonscientific.com

Wombaroo Food Products, PO Box 151, Glen Osmond SA, Australia 5064; 08-8379-1339; wombaroo@adelaide.on.net

Zoologic Milk Matrix Nutritional Components: PetAg Inc., 261 Keyes Ave., Hampshire, IL 60140; 1-800-323-0877, 1-800-323-6878; www.petag.com

ZuPreem Feline Diet:. Premium Nutritional Products, Inc., PO Box 2094, Shawnee Mission, KS 66202; 1-913-438-8900; FAX 1-913-438-1881; www.zupreem.com

REFERENCES

1975. Composition of Foods; Raw, Processed, Prepared. Watt BK, Merril AL, editors. Washington D.C.: United States Department of Agriculture.

1985. Infant Diet/Care Notebook. Silver Sprigs. MD: American Association of Zoological Parks and Aquariums.

1996. Status Survey and Conservation Action Plan, Wild Cats. Nowell K, Jackson P, editors. Gland, Switzerland: IUCN/SSC Cat Specialist Group.

Anonymous. 1982 Mother's Milk Is Nature's Most Perfect Food, Then Come Borden Milk Replacers. Composition of Animal Milks. Borden, Inc Pet/Vet Products, Elgin, Il.

Abrams J. 1950. *Linton's animal nutrition and veterinary dietetics.* Edinburgh: W. Green and Son.

Ben Shaul DM. 1962. The composition of the milk of wild animals. *International Zoo Yearbook*: Zoological Society of London. p 333–342.

Burton MS, Gillespie DS, Rogers QR, Morris P. A taurine reponsive dilated cardiomyopathy in a snow leopard and plasma taurine levels in exotic cats; 1988. *Proceedings of the American Association of Zoo Veterinarians.* p 199–200.

Casal ML, Jesyk PF, Giger U. 1996. Transfer of colostral antibodies from queens to their kittens. *American Journal of Veterinary Research* 57(11):1653–8.

Ewing MA. May 1984. Felid Infant Diets and Dietary Formulations Used In Hand-Rearing Cubs. San Marcos, TX: Southwest Texas State University. 158 p.

Howard J, Rogers QR, Koch SA, Goodrowe KL, Montali RJ, Bush M. 1987. Diet-induced taurine deficincy rettinopathy in leopard cats (*Felis bengalensis*); *Proceedings of the American Association of Zoo Veterinarians.* p 496–498.

Jenness R, Sloan R. 1970. The Composition of Milks of Various Species: A Review. *Dairy Science Abstract* 32(10):599–612.

Levy JK, Crawford PC, Collante WR, Papich MG. 2001. Use of adult cat serum to correct failure of passive transfer in kittens. *Journal of American Veterinary Medical Association* 219(10):1401–1405.

Madigan JE. 1997. Daily Nursing Care. In: Madigan JE, editor. *Manual of Equine Neonatal Medicine.* 3rd ed. Woodland, CA: Live Oak Publishing. p 92–94.

McManamon R, Hedberg G. 1993. Practical tips in nursery rearing of exotic felids. *Journal of Small and Exotic Animal Medicine* 2(3):137–140.

28
Elephants

Karen A. Emanuelson and Colleen E. Kinzley

NATURAL HISTORY

The average birth weight of an African elephant calf (*Loxodonta africana*) is 100–120 kg, and that of an Asian elephant calf (*Elephas maximus*) is 90–110 kg. Most wild elephant populations show an annual reproductive cycle that corresponds to the seasonal availability of food and water. Typically females are reproductively viable in the second half of the rainy season and the first months of the dry season. Captive elephants are not driven by the seasons and females typically cycle every 14–16 weeks. The average gestation period is 22 months, but some pregnancies can last 24 months. Calves are milk dependent for the first two years and will often suckle to the age of four or five.

RECORD KEEPING

Daily records that allow for the 24-hour tabulation of input/output will translate easily into weekly and monthly summaries that make it easier to monitor trends in feeding and stool production. Other information that should be included is vital signs, sleeping periods, and behavior. Documentation of body development, eruption of molars and tusks, and behavioral learning stages of the calf would be valuable additions to the knowledge of elephants. Complete medical records including clinical notes, prescriptions, and diagnostic test results should be updated frequently by the veterinarian.

EQUIPMENT

Planning should include the acquisition of supplies several months in advance of the anticipated birth date. Supplies needed include bovine bottles and nipples, elephant milk replacer, human breast pump, walk-on heavy-duty scale, elephant plasma, and elephant colostrum, if available (see more under Assessment below). A portable radiology unit and an oxygen-administration system are advisable. A 300 MA radiology unit is necessary for all but the distal extremities.

CRITERIA FOR INTERVENTION

Planning for any elephant birth should include plans for possible need to hand raise the calf, or supplement the calf's diet. There are many possible scenarios that would necessitate hand rearing or supplementing a calf, such as aggression from the dam, death or illness of the dam, poor milk production, a weak or undersized calf, and others. Very few elephants have been hand raised from birth. In the eleven reported cases of calves entirely hand raised from birth only five survived past infancy. Five other cases reported successful reintroduction to the dam after a period of up to ten days of bottle-feeding the calf (Kinzley 1997).

ASSESSMENT OF THE NEONATE AND INITIAL CARE

Suggested medical protocol for a rejected or orphaned elephant calf less than 24 hours of age is as follows: Assess immediate needs by evaluating respiration, heart rate, and mucous membrane perfusion. Administer emergency therapy or oxygen therapy immediately if needed. Normal body temperature is 97.5–99°F (36–37.2°C). If the body temperature is less than 97.5°F (36°C), use heat sources such as heat lamps and/or heating blankets to bring the temperature back to normal range. Collect blood samples for complete blood count and serum chemistry analysis (STAT), qualitative IgG test, and serum electrophoresis. Save extra serum and freeze.

Draw blood for aerobic/anaerobic culture if the calf is weak and/or placentitis is present. Weigh the calf. Administer elephant colostrum if available, two to ten liters orally, preferably by bottle-feeding (Fowler 1978). The calf is unlikely to consume more than 0.5 liters in a single feeding. The colostrum should be given when the calf is less than 6–12 hours old, if possible, and no more than 24 hours old. Bovine colostrum may be substituted if elephant colostrum is not available. Assess fluid balance. Insert IV catheter if fluid therapy or plasma therapy is indicated. If the calf has not received colostrum, elephant plasma is the preferred fluid. If the calf has received colostrum, use LRS and/or plasma. Perform a thorough physical examination, including examination of the umbilicus, and assess maturity. Examine the placenta to see if it is complete or incomplete. Save appropriate samples of it for culture and sensitivity, and histopathology. Evaluate lab data and physical exam, decide upon appropriate antibiotic, plasma, fluid, and dextrose therapy. Give tetanus prophylaxis, umbilical care, and vitamin E injection.

Normal vital signs are not well established, but are briefly summarized in the AZA *Elephant Husbandry Notebook* (Kinzley and Emanuelson, in press). Normal hematologic and serum chemistry values have been reported (Allen et al. 1985; Heard, Jacobson, and Brock 1986).

MILK REPLACER AND SUPPLEMENT

Grober's Elephant Calf Milk Replacer (Grober) is the most commonly used elephant milk replacer. Nutricia Elephant Calf Milk Replacer has been used in Israel and the Netherlands (Kinzley 1997). Several human infant formulas have also been used to bottle-feed calves, including most commonly Wyeth's SMA Goldcap (also known as S26; manufactured in England) or Enfamil. Grober produces both African and Asian elephant milk replacer, which have been formulated from the analysis of milk collected from lactating females. The African formula has 750 kcal/liter, the Asian formula 1215 kcal/liter, and Enfamil, the most commonly used human infant formula, has 666 kcal/liter. In some cases additional dietary supplementation may be provided. Desiccated coconut and butterfat have been added to increase the fat in the diet (Sheldrick 1993). Vitamin and mineral supplements are commonly used (vitamins B and E, and calcium). In many cases rice water and glutinous rice broth have been used when mixing the formula to alleviate diarrhea.

NURSING TECHNIQUES

Most often a bovine calf nurser is used for bottle-feeding, with the nipple openings slightly enlarged to allow a steady drip when tipped (see Fig. 28.1). A rubber band is placed between the nipple and the bottle rim to allow air to escape. One method that has been used when trying to get a calf to nurse from the dam is to use an IV line attached to a fluid bag containing milk, with the end of the IV line attached to the caretaker's fingers so the calf could be more easily led to the dam's teat.

Initially, when being fed by a caretaker, some calves may struggle with finding a comfortable

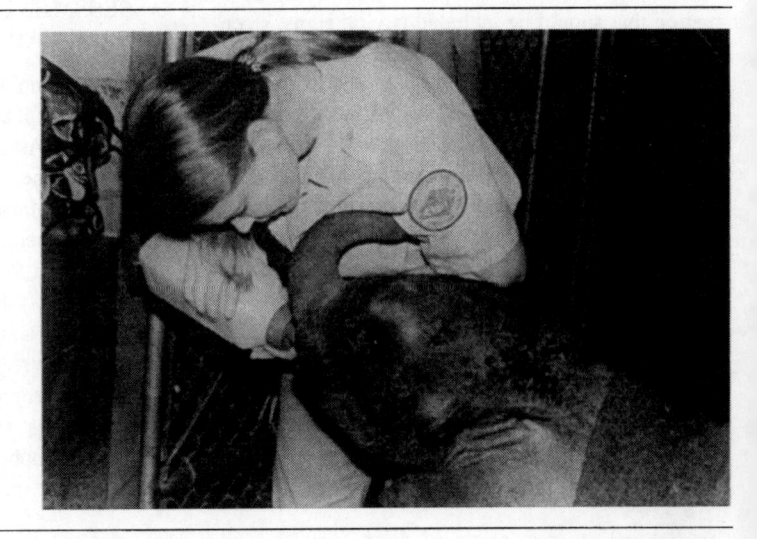

Figure 28.1 Elephant calf nursing on bovine calf nurser.

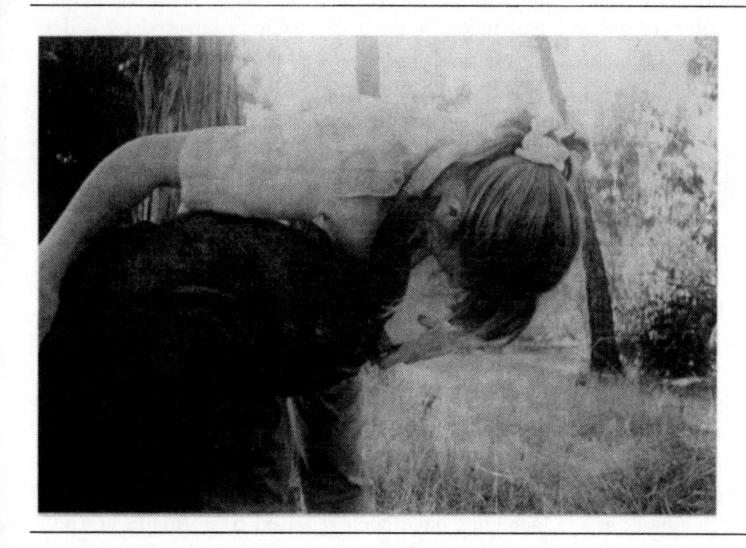

Figure 28.2 Elephant calf with trunk on keeper's neck.

nursing position and will not nurse well until they do. They seem to need to have their trunks up against something. Some calves need intimate contact with the keeper and will come to rest their trunk at the underarm, face, or neck (see Fig. 28.2). Some caretakers have had success with hanging a piece of canvas for the calf to push up against to nurse (Sheldrick 1993). Once a calf finds a comfortable position, it will be reluctant to nurse until it is in that position. Covering the calf with a blanket pulled just over the ears so the front of the face is visible, may also comfort very young calves. Thin blankets or sheets may be used in warmer weather. Newborn elephants often have difficulty lying down and have been observed shuffling around the enclosure until they stop and begin falling asleep. At some point they just collapse or tip over. They may also need help in getting up. Large canvas sleeping cushions, straw bedding, or whole bales for the calf to lean against and slide down should be provided.

MILKING THE DAM

If possible, the dam should be milked so the calf can receive colostrum, and then milked to supplement formula feeding. Milking methods include hand milking, manual human breast pump, and electric human breast pump. Manual milking is similar to that used in goats: squeeze the teat at the top with the thumb and forefinger then squeeze the other three fingers in succession. Human lactation consultants can assist with instruction on use of the human breast pump. Oxytocin may be given intramuscularly approximately five minutes before pumping to facilitate milk letdown. Oxytocin has also been administered to facilitate milk letdown that appeared to be deficient when a calf was nursing. The amount of milk that can be collected in the first 24 hours varies widely: from 300–4000 ml approximately, although up to 10 liters is theoretically possible. In some cases, the dam may only be able to be milked once to collect colostrum. Frequent milking and the use of oxytocin should dramatically increase the amount of milk collected. One zoo milked their elephant cow every three hours and used oxytocin each time, with average collections of 1080 ml per milking during the first week (Kinzley 1997).

The breast pump is usually used for approximately 10–20 minutes per breast. Rest periods, warm-water packs, and massage have been used during milking to increase the volume of milk collected. Milking has also been used to collect samples from a nursing mother over the course of lactation for the development and modification of formula.

AMOUNTS TO FEED

Calves weighing 100 kg (220 lb) should receive between 6000 and 8000 kcal per day and calves weighing 200 kg (440 lb) should receive between 16,000 and 20,000 kcal per day. To meet this requirement, the Grober Asian formula should be fed at a rate of 5–6.6 liters/day, and 13.2–16.5 liters/day, respectively. The African formula requires a rate of 8–10.7 liters/day and 21.3–26.7 liters/day, respectively. At these weights a calf would require at 9–12 liters and 24–30 liters of the

Enfamil formula per day. One recommendation is that newborns should receive at least 8 liters (2 gallons) of formula per day, but may receive as little as 5 liters/day for up to two days (Sheldrick 1993).

Overfeeding is probably not a concern in elephant calves. The calf should gain 0.5–1.4 kg (1–3 lb) per day, averaging 0.9 kg (2 lb) of weight gained per day during the first year of life.

FREQUENCY OF FEEDING

Calves should be fed on demand initially. The feeding interval for very young calves is generally every one to two hours, around the clock. At three months of age, the frequency of nighttime feedings may start to be gradually reduced, depending upon the demands and growth rate of the calf. Some caretakers begin gradually shifting to an every-three-hours feeding schedule during the daytime at this time; or, the calf may continue to be fed on demand. At one year of age, the bottle-feeding should be every four hours during the hours of daylight, with one to two night feeds if the calf is hungry. Over about 15 months of age, an elephant calf should be taking in solid foods in sizeable quantities, and the milk can be eased out with three bottle feeds a day only, providing that sufficient solid foods are on hand for the calf at night (see Tips for Weaning below) (Sheldrick, Personal communication, 2001).

CARETAKERS

The team of caretakers for the calf should consist of a carefully selected, consistent group of approximately five to eight people, starting the first day of hand rearing. It is very important that the calf not always be fed by just one or two particular caretaker(s), because the calf may become so attached to those individuals that it will become extremely distressed by even brief separations from them, and may refuse to feed without their presence.

NURSERY LOCATION

Planning should include the development of a nursery. It will need to be safe from the adult elephants but allow for visual, auditory, and olfactory contact with them. Chain-link fence works well as a barrier for the calf but the smaller links (1 in x 1 in) are necessary to prevent the calf from pulling its trunk through the fence. Generally, the nursery area should be kept at about 18°C (65°F) in winter, but a very young or ill calf may require a warmer temperature. Blankets and heavy bedding may help to offset the cold. The space should have drainage for hosing; calves will produce large volumes of urine and feces. A layer of shavings covered by a deep straw bedding works well to insulate the calf and to absorb urine and feces between cleanings. A service area with electricity, water, and storage space should be nearby.

IMMUNE STATUS AND FAILURE OF PASSIVE TRANSFER (FPT) OF IMMUNOGLOBULINS

Elephants have long been thought to have no placental transfer of immunoglobulins, only passive transfer through colostrum after birth. Recent findings suggest further work is needed in this area (Parrot and Dierenfeld 1996). At this time it is still assumed that it is essential for a newborn calf to receive either colostrum, plasma, or both. Elephant neonates have been reported to normally consume 2–10 liters of colostrum, with nursing beginning as early as 30 minutes after birth (Kinzley 1997). This volume is therefore the amount to strive for when giving colostrum to a newborn elephant that has not nursed from the mother, however some calves may not drink more than a total of 2 liters in the first day of life. Colostrum can be stored at –20°C (–4°F) for at least one year in equids and it is assumed this also holds true for elephant colostrum (Smith 1996).

Information on evaluating the immune status of an elephant calf is limited. Tests that should be performed on any calf that is to be hand reared are total protein, globulins, serum electrophoresis, and a qualitative immunoglobulin test such as the zinc turbidity test. Electrophoresis will probably become the most reliable of these tests as more information is gathered (Kinzley and Emanuelson, in press).

Elephant plasma should be collected well in advance of the earliest expected calving date. The sterile plasma may be stored at –20°C for 6 months, and at –70°C for 12 months. The donor elephant should preferably not be the mother due to the potential for isoantibodies, should be healthy, and should be herpesvirus negative by whole blood PCR tests performed with each plasma collection (Fowler 1986; Smith 1996). It is preferable to collect plasma from elephants on-site, as it more likely offers resistance to local infectious agents.

The volume of elephant plasma that should be administered to a calf in cases of failure of passive transfer (FPT) is not known, but it is likely that amounts similar to that required for the foal are necessary. Foals are given 40–80 ml/kg IV over a two- to four-day period (Smith 1996). For a 100-kg elephant calf, this would total 4–8 liters. This amount is too large for one administration, especially for a calf with normal hydration. About 10–20 ml/kg is a reasonable amount to give as one IV bolus over 30 to 60 minutes. Note that the volumes administered to elephant calves to date have been lower than recommended equine amounts: 1.5 liters or less. Elephant plasma may also be given orally during the first 24 hours after birth (first 6 to 12 hours preferred), but the antibody content is likely to be lower than that found in colostrum. Therefore a larger volume must be given to approach a similar absorption. Colostrum or plasma may have a local protective effect on the gut even if GI absorption is closed.

COMMON MEDICAL PROBLEMS

Diarrhea

Loose stools in a variety of colors may be "normal" for formula-fed infants. Stool that is unusually odorous, separated into chunks and liquid, or very liquid, is abnormal. The frequency of stool production, and the appearance of the stool that is considered normal for one particular calf, is helpful for determining the extent of diarrhea when it occurs. Changes in formula are used to manage mild diarrhea that occurs without any additional clinical signs. Options are to dilute the formula 25% to 50% for one to three days; to discontinue the formula and substitute water, electrolyte solution such as Pedialyte, rice water, or rice milk for one to two days; alternate each formula feed with a feed of electrolyte solution for one to three days; or to change to a different formula. When diarrhea is severe, or accompanied by other clinical signs such as lethargy, weakness, reduced appetite, colic, or dehydration, diagnostic evaluation as well as treatment is necessary. Recommended diagnostic tests include a complete blood count; serum chemistry analysis; urinalysis; aerobic/anaerobic fecal culture for a variety of potential pathogens including *Salmonella, Clostridium, Campylobacter,* enterotoxigenic *Escherichia coli, Pseudomonas,* and others; fecal examination for parasites; and a fecal cytology smear. Additional diagnostic tests to consider include herpesvirus PCR, blood culture, fecal exam for cryptosporidia and giardia, fecal electron microscopy or other evaluations for viruses, and abdominal radiographs. Note that blood collection, and also positioning for X rays, can be very stressful for elephant calves, so the necessity for these should be carefully considered. Treatment options for diarrhea include dietary changes as above, with emphasis on oral electrolyte fluids, Kaopectate orally, antibiotic therapy, intravenous fluid therapy, and antiparasitic therapy when appropriate.

Constipation

Constipation has been reported in mother-reared and hand-reared calves (Kinzley 1997). This may occur following a stressful event or abrupt diet change. Signs include listlessness, anorexia, abdominal contractions with no defecation (straining), absence of defecation, and rubbing hindquarters against the walls.

Treatments to consider are enemas (may be necessary to be given daily); antibiotics, corticosteroids, and vitamin B_{12} if the calf is weak; and oral cathartics such as mineral oil, but these should be used with caution in very young animals as they could cause further abdominal discomfort and/or diarrhea.

Metabolic Bone Disease/Rickets

Metabolic bone disease/rickets has occurred in young growing elephants fed a diet with an imbalanced calcium:phosphorus ratio, or chronic intestinal malabsorption (Fowler 1978; Richman 2000). The recommended dietary calcium and phosphorus levels have not been established, but multiple elephant milk and formula analyses have been reported (Kinzley 1997). Access to sunlight may also be important in the prevention of this disease, as a source of vitamin D, which is necessary for calcium absorption. Diagnostic evaluation may include evaluating serum calcium and phosphorus levels, radiology, and formula analysis. Treatment would involve correcting the dietary imbalance, vitamin D injection in some cases, access to sunlight, and care with regard to body weight and type of exercise (or any activity that could lead to pathologic fracture).

Herpesvirus Infection

Twenty-two cases of the disease have occurred, 19 of these cases have been in young Asian elephants. The disease is acute to peracute, and often rapidly fatal. Recently, six young elephants with the disease were treated with the oral antiherpes medication, famciclovir (Famvir, Smith Kline Beecham), and of these cases three have survived. Two of the cases that survived received famciclovir rectally (Richman 2000). A whole blood PCR test is available upon special request (Dr. Laura Richman, Johns Hopkins Medical School, Baltimore, MD).

Results from this test may not be received for one to two days. Treatment may therefore need to be initiated immediately based solely on history and clinical signs. Symptoms include lethargy; weakness; reduced appetite; diarrhea or lack of stool production; cyanosis of the tongue tip or diffuse swelling and cyanosis of the entire tongue; swelling around the face, trunk, and front limbs; elevated heart rate; collapse; and sudden death. Not all of these symptoms have been seen in each case of herpesvirus infection, and in older animals the symptoms have appeared to be less specific. It is advised that at least a three-day supply of famciclovir be kept on hand at the zoo when young calves are present. Famciclovir has been used at doses ranging from 6 mg/kg every 12 hours, to 12 mg/kg every 8 hours, orally or rectally. The initial treatment protocol for herpesvirus infection is under review and should be discussed with the veterinarian. It is recommended that hand-reared calves be trained to allow a physical examination, especially of the oral cavity.

Sunburn

Elephants are susceptible to sunburn, especially on the head. Ensure that adequate shade is available during outdoor time. Sunscreen has been used on calves, however effectiveness is uncertain and there could be some potential for allergy, so covering the calf with sheets, and keeping it in the shade are better options. Treat sunburn with a soothing cream such as vitamin E cream and restricted access to sunlight until healed.

Skin Dryness

Skin dryness has been noted in hand-raised calves, which can cause a marked pruritus. Treat by applying a mixture of lanolin and mineral oil (1 lb lanolin added to 1 gal mineral oil) to the calf's skin once to three times weekly after gently bathing the calf with warm water. It may be advisable to test the calf for allergy to the mixture by applying a small amount to the skin the first time it is used.

Umbilical Infection

Umbilical infections have been reported in elephants, including one fatality (Mikota, Sargent, and Ranglack 1994). The newborn elephant has an open umbilical sheath that can be mistaken for an umbilical cord. The cord (umbilical artery and veins) actually retracts inside the sheath into the abdomen. When disinfecting the umbilical sheath, use a syringe to deliver the disinfectant into the open umbilical sheath, as just dipping the structure may not be adequate (Schmitt 2000). Serious umbilical infection may be more likely in a calf that is immunocompromised by FPT, stress, or other factors. Diagnostic evaluation includes aerobic and anaerobic culture and sensitivity. Treatment in mild cases consists of cleansing, gentle debridement, and antiseptic flush with dilute Betadine or Nolvasan once to twice daily. In more advanced cases, or particularly in cases of FPT, add topical antibiotic irrigation and systemic broad-spectrum antibiotic therapy.

Trauma

An infant that has been rejected may have received traumatic wounds from the mother, from other elephants, or by birth accident. Diagnostic evaluations include physical examination, aerobic and anaerobic culture and sensitivity of any infected wounds, CBC, chemistries, radiology. An x-ray generator of 300 MA or greater will be necessary for all but the distal extremities. Anesthesia may be required to x-ray a calf that is not depressed or weak.

FLUID THERAPY

Adult elephant fluid requirement is approximately 30–50 ml/kg/day (Fowler 1978). The infant requirement is likely to be higher. One calf was reported to have an average milk consumption of 108–138 ml/kg/day, which continued up to 11 months of age (Kinzley 1997). Active disease and fluid losses may increase fluid requirement to two to four times maintenance.

Subcutaneous fluid administration is not a good option for therapy due to limited SQ space. Fluid is well absorbed by the oral route, and this should be used whenever possible, although clear fluids such as electrolyte solutions should not completely replace milk for more than two days due to caloric reduction. Intravenous fluid therapy is used when marked dehydration is present, especially if the calf is anorexic. It is difficult to maintain an IV catheter in an infant for continuous infusion. One option is to give fluid by intermittent IV bolus. As a guideline, no IV bolus should exceed 40 ml/kg, 20 ml/kg being preferred; and the fluids should be given as slowly as possible, over a 30- to 60-minute period. Anesthesia should be considered if the calf is extremely stressed by restraint for IV fluid administration.

IV catheterization may be accomplished with an 18-gauge or 20-gauge catheter placed in the medial saphenous vein or ear vein. Sloughing may occur with the injection of medications other than fluids into the vasculature of the ear. It may be difficult to thread an over-the-needle catheter through the skin on the hindlimb. Butterfly catheters may also be used but are difficult to keep in place, even for short periods. Use buffered 2% lidocaine infused into the tissue over the vein for catheter placement. Suture or apply surgical adhesive to help keep the catheter in place.

Lactated Ringer's is a suitable fluid solution for most cases. Do not add potassium chloride if the fluids are given as a rapid IV bolus. Glucose may be added to make a 2.5% or 5% solution if the blood glucose is reduced below 60–80 mg/dl.

ANTIBIOTIC THERAPY

Commonly used antibiotics include ampicillin, amoxicillin, penicillin G procaine, and ceftiofur in less-severe infections; amikacin or gentocin can be added in more-severe cases, when hydration is maintained, and if possible serum levels are measured. Avoid fluoroquinolones and tetracyclines.

VACCINATIONS

Tetanus toxoid, a vaccination for *Clostridium tetani*, has been given to adults, subadults, and neonates at multiple zoological institutions. Give 1 ml IM, with the first dose at three months of age, and the second dose at four months of age. Consider an initial dose as early as the first day, if calf has not received colostrum.

Tetanus antitoxin has been administered in adults and could be considered for use in a neonate with lesions likely to become contaminated with *Clostridium*. However, note that fatal serum hepatitis has occurred following administration of tetanus antitoxin to horses. Uncommon vaccinations such as those for other clostridial diseases, encephalomyocarditis virus, and rabies; and signs and treatment for adverse reactions to vaccinations should be discussed with the veterinarian.

PHYSICAL AND BEHAVIORAL DEVELOPMENT

Physical development of hand-raised calves should follow closely that of mother-raised calves. If a hand-raised calf is not able to spend an adequate amount of time with other elephants, normal behaviors may be absent or slow to develop. The caretakers may encourage some behaviors like dusting, eating solid foods, mud wallowing, swimming, and play behaviors. Further study is needed to determine the effect of hand raising on the calf's communication and social skill once it is integrated into a herd (Fig 28.3).

SOLID FOODS

Although hand-raised calves experiment with solid foods at an early age, they develop normal feeding habits much more slowly than mother-raised calves. Small amounts of solid food such as hay and other adult elephant feeds may be offered to the calf beginning at one or two months of age. Calves are

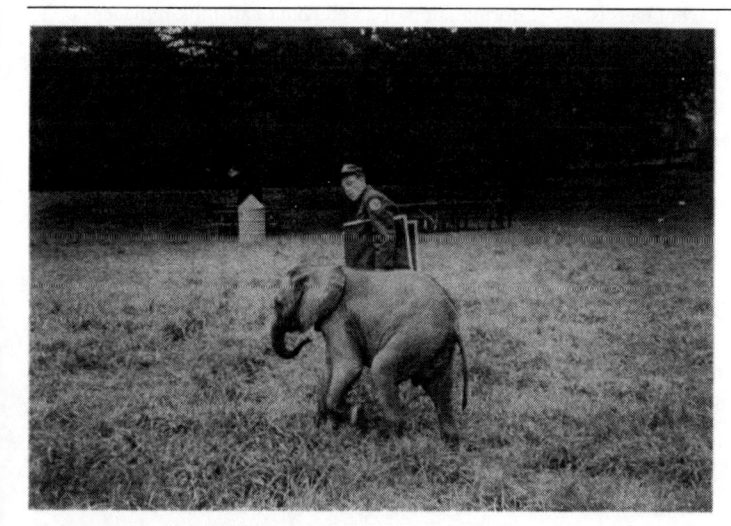

Figure 28.3 Elephant calf on walk with caretaker.

often are most interested in tasting foods being eaten by their caretakers. Caretakers might be able to generate more interest in appropriate foods by pretending to eat them with the calf. As with mother-raised calves, weaning, and consequently hunger, may increase the calf's appetite for solid food. It has been recommended that young calves be encouraged to ingest small amounts of healthy, screened, adult elephant feces on a regular basis (Sheldrick 1993).

TIPS FOR WEANING

Very little information has been reported on weaning of hand-raised calves. Mother-raised calves are weaned between the ages of four and five years, which is usually when the next calf is born. However, after the age of two, the volume of milk they consume begins to gradually decrease (Moss 1992).

Many hand-raised African calves have been successfully weaned at the Sheldrick Wildlife Trust orphanage in Kenya. They describe their process for weaning as follows: when the calf is four to six months of age, milled whole barley, oatmeal cereal, and desiccated coconut are added to the calf's formula (they use Wyeth's SMA Goldcap/S26). One tablespoon of each ingredient is added initially, then the amounts are gradually increased until the formula becomes the consistency of porridge. This introduces an appropriate type of fat, and more solid foods to their diet. At nine months, the calf should be receiving the largest volume of formula at about 28 liters/day. After this point, the amount of formula is very gradually decreased. At one year, either bottles are mixed with half S26 formula and half skim milk, or a skim-milk-based milk replacer is used instead of S26, with *no* antibiotics added. Coconut continues to be added to the formula. After two years of age, the formula and skim milk are gradually replaced with water, but the calf is still bottle-fed until the age of five years. Enabling the calf to nurse as it would if it were mother-raised may be important for both the physical and psychological health of the calf (Sheldrick 1993).

SOURCES OF PRODUCTS MENTIONED

Grober Company, Cambridge, Ontario, Canada; Phone: 519-622-2500, 1-800-265-7863; www.grober.com

Smith Kline Beecham, Philadelphia, PA

REFERENCES

Allen J. L., E. R. Jacobson, J. W. Harvey, and W. Boyce. 1985. Hematologic and serum chemistry values for young African elephants (*Loxodonta africana*) with variations for sex and age. *Journal of Zoo and Wild Animal Medicine* 16(3): 98–101.

Fowler, M. E. 1978. *Zoo and wild animal medicine*. Philadelphia, PA: Saunders.

———. 1986. *Zoo and wild animal medicine*. 2d ed. Philadelphia, PA: Saunders.

Fowler M. E., and E. M. Miller, 1999. *Zoo and wild animal medicine: Current therapy 4*. Philadelphia, PA: W.B. Saunders Co.

Heard, D. J., E. R. Jacobson, and K. A. Brock. 1986. Effects of oxygen supplementation on blood gas values in chemically strained juvenile African elephants. *Journal of the American Veterinary Medical Association* 189(9): 1071–74.

Kinzley, C. E. 1997. *The elephant hand raising notebook*. Available on request from the Oakland Zoo, Oakland, CA; 1-510-632-9525, ext. 161.

Kinzley, C. E., and K. A. Emanuelson. Hand-rearing elephants. In *Elephant husbandry notebook* (in press).

Mikota, S. K., E. L. Sargent, and G. S. Ranglack. 1994. *Medical management of the elephant*. West Bloomfield, MI: Indira Publishing House.

Moss, C. 1992. Elephant calves: The story of two sexes. In *Elephants*, edited by J. Shoshani. Emmaus, PA: Rodale Press.

Oosterhuis, J. E. 1992. The birth and attempted hand rearing of an Asian elephant calf. *Proceedings of the American Association of Zoo Veterinarians*. Oakland, CA.

Parrott, J. J., and E. S. Dierenfeld. 1996. Analysis of African elephant mature milk in early lactation and formulation of an elephant calf milk replacer. *Proceedings of the American Association of Zoo Veterinarians*. Puerto Vallarta, Mexico.

Richman, L. K. 2000. Phone conversation with author.

Schmitt, D. 2000. Phone conversation with author.

Sheldrick, D. 1993. Raising infant orphaned elephants. Nairobi, Kenya: David Sheldrick Wildlife Trust.

———. 2001. Phone conversation with author.

Smith, B. P. 1996. *Large animal internal medicine*. 2d ed. St. Louis, MO: Mosby Year Book, Inc.

29
Nondomestic Equids

Terry Blakeslee and Jeffery R. Zuba

INTRODUCTION

The successful hand rearing of the nondomestic equid foal is dependent upon many factors. This includes accurate record keeping, dedicated and experienced animal care personnel, facilities appropriate for the species, unique husbandry practices, and quality veterinary care. The size, disposition, and value of these nondomestic equine neonates make them a challenge to hand raise. Attempts are always made to allow the mare to raise her offspring but at times intervention is necessary. Generally, these foals have only been hand raised due to maternal neglect or medical problems that may compromise the foal's health and survival. If appropriate, debilitated neonates are treated, stabilized, and reintroduced to their mare to allow natural rearing to occur.

The San Diego Wild Animal Park (SDWAP) currently exhibits six species of nondomestic Equidae. The Przewalski's horse (*Equus przewalskii*), Grevy's zebra (*Equus grevyi grevyi*), Hartmann's mountain zebra (*Equus zebra hartmannae*), and Somali wild ass (*Equus africanus*) have been hand raised at this institution (see Table 29.1). There is a paucity of information on the protocols and practices for hand raising these species. Fortunately, there are excellent references as well as a Chapter 4 in this book, available on the domestic equine neonate, which are readily applicable to their nondomestic relatives (Koterba, Drummond, and Kosch 1990; Madigan 1997; Orsini and Divers 1998).

RECORD KEEPING

Maintain a daily log of formula intake, body weights, and fecal output and consistency. Horses

Table 29.1 Biological Data for Hand-Raised Nondomestic Equidae at the SDWAP

	Przewalski's horse	Grevy's zebra	Hartmann's mountain zebra	Somali wild ass
Birth weight (kg)	Avg:23.2 Range: 18.6–28 N = 8	Avg: 37.5 Range: 29.5–47 N = 6	Avg: 36.8 Range: 30.5–40.9 N = 5	Avg: 24.1 Range: 22.8–25.5 N = 2
Seasonal births	no	no	no	no
Daily weight gain (kg)	Avg: 0.7 Range: 0.1–2.2 N = 1	Avg: 0.6 Range: 0.5–1.5 N = 1	Avg: 0.62 Range: not available N = 1	Avg: 0.52 Range: 0.1–1.3 N = 2
Age at weaning	4 1/2 months	4 1/2 months	4 1/2 months	4 1/2 months

urinate and defecate without the assistance of physical stimulation. Body temperature should be obtained twice daily for the first several days, longer if the foal's condition is compromised. This can be accomplished using a rectal thermometer while the foal is nursing its first and last bottle of each day. Note exercise times and behavioral changes. Weigh daily for two weeks, every other day for an additional two weeks, twice a week until three months of age, and once a week until weaned. Weights may be obtained by leading the foal onto a platform scale with the formula bottle.

EQUIPMENT

The following items should be on hand: a pliable, 1-liter polyethylene laboratory bottle (Fisher) with a narrow mouth, an artificial lamb's nipple with a small crosscut opening, 1- and 2-liter calf bottles, a slender calf nipple with a small crosscut opening (Nasco), large containers with screw tops for storing formula, large cooking pot, hot plate, refrigerator, sink, disinfectant, bottle brush, measuring cups, gram scale, and walk-on platform scale. Any type of room heater and electric blanket may be needed.

CRITERIA FOR INTERVENTION

All four species should be on their feet approximately 30 minutes after birth. The foal should become strong enough to keep up with the dam. Should the foal's legs appear weak, consider applying external support, such as splints or wraps, which will allow it to keep up with the dam. Nursing should be seen frequently and within the first several hours. It is common to see the foal sleeping in lateral recumbency. A problem is indicated if the foal is seen alone for extended periods when awake, appears weak, or is having trouble keeping up with the dam. Any deviation from the normal rectal body temperature of 100.5–102.5°F (38.0–39.2°C) may be an indication of poor health. The stool should be tan or yellowish in color and the consistency of stiff putty or firmer. A healthy foal may not have a stool for the first 24 to 48 hours. For foals with diarrhea, a fecal sample should be submitted for culture of enteric pathogens and internal parasite screen.

The dam's history in raising foals should be considered as well as her current attentiveness toward the foal. If the dam's attentiveness is in question, nonintervention is strongly recommended, allowing a strong bond to develop. Aggression from the stallion should be of immediate concern. A breeding Przewalski's horse stallion, new to the collection, should not be introduced to a group of pregnant mares, as he will kill offspring he did not sire. This is also thought to be true of Grevy's zebra.

INITIAL CARE AND ASSESSMENT

Upon arrival at the nursery, the foal should be weighed, its temperature obtained, and the umbilicus dipped in 3% iodine. The iodine treatment is continued until the umbilicus is dry and healed. Body temperatures are obtained twice daily for the first week. Ideally, a complete veterinary exam is given upon arrival. In a weak or debilitated foal, blood is collected from a neck vein and analyzed for a complete blood count, biochemical profile, and immunoglobulin levels using an Equi-Z test (V.M.R.D). At 24 hours after the first nursing, blood is collected from a healthy foal, or repeated for the debilitated foal, and analyzed for immunoglobulin levels.

If the foal is hypothermic, wrap it in an electric blanket and place it in a warm room. Take care not to raise the body temperature too rapidly. Bottle-feeding should not be attempted when the body temperature is below 96°F (35.5°C), as formula may not be digested due to decreased gastrointestinal motility. Subcutaneous fluids may be given to a normothermic foal, using 2.5% dextrose in 0.45% NaCl, if the foal is mildly dehydrated. Intravenous administration of fluids or total parenteral nutrition may be indicated, using the jugular vein, in the clinically dehydrated foal or when there is the assumption that no nursing will occur within the next 24 hours in a debilitated animal. In addition, when a debilitated foal is known not to have nursed from its dam, intravenous equine plasma administration is considered.

During the first week, attempts should be made to keep the foal in a clean environment. This will decrease the chance of an overwhelming infection in an immunologically naive or debilitated foal. Wear separate coveralls, disposable gloves, and booties when caring for the foal, especially when working with other species. Wash the bottle and nipple in a disinfectant after every feeding. Change the bedding and disinfect the stall daily.

FORMULAS AND SUPPLEMENTS

Equine milk is similar to rhino milk in that it is low in fat, solids, and proteins, but high in carbohydrates (Oftedal and Iverson 1995). The formula is commercial, fresh, nonfat, and 1% low-fat cow's milk, powdered edible grade lactose (AMPC), and tap water, in a ratio of 9:9:1:3. This is an example formula: 900 ml nonfat milk, 900 ml 1% low-fat milk, 100 g of lactose powder, and 300 ml water. First, reconstitute 100 g of lactose powder in 300 ml (300 g) of water, heating and stirring this mixture in order to dissolve the lactose completely. This lactose solution now becomes four parts (400 g) of the formula, and when cooled, is added to the 900 ml of nonfat and 900 ml of low-fat cow's milk. At our facility, the lactose solution is made in large batches and refrigerated for a maximum of four days. When measuring from a large batch, the amount is measured in weight rather than volume, since the addition of lactose powder to water causes the water to become more dense. The same formula ratio is used until the foal is weaned. A liquid iron supplement such as ViSorbin (Animal Health) may be added to the morning bottle. The dosage is 0.33 ml/kg of body weight until the foal is approximately two months of age, at which time the dosage is held constant.

Reagent grade powdered dextrose (Sigma) may be used as a substitute if lactose is unavailable. Lactose is preferred, as it is the type of sugar found in horse milk. The powder may be stored at room temperature, however, the lactose-water solution must be refrigerated. Prepared formula, which may be made in batches, must be refrigerated and used within two days.

Equine, as other ungulates, may have a tendency to eat dirt. This may be an indication of inadequate formula intake or, in older foals, the interval between bottle-feedings may be too large. If there is concern, a psyllium product such as Equi-Aid (Equi-Aid) may be added to the bottles (5 cc/4.5 kg of body weight) to facilitate the passage of dirt through the foal's system.

WHAT TO FEED INITIALLY

A newborn should be fed horse's or cow's colostrum for the first 24 hours of nursing to provide important factors such as immunoglobulins. At the time the foals discussed in this chapter were raised, the availability of equine colostrum from a reliable source was in question. However, since that time, several commercial companies have made equine colostrum and colostrum replacers available. These sources may be found on the internet. To date, the authors have not had the opportunity to apply these products in rearing nondomestic equids. Do not overheat colostrum, as this may destroy important immunoglobulins and proteins.

A mixture of colostrum and formula, as described below, is offered at a ratio of 1:1 for the following 24 hours. Continue feeding formula with the addition of 10% colostrum until the foal is one month of age, at which time the colostrum may be discontinued. Long-term feeding of colostrum provides nutrients and local immunity to the gastrointestinal track on a daily basis.

Commercially available cow's colostrum replacer, such as Colostrum Plus (Jorgensen) may be used when fresh or frozen horse or cow's colostrum is unavailable. It should be mixed with formula in a ratio of 1:1 and fed for the first 48 hours. The replacer is handled similarly to fresh colostrum, therefore is added as 10% of the formula for the first month. If colostrum or colostrum replacer is not available, use full-strength formula.

NURSING TECHNIQUES

The formula temperature should feel warm to the wrist. It appears that foals are sensitive to formula temperature and seem to prefer the formula a little cooler than most other ungulates. As it is difficult to acquire calf nipples that are soft and supple, a supple lamb's nipple affixed to the laboratory bottle may be used initially to encourage nursing (Fig. 29.1).

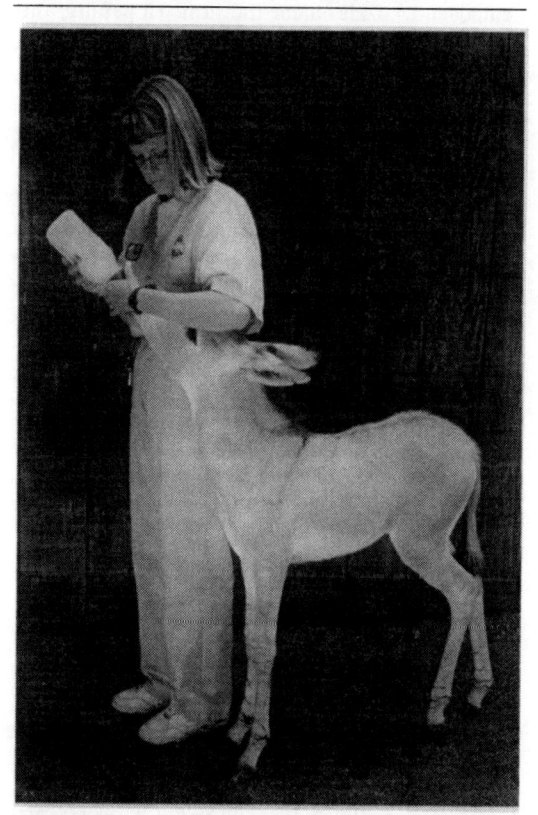

Figure 29.1 Feeding a one-month-old Somali wild ass.

A small crosscut, 0.3 cm in each direction, in the nipple is recommended. Foals tend to aspirate easily during nursing. Signs of aspiration include coughing, nasal congestion, or milk running from the nose. Aspiration of formula may result in pneumonia. When these symptoms appear, the crosscut is probably too large. Keeping the foal's head low, approximately in line with its body as it nurses, also helps to prevent aspiration. When the crosscut is too small, the foal may tire of sucking before consuming an adequate amount of formula. If the foal does not nurse continuously, the formula may be the wrong temperature. Once the foal is nursing well, switch to a calf bottle and nipple, if possible, as larger bottles will be needed as formula consumption increases. Since the foal becomes familiar with the rate of flow and feel of its nipple, only one nipple should be used. Tube feeding has never been found to be necessary at this facility.

It is more important with this species than with most other ungulates to approximate the nursing posture up under the dam in order to stimulate nursing. The keeper should stand with his arm slightly out from his side, allowing the foal to come from behind and nuzzle under the arm. Hopefully, this will stimulate searching behavior for the nipple. A foal does not like the entire nipple, but just the tip, in its mouth.

The foal will need to be restrained during initial feedings if it does not take the nipple on its own. Stand next to the foal, facing the same direction. Put its head under your arm. While supporting the chin with that hand, introduce the nipple and hold the bottle with the other. You may have to hold the foal's lips firmly around the nipple while moving the nipple in and out slightly, to encourage nursing. Use at least one more person to keep the foal from backing away, as it will probably fight this procedure until nursing begins. Be watchful around Grevy's zebras, as they are powerful kickers.

Have on hand a variety of nipples that are more supple or shaped differently, to try if the initial nipple is not accepted.

AMOUNTS TO FEED AND FREQUENCY

Foals do not need to be fed around the clock. Feedings may be offered every two hours from 6 A.M. until 6 P.M., a total of seven feedings per day. However, since equine are adapted to consume smaller amounts of milk over longer periods, the foal may not finish the entire bottle when first offered. The unfinished portion must be refrigerated, then reheated and offered again one-half to one hour later. Measure and discard any formula not consumed after it has been reheated once. Offering smaller quantities every hour, measuring and discarding the unfinished formula, would be an alternative to reheating unfinished formula. The daily amount offered is determined by body weight, beginning at approximately 10%, divided equally among the seven feedings. This amount is reassessed every morning and increased to account for daily weight gains and appetite until the foal is consuming approximately 16 to 18% of its body weight at two weeks of age. However, do not exceed the stomach capacity, which is calculated by multiplying the body weight in kg by 50. For example, a 20-kg foal will have a stomach capacity of about one liter. It is recommended not to exceed 80% of its stomach capacity; which for this example would be 800 cc. An additional feeding may be necessary if weight gains are not sufficient and appetite does not warrant an increase in the current bottles. A low body temperature may also be an indication that the foal is not consuming enough formula.

After three weeks of age, the foal's appetite may dictate decreasing the percentage of daily intake to approximately 11 to 14% of its body weight, provided its weight gains continue to remain constant. Weight gains seem to be the most important parameter to monitor. With the total daily volume remaining constant, feeding frequency should be decreased to five times per day at approximately four weeks of age, four times per day at two months, and finally, three times per day when the foal is three months old. Continue offering unfinished bottles one-half to one hour later. If dirt eating appears or increases at this time, return to four feedings per day. This time schedule then continues until weaning. Formula increases are discontinued at approximately two months of age, as the foal is usually eating solids by this age.

HOUSING

An air temperature of 60–85°F (15.5–29.4°C) is satisfactory for a healthy foal. Plan to use a heater at night if the air temperature is expected to drop below 60°F. For a hypothermic or debilitated foal, a constant temperature of 80–85°F (26.7–29.4°C) is recommended. The bedding should be placed over a nonskid surface. A thick layer of sudan hay is a good choice for bedding. Other types of hay or wood shavings would also be appropriate.

A large exercise yard is important for physical

and mental development. A healthy foal should be exercised approximately 30 minutes, twice daily, which includes some running. This daily exercise encourages normal defecation. A keeper will need to run along with the foal as it will not usually exercise on its own, even as it grows older. Be careful—wild equine neonates like to kick up their heels as they run by the keeper. If another equine is being raised at the same time, they may be placed together at one week of age, or earlier if the foal is strong and healthy, with keeper supervision. The initial introduction should take place in an area large enough to allow some distance between the two animals until they become accustomed to one another. The two may need to be separated overnight until a bond has developed. This may take approximately one week. When another equine neonate is not available, a large ungulate neonate might be an option as a companion. Two animals will be more likely to exercise without a keeper's prompting. A companion animal will also discourage the foal from becoming dependent on keepers for comfort and security.

TIME TO WEANING

Equine tend to eat solids at a young age and may be weaned as early as four to four and one half months. At approximately 11 weeks of age, the midday bottle is decreased daily over two weeks' time, until approximately 240 ml remain, at which time it is deleted. As an example, for a foal receiving 2.25 liters of formula per bottle, the middle bottle would be decreased 155 ml every other day. The two remaining bottles are then decreased simultaneously, every other day, by the same amount as the midday bottle had been decreased, 155 ml in our example. This takes an additional four weeks, at which time both are deleted. An alternate method, especially if the foal is still on four feedings per day, is to decrease all bottles equally over a six-week period and delete them all at the same time. Decreasing the formula to a small amount helps the foal to stop expecting a bottle once it is deleted.

TIPS FOR WEANING FROM FORMULA TO SOLID FOOD:

Offer one-fourth-inch, low-fiber 16% ADF herbivore pellet (O.H. Kruse), a high-milk-content pellet (Perfection Brand Milk Pellet also available from O.H. Kruse), a grain and molasses feed, and rolled corn and barley at two weeks of age. Foals seem more apt to eat out of a food tub when it is hung from a wall, approximately 760 cm from the ground. Once the foal begins eating solids well, the corn and barley are discontinued, the milk pellet and grain and molasses feed is held at a small amount, with unlimited amounts offered of the low-fiber pellet. Alfalfa hay is offered along with grass hays, such as sudan and bermuda, to encourage the intake of hay. Once the foal begins to consume a significant amount of alfalfa, it is eliminated as it is thought to precipitate enterolyths. At weaning time, the milk pellet is deleted and the low-fiber pellet is gradually replaced with a high-fiber 25% ADF herbivore pellet (O.H. Kruse). Carrots may be offered as treats.

COMMON MEDICAL PROBLEMS

There are many medical conditions documented at the SDWAP when hand raising nondomestic equid species. In general, it appears that these neonates are susceptible to the same diseases and problems common to their domestic equine counterpart. Treatment of infections with antibiotics and other appropriate medication is administered as would be in the domestic equine. As stated previously, there are many veterinary text books and journals available that provide this important information.

Musculoskeletal problems include fetlock joint laxity and contracture, gore wounds, fractured bones, and conformational defects such as angular limb deformities and uneven hoof wear. Bacterial infections of the umbilicus (omphalitis), bloodstream (sepsis), joints, respiratory system (pneumonia), and gastrointestinal system (enteritis) have been diagnosed in neonatal foals at the SDWAP.

Gastrointestinal disease appears to be the most frequent problem in the equine species hand raised at our institution. Clinical diarrhea in the neonatal foal may be caused by infection, stress, or formula intolerance. Since infectious enteritis is a potentially fatal problem, a rectal culture is submitted to screen for enteric pathogens immediately. Due to the ability to infect humans, zoonotic bacterial enteric infections such as *Campylobacter* spp. and *Salmonella* spp., when identified, are treated aggressively. These foals are isolated, treated with appropriate antibiotics, and cultured three times during the week following treatment to ensure they are negative for these enteric pathogens. In cases of persistent diarrhea, an oral electrolyte solution such as Biolyte (Pharmacia and UpJohn) or Pedialyte (Ross) may be offered in place of formula for 24 hours to allow the gastrointestinal tract to rest.

Formula is then gradually provided back to full strength over a two- to four-day period, alternating electrolyte solution with formula bottles. Do not dilute the formula with the electrolyte solution, as it has been shown to inhibit the formation of milk clots in the stomach, which are necessary for proper digestion. It is thought that by alternating formula bottles with electrolyte bottles, the milk has enough time to clot. This is a way of gradually reintroducing formula after gut rest. If a more extended reintroduction is desired, a formula bottle may be offered every third or fourth feeding. A psyllium product such as Equi-Aid, provided at manufacturer-recommended doses, may also be added to every bottle to improve stool consistency. If inappetence is accompanied by loss of energy or vitality in the foal, sickness must be considered.

The susceptibility of domestic foals to stress-induced gastric ulcers warrants the use of preventative ulcer medications, such as sucralfate, cimetidine, and omeprazole, and are commonly provided at our institution. Teeth grinding is abnormal and may be an indication of pain. Constipation may occur if adequate exercise is not routinely provided or if insufficient fluid intake has occurred. A warm-water enema should be considered if this continues for more than 24 hours or there is evidence of straining to defecate. Internal parasite infections such as *Giardia* spp. have been identified and may have caused clinical diarrhea in one foal.

We have not diagnosed any of the common domestic equine viral diseases in our nondomestic neonatal foals but they are assumed to be susceptible. Vaccines intended for use in the domestic equine such as Cephalovac (Boehringer Ingelheim) have been safely used at manufacturer-recommended doses and administration intervals in our equine species at the SDWAP. However, the efficacy of such vaccines has not been proven.

The neonatal foal that has not received mare's colostrum will be deficient of important maternal antibodies necessary to combat infections while the neonate's immune system is developing. The term "failure of passive transfer" (FPT) is used to describe this condition and typically represents a medical challenge. Since these FPT foals are sometimes also found to be hypothermic, hypoglycemic, and potentially in shock, standard equine critical care medical procedures and protocols are instituted immediately (Koterba et al. 1990; Madigan 1997; Orsini and Divers 1998). As in all of our nondomestic hoofstock neonate species, the administration of intravenous conspecific plasma is ideal and found to be clinically rewarding. The SDWAP has frozen plasma from over one hundred nondomestic hoofstock species available for the FPT neonate.

INTEGRATION BACK INTO THE GROUP OR TO A HOLDING PEN

Hand-raised Przewalski's horse and Grevy's zebra colts should not be placed back into a herd containing a breeding sire, however, they can be placed with a group of adult females. Hand-raised fillies may be placed in a herd with a breeding sire or a group of females only. Adult female Grevy's zebras may be a threat to a young hand-raised animal of either sex and should be closely monitored. Foals and the herd should have visual access to each other for at least one week prior to any introduction. A hand-raised Somali wild ass has not been reintroduced to the herd at this institution, however, we would follow the same guidelines.

ACKNOWLEDGMENTS

Our thanks to Mark S. Edwards, Ph.D., Nutritionist, Zoological Society of San Diego, San Diego, CA, and Denise Wagner, Mammal Keeper, San Diego Wild Animal Park, Escondido, CA.

SOURCES OF PRODUCTS MENTIONED

AMPC, Inc., 2325 North Loop Dr., Ames, IA 50010

Animal Health, Exton, PA 19341, Division of Pfizer, Inc., New York, NY 10017

Boehringer Ingelheim Animal Health, Inc., St. Joseph, MI 64506

Equi-Aid Products, Inc., Phoenix, AZ 85027

Fisher Scientific, Inquiry Department, 600 Business Center Dr., Pittsburgh, PA 15205-9913; 1-412-490-8300; www.fishersci.com

Jorgensen Laboratories, Inc., Loveland, CO 80538; 1-800-525-5614

Nasco Farm and Ranch, 4825 Stoddard Rd., Modesto, CA 95356-9318; 1-209-545-1600; www.nascofa.com

O.H. Kruse Grain and Milling, 321 South Antonio Ave., Ontario, CA 91762; 1-800-729-5787

Pharmacia and UpJohn Co., Kalamazoo, MI 49001

Ross Products Division, Abbott Laboratories, Columbus, OH 43215-1724; 1-800-986-8510; www.abbott.com, www.ross.com

Sigma Chemical Co., PO Box 14508, St. Louis, MO 63178

V.M.R.D., Inc., PO Box 502, Pullman, WA 99163

REFERENCES

Koterba, A. M., W. H. Drummond, and P. C. Kosch. 1990. *Equine clinical neonatology.* Philadelphia, PA: Lea & Febiger.

Madigan, J. E. 1997. *Manual of equine neonatal medicine.* 3d ed. Woodland, CA: Live Oak Publishing Company.

Naylor, J. M. 1999. Oral electrolyte therapy. In *Fluid and electrolyte therapy. Veterinary clinics of North America: Food animal practice.* 15(3): 487–504.

Oftedal, O. T., and S. J. Iverson. 1995. Comparative analysis of non-human milks. In *Handbook of milk comparison*, edited by R. G. Jensen. San Diego, CA: Academic Press.

Orsini, J. A., and T. J. Divers. 1998. *Manual of equine emergencies: Treatment and procedures.* Philadelphia, PA: Saunders.

30
Rhinoceros

Terry Blakeslee and Jeffery R. Zuba

INTRODUCTION

The rhinoceros calf presents several challenges for those involved with the hand rearing of this unique species. Large size at birth, rapid growth, disposition, facility requirements, value to the collection, and lack of information on specific nutritional needs are a few of the difficulties that must be addressed. As with all of the species hand raised at the San Diego Wild Animal Park (SDWAP), success is dependent upon accurate record keeping, dedicated and experienced animal care personnel, unique husbandry practices, and quality veterinary care.

The SDWAP has hand raised East African black (*Diceros bicornis michaeli*) and southern white (*Ceratotherium simum simum*) rhinoceros neonates (Table 30.1) due to maternal neglect or medical problems that compromised the calves' health. If possible, attempts are made to reintroduce a transiently debilitated calf to its mother following a period of treatment and stabilization in our nursery.

Since there is a lack of information on hand raising members of the Rhinocerotidae family, we rely on veterinary reference material available for the domestic equine neonate as both animals are members of the order Perissodactyla (Orsini and Divers 1998; Madigan 1997; Koterba, Drummond, and Kosch 1990). However, this association is made with caution since there are notable differences. For instance, analysis of rhinoceros mother's milk is somewhat different from that of the horse, therefore, replacement milk formula must reflect this disparity (Oftedal and Iverson 1995).

RECORD KEEPING

Accurate record keeping is extremely important. Maintain a daily log of formula intake, body weight, body temperatures, and fecal output and consistency. It is helpful to have this information in a format such that one month's statistics may be viewed on one page. Note exercise times and behavioral changes each day. Rhinoceros calves should urinate large amounts daily without the assistance of physical stimulation. Weigh the calf at the same time each day for two to four weeks, every other day

Table 30.1 Biological Data for Hand-Raised Rhinocerotidae at the SDWAP

	East African black rhinoceros	Southern white rhinoceros
Birth weight (kg)	Avg: 35.5 Range: 23.3–48.6 n = 6	Avg: 62.7 Range: 43.1–78.6 n = 5
Seasonal births	No	No
Daily weight gain (kg)	Avg: 0.87 Range: 0.1–3 kg/day n = 2	Avg: 1.4 Range: 0.4–3 kg/day n = 2
Age at weaning	Range: 12–15 months	Range: 12–15 months

until two months of age, twice a week until three months of age, and once a week until five to six months of age. Weights may be obtained by leading the calf onto a platform scale while it is nursing on a bottle.

EQUIPMENT

The following items should be on hand:

Pliable, 1-liter polyethylene laboratory bottle with a narrow mouth (Fisher)
Artificial lamb's nipple with a crosscut opening (any local ranch supply store)
Calf bottles and calf nipples (Nasco)
Large containers with screw tops for storing formula
Large cooking pot, hot plate, large refrigerator, sink, disinfectant, and bottle brush
Measuring cups, gram scale, walk-on platform scale
Large stuffed animal to serve as a companion

In addition, a radiant room heater, or other safe heating system, and an electric blanket may be needed.

CRITERIA FOR INTERVENTION

A newborn rhinoceros should be up and walking within approximately one hour after a normal birth. Following a dystocia, the dam may be too exhausted to clean and care for the calf immediately. Similarly, calves weak from a dystocia or breach birth may also take longer to stand. This, however, does not mean that intervention is necessary. Close monitoring is warranted. Nursing should be seen frequently and within the first five hours. The dam often lies on her side while nursing the calf. At this institution, southern white rhinoceros are allowed to calve in a large exhibit area where the dam will take the calf for long walks, usually beginning the day of birth. The calf should be with the dam constantly and touching her while sleeping. A problem is indicated if the calf is seen alone for extended periods, appears weak, or is having trouble keeping up with the dam.

If the dam and calf can be safely separated, daily weights of the calf should be obtained. Normal daily weight gains are representative of nursing success. Calves with suboptimal weight gains have been provided with supplemental bottle-feedings, however this is dependent on the disposition of the calf and dam. The stool should be gray or yellowish gray in color and the consistency of stiff putty. A healthy calf may not have a stool for the first 24 to 48 hours. For all calves with diarrhea, a fecal sample should be submitted for culture of enteric pathogens and internal parasite screen. Daily observations of the calf's stamina are important, as its condition may decline rapidly. Any deviation from the normal rectal body temperature of 98.5–100°F (36.9–37.8°C) is likely an indication of poor health.

INITIAL CARE AND ASSESSMENT IN THE NURSERY

Upon arrival at the nursery, the calf should be weighed, its temperature obtained, and the umbilicus dipped in 3% iodine. The iodine treatment is continued until the umbilicus is dry and healed. Body temperatures are obtained twice daily for the first week. This may be accomplished using a rectal thermometer while the calf is nursing its first and last bottle of each day. Ideally, a complete veterinary exam is given at this time. In a debilitated calf, blood is collected from an ear or leg vein (medial saphenous or cephalic) and analyzed for a complete blood count, biochemical profile, and immunoglobulin levels. At 24 hours after the first nursing, blood is collected from a healthy calf or repeated for a debilitated calf and analyzed for immunoglobulin levels.

If the calf is hypothermic, wrap it in a heating blanket and place it in a warm room. Care must be taken not to raise the body temperature too rapidly. Bottle-feeding should not be attempted when the body temperature is below 96°F (35.5°C) as formula may not be digested due to decreased gastrointestinal motility. Intravenous administration of fluids or total parenteral nutrition may be indicated in a nonnursing animal to maintain hydration or caloric needs. In rhinoceros, an intravenous catheter is placed in an ear vein, supported by a rolled gauze pad placed inside the pinnae, and taped around the ear. If the calf has failed to nurse from its dam and appears weak or debilitated, intravenous rhinoceros plasma administration is considered.

During the first week, every attempt should be made to keep the calf in a clean environment. This will decrease the chance of an overwhelming infection in an immunologically naive debilitated calf. Wear separate coveralls, disposable gloves, and booties when caring for the rhinoceros, especially when working with other species. Wash the bottle and nipple in a disinfectant after every feeding. Change the bedding and disinfect the stall daily.

WHAT TO FEED INITIALLY

If it is possible to obtain milk from the dam, offer her milk for as long as possible, following the guidelines described under Amounts and Frequency of Feeding below. As it is difficult to milk a sufficient amount from the dam, you may have to supplement her milk with cow's colostrum, which may be available from a local dairy. When the dam's milk is not available, offer cow's colostrum for the first 24 hours to provide important factors such as immunoglobulins. Rhinoceros calves seem to prefer their formula at approximately 99°F (37.2°C). Do not overheat colostrum as this may destroy important immunoglobulins and proteins. A mixture of cow's colostrum and formula, as described below, is offered at a ratio of 1:1, for the following 24 hours. Continue feeding formula with the addition of 10% colostrum until the calf is one month old, at which time the colostrum may be discontinued. Long-term feeding of colostrum provides nutrients and local immunity to the gastrointestinal tract on a daily basis.

Commercially available cow's colostrum replacer such as Colostrum Plus (Jorgensen) may be used when fresh or frozen cow's colostrum is unavailable. It should be mixed with formula in a ratio of 1:1 and fed for the first 48 hours. The replacer is handled similarly to fresh colostrum, and therefore is added as 10% of the formula for the first month. If cow's colostrum or colostrum replacer is not available, begin full-strength formula.

FORMULAS AND SUPPLEMENTS

Rhinoceros milk is high in carbohydrates, low in solids and proteins, and very low in fat (Oftedal and Iverson 1995). Fresh nonfat and 1% low-fat cows milk, powdered edible grade lactose (AMPC), and tap water or bottled water are used in a ratio of 27:9:1:1. This is an example formula: 2700 ml nonfat milk, 900 ml 1% low-fat milk, 100 ml water, and 100 g lactose powder. First, reconstitute 100 g lactose powder in 100 ml (100 g) water, heating and stirring this mixture in order to dissolve the lactose completely. This lactose solution now becomes two

Table 30.2 Rhino Formula and Guidelines used at the San Diego Wild Animal Park

Age	Formula	Ratios	Feedings per day[1]
1 day old	100% cow's colostrum		7 times, every 2 hrs
2 days old	NFC:LFC:Lactose:H_2O w/ 50% colostrum	27:9:1:1[2]	7 times, every 2 hrs
3 days to 1 month, early lactation formula	NFC:LFC:Lactose:H_2O w/ 10% colostrum	27:9:1:1	7 times, every 2 hrs
1 to 3.5 months, early lactation formula	NFC:LFC:Lactose:H_2O	27:9:1:1	5 times, every 3 hrs[3]
3.5 to 6 months, midlactation formula	NFC:LFC:Lactose:H_2O	27:9:1:2	4 times
6 to 9 months, midlactation formula	NFC:LFC:Lactose:H_2O	27:9:1:3	3 times
9 to 12 months, midlactation formula	NFC:LFC:Lactose:H_2O	27:9:1:4	3 times
12 to 15 months, late lactation formula	NFC:LFC:Lactose:H_2O	27:9:1:6	2 times
15 to 16 months, late lactation formula	NFC:LFC:Lactose:H_2O	27:9:1:8	2 times

Note: NFC = Liquid nonfat cow's milk (skim milk); LFC = Liquid low-fat cow's milk (1% fat); Lactose—powdered, edible grade dextrose (reagent grade) may be substituted for the lactose.
[1]Day consists of a twelve-hour period from 6 A.M. to 6 P.M.
[2]27 parts NFC to 9 parts LFC to 1 part lactose to 1 part water.
[3]At roughly two months of age the calf can go to 4 times per day.

parts (200 g) of the formula, and when cooled is added to the 2700 ml of nonfat and 900 ml of lowfat cow's milk. At our facility, the lactose solution is made in large batches and refrigerated for a maximum of four days. When measuring from a large batch, the amount is measured in weight rather than volume, since the addition of lactose powder to water causes the water to become more dense. As the calf grows, the lactose solution becomes less concentrated (Table 30.2).

Reagent grade powdered dextrose (Sigma) may be used as a substitute if lactose is unavailable. Lactose is preferred as it is the type of sugar found in rhinoceros milk. The powder may be stored at room temperature, however, the lactose-water solution must be refrigerated. Prepared formula, which may be made in batches, must be refrigerated and used within two days. A liquid iron supplement such as ViSorbin (Animal Health) may be added daily to the first bottle. The dosage is 0.33 ml/kg of body weight until the calf weighs 120 kg, at which time the dosage is held constant at approximately 40 ml/day.

Rhinoceros calves, as other ungulates, have a tendency to eat dirt, which may be an indication of inadequate formula intake. If the calf's appetite does not dictate an increase in formula or an increase does not solve the problem, a psyllium product such as Equi-Aid (Natural Psyllium Fiber, Equi-Aid) may be added to every bottle for several days, as prescribed by the manufacturer, to facilitate the passage of dirt through its system. The intake of dirt should not be allowed as impaction of the digestive tract may occur.

NURSING TECHNIQUES

Rhinoceros calves prefer their milk cooler than many other ungulates or, as stated earlier, approximately 99°F (37.2°C). As calf nipples are often too stiff, a supple lamb's nipple affixed to the laboratory bottle may be used initially to encourage nursing. A crosscut, 0.6 cm in each direction, for an opening is preferred over a single hole, which may contribute to aspiration. Signs of aspiration may include coughing, nasal congestion, or milk coming from the nose. If these symptoms appear, the crosscut is too large. A small amount of milk dripping from its mouth as the calf nurses may be normal. Conversely, if the calf nurses well, but appears to tire before the milk is consumed, the crosscut may need to be enlarged. If the calf does not nurse continuously, the formula may be the wrong temperature. Once the calf is nursing well, begin using a calf bottle and nipple, as larger bottles will be needed as the young rhinoceros grows (see Fig. 30.1). When it takes more than one bottle per feeding, multiple nipples and bottles may be used, as rhinoceros are not selective about their nipples. Tube feeding has not been used at this institution.

The calf will probably take the nipple on its own if it has not previously nursed from the dam. If it refuses the nipple, the calf may need to be restrained during initial feedings. Kneel next to the calf, facing the same direction. Put its head under your arm.

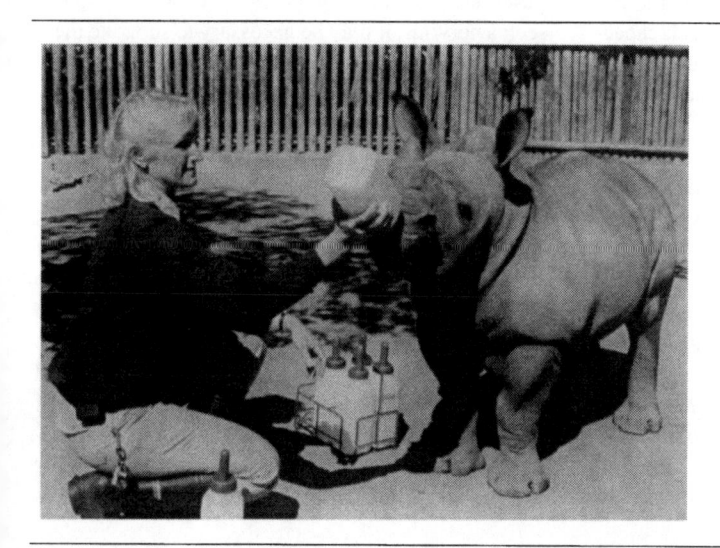

Figure 30.1 Feeding a 6.5-month-old southern white rhinoceros calf.

While supporting the chin with that hand, introduce the nipple and hold the bottle with the other. You may have to hold the calf's lips firmly around the nipple while moving the nipple in and out slightly to encourage nursing. Use at least one more person to keep the calf from backing away, as it will probably fight this procedure until nursing begins. Try nipples that are more supple or shaped differently if the calf continues to resist nursing.

Rhinoceros calves have limited venipuncture sites available for blood collection. Therefore, desensitization of the calf's ears by routine touching and manipulation during nursing increases the chances of obtaining a blood sample from this site without immobilizing the calf.

AMOUNTS AND FREQUENCY OF FEEDING

Rhinoceros do not need to be fed around the clock. Feedings may be offered every two hours from 6 A.M. until 6 P.M., for a total of seven feedings per day, for the first month. The amount is determined by the body weight, beginning at 9–10% divided among the seven feedings. After the first day or two, begin increasing the amount daily, offering 15–20% of its body weight per day by approximately seven to ten days of age.

The amount is adjusted daily to account for weight gains and appetite. A low body temperature may be an indication of insufficient formula intake. When the calf is still hungry following the last bottle of the day, the daily volume is increased and equally divided between all the bottles. It is recommended not to exceed 80% of the stomach capacity. It is estimated that the stomach capacity in a rhinoceros is approximately 5% of its body weight. For example, a 54 kg calf would have a stomach capacity of approximately 2.7 liters. Eighty percent of this volume is 2.2 liters. This example calf should not receive more than this volume at one feeding. A healthy calf should finish every bottle. If inappetence occurs and it is not due to overfeeding, sickness must be considered, especially when it is accompanied by depressed vitality.

With the total daily volume remaining constant, feeding times decrease to five times per day at approximately one month of age, four times a day at two months, and three times a day at four months of age. This feeding schedule is then continued until weaning. Increases are made until the calf is six months old, at which time the amount, approximately 11 liters per feeding, stays constant until weaning begins at one year. Limiting formula intake encourages the consumption of solid foods.

HOUSING

An air temperature of 60–85°F (15.6–29.4°C) is satisfactory for a healthy calf. A heater should be used at night, if the air temperature is expected to drop below 60°F. For a hypothermic or debilitated calf, a constant temperature of 80–85°F (26.7–29.4°C) is recommended. Sudan grass or any type of soft hay is a good choice for bedding. Wood shavings would not be suitable as the calf often lies with its lips on the ground. Shavings might adhere to its lips and be ingested.

As rhinoceros calves require physical contact with the dam for security, placing a large stuffed animal in with the calf has been observed to provide comfort and companionship. If another large ungulate neonate is available, it may be placed together with the rhinoceros calf after it has reached one week of age, replacing the stuffed animal. When this is not an option, a young or adult domestic goat or sheep could be utilized as a companion. The developing bond may take a week. The initial introduction may need to be of limited time with supervision until they each become accustomed to one another. The time limit and success of this introduction depends on the size of the area in which they are introduced and the temperament of each animal. Often other species are frightened of rhinoceros calves. An area large enough to allow a safe retreat by one of the animals is helpful, but not so large that they can completely ignore each other. They may be left together all day if signs of stress are not observed in either animal. If one of the animals seems nervous, it may be necessary to separate them overnight, replacing the companion with the stuffed animal, until a bond has formed. A companion animal also discourages the rhinoceros from becoming dependent on keepers for security and companionship.

A large exercise yard is important for physical and mental development. A healthy newborn calf should be walked for 30 minutes, twice daily. The first few days, the calf may be allowed to explore on its own with a keeper nearby for emotional security. If it will not venture out on its own, the keeper will have to lead. Rhinoceros calves love to run and will probably do so at three to four days of age, following the keeper initially, but then on its own. This daily exercise encourages normal defecation. It is common for the newborn calf to be uncoordinated for the first few days, often tripping over its own feet. Generally, young rhinoceros are hesitant in stepping up onto different levels. Therefore, it may be necessary to construct a dirt ramp if you need the calf to step up over a threshold.

At one to two weeks of age, toys are provided to allow the calf to exercise its natural behavior of head butting. While it is normal and may seem cute for the animal to practice this behavior on the keeper, due to the potential danger, this behavior should be discouraged. Items the calf can use to practice this behavior include two electric cart tires bolted together in order to keep them upright and rolling, large plastic trash cans, boomer balls, or any other object the calf can push around without the risk of wedging its head inside the object.

TIME TO WEANING

Calves may be weaned as early as 12 months, however 15 months is optimal. At 12 months of age, the midday bottle is decreased daily over a one-month period to approximately 960 ml, at which time this feeding is deleted. The remaining two bottles are then decreased simultaneously over a two-month period, also to approximately 960 ml, at which time both bottle-feeds are deleted. By decreasing the formula to a small amount, the calf will stop expecting a bottle more quickly, once it is deleted.

TIPS FOR WEANING FROM FORMULA TO SOLID FOOD

The transition to solid food may best be accomplished by raising the calf with another large ungulate such as an eland, *Taurotragus oryx pattersonianus,* an Indian gaur, *Bosgaurus b. bosgaurus,* or a water buffalo, *Bubalus bubalis.*

Since these animals usually begin eating solids at an age earlier than a single, lone rhinoceros, their presence stimulates the intake of solids by the rhinoceros. Offer one-fourth-inch, low-fiber 16% ADF herbivore pellets (O.H. Kruse), a small portion of rolled corn and barley, a grain and molasses feed, and a high-milk-content pellet (Perfection Brand Milk Pellet, also available from Kruse). The different food types are kept separate in the tub to better monitor consumption. When the calf's favorite food item is identified, mix the items to encourage consumption of all items. Solid food items and water should be provided at two to four weeks of age. Alfalfa and grass hays are offered to both species of rhinoceros and acacia browse to the black rhinoceros because these animals are browsers.

A rhinoceros calf may be very reluctant to eat solids when living alone. To encourage the intake of solids, pellets are placed in its mouth after every bottle-feeding, beginning at approximately one month of age. After the calf has been eating pellets regularly, at approximately four months of age, delete the rolled corn and barley and molasses feed. At approximately six months of age, begin adding one-half-inch high-fiber 25% ADF herbivore pellets (O.H. Kruse) and delete the milk pellet. Cut carrots, yams, and apple may also be added daily.

COMMON MEDICAL PROBLEMS

Many medical conditions have been identified in the rhinoceros neonate with most being similar to other hoofstock species hand raised at our institution. As mentioned above, the domestic equine is used as a prototype species for baseline veterinary medical information so, when necessary, the choice and dose of antibiotics and other medications are prescribed according to the equine literature. Several of the maternally neglected calves hand raised at the SDWAP were found clinically weak, hypothermic, and hypoglycemic. Treatment was instituted according to protocols and procedures used in equine emergency and critical care medicine. Fortunately, these calves must have obtained colostrum prior to being abandoned since their immunoglobulin status was within expected range using a standard serum immunoglobulin test such as Equi-Z (V.M.R.D.). If an animal has not received colostrum and is therefore deficient in maternal antibodies found in this mother's first milk, the term "failure of passive transfer" (FPT) is used to describe this condition and typically represents a medical challenge. The SDWAP has frozen plasma stored and available from over one hundred nondomestic hoofstock species including our rhinoceros. Intravenous conspecific plasma is routinely provided to any neonate identified as being colostrum deprived at our institution. If a rhinoceros calf is identified as FPT, administration of intravenous conspecific plasma would be instituted immediately as it would be to a similarly affected foal. Unfortunately, rhinoceros calves have limited sites available for venous access if an intravenous catheter is necessary. The central ear vein appears to be the best choice and will require creative catheter management for it to remain patent, as described earlier.

One black rhinoceros calf was found abandoned by its mother and presented with weak fetlock joints resulting in severe lameness and inability to walk. This animal was successfully managed by application of fiberglass casts to the affected front limbs for three days to provide temporary external support.

Gastrointestinal disease appears to be a frequent problem when hand raising rhinoceros calves. Diarrhea may be caused by bacterial or parasite infection, stress, or formula intolerance in individual animals. When a case of clinical diarrhea is noted, a rectal swab is obtained and submitted for enteric pathogen culture immediately. A fecal sample is also submitted for parasite screen. *Campylobacter coli* and *Salmonella* spp., both known pathogens, have been identified in our rhinoceros calves with diarrhea. Due to the ability to infect humans, these zoonotic bacterial enteric infections are treated aggressively. Calves were isolated, treated with appropriate antibiotics, and then cultured three times during the week following treatment to ensure a negative pathogen status.

The susceptibility of the domestic equine foal to stress-induced gastric ulcers warrants the consideration and use of preventative ulcer medications such as sucralfate, cimetidine and omeprazole in the similarly affected rhinoceros calf. One white rhinoceros calf seemed to be adversely affected by the removal of a companion animal resulting in clinical diarrhea and possibly dehydration. Digested blood was also found in a fecal sample. Gastric ulcer medication was prescribed and the animal's condition and stool consistency quickly returned to normal. In cases of persistent diarrhea of any cause, an oral electrolyte solution such as Biolyte (Pharmacia and UpJohn) or Pedialyte (Ross) may be provided in place of formula for 24 hours, to rest the intestinal tract. Formula is gradually increased over a two- to four-day period, alternating electrolyte bottles with formula bottles. Do not dilute the formula with the electrolyte solution, as it has been shown to inhibit the formation of milk clots in the stomach, which are necessary for proper digestion (Naylor 1999). Alternating formula bottles with electrolyte bottles gives the milk the necessary time to clot. If a more gradual reintroduction is desired, a formula bottle may be offered every third or fourth feeding.

Other gastrointestinal medications, such as psyllium, have been successfully provided as prescribed by the product manufacturer. Constipation of unknown origin has been diagnosed in our calves and has been treated with positive results with occasional warm-water enemas. In our experience, it appears important to provide daily exercise to the rhinoceros calf to encourage regular bowel movements. Constipation may also indicate an increase in formula quantity is needed. One black rhinoceros calf was found to eat a considerable amount of dirt when allowed access to its exercise yard. This animal was placed on daily psyllium, was monitored during exercise, and had significant evidence of dirt in feces for over one week.

INTEGRATION BACK INTO THE GROUP

The introduction into an adult group should be slow and methodical, as a rhinoceros calf is easily stressed and may become susceptible to disease. Signs of stress may include depression, anxiety, decreased sleep times, increased vocalizations, and diarrhea. It is important to make an emotionally smooth transition to a new temporary location adjacent to its permanent home.

It is best if the calf's companion animal accompanies it to the new location. Once the rhinoceros becomes acclimated to its new home, taking one to two weeks, the companion animal, if present, should be removed during the day but put back at night to offer comfort, allowing the calf to sleep well. Typically, this transition period will take an additional one to two weeks. The companion can then be removed permanently. However, the more time and patience allowed for this process, the more likely the transition will be safe and healthy for the calf. The calf may look as though it is adjusting well sooner than expected and it may be tempting to move through this process more quickly. However, the calf may develop diarrhea, and the entire process will have to be started over. Once the rhinoceros is comfortable in its new area, you can then begin introducing it to other rhinoceros.

The actual introduction of the calf into the rhinoceros herd depends on numerous factors including facilities, number and disposition of animals, and amount of keeper supervision available. It is best if a docile herd member is allowed to bond with the calf initially in the calf's familiar surroundings, continuing to separate the calf overnight. Ideally, this should take one to two weeks, depending on their dispositions. At that point they can be introduced together into the herd once they are familiar with each other.

This institution has not hand raised an Indian rhinoceros, but would follow the same protocol.

ACKNOWLEDGMENTS

Our thanks to Mark S. Edwards, Ph.D., Nutritionist, Zoological Society of San Diego, San Diego, CA, and Denise Wagner, Mammal Keeper, San Diego Wild Animal Park, Escondido, CA.

SOURCES OF PRODUCTS MENTIONED

AMPC, Inc., 2325 North Loop Dr., Ames, IA 50010

Animal Health, Exton, PA 19341, Division of Pfizer, Inc., New York, NY 10017

Equi-Aid Products, Inc., Phoenix, AZ 85027

Fisher Scientific, Inquiry Department, 600 Business Center Dr., Pittsburgh, PA 15205-9913; 1-412-490-8300; www.fishersci.com

Jorgensen Laboratories, Inc., Loveland, CO 80538; 1-800-525-5614

Nasco Farm and Ranch, 4825 Stoddard Rd., Modesto, CA 95356-9318; 1-209-545-1600; www.nascofa.com

O.H. Kruse Grain and Milling, 321 South Antonio Ave., Ontario, CA 91762; 1-800-729-5787

Pharmacia and UpJohn Co., Kalamazoo, MI 49001

Ross Products Division, Abbott Laboratories, Columbus, OH 43215-1724; 1-800-986-8510; www.abbott.com, www.ross.com

Sigma Chemical Co., PO Box 14508, St. Louis, MO 63178

V.M.R.D., Inc., PO Box 502, Pullman, WA 99163

REFERENCES

Koterba, A. M., W. H. Drummond, and P. C. Kosch. 1990. *Equine clinical neonatology*. Philadelphia, PA: Lea & Febiger.

Madigan, J. E. 1997. *Manual of equine neonatal medicine*. 3d ed. Woodland, CA: Live Oak Publishing Company.

Naylor, J. M. 1999. Oral electrolyte therapy. In *Fluid and electrolyte therapy. Veterinary clinics of North America: Food animal practice*. 15 (3): 487–504.

Oftedal, O. T., and S. J. Iverson. 1995. Comparative analysis of non-human milks. In *Handbook of milk comparison*, edited by R. G. Jensen. San Diego, CA: Academic Press.

Orsini, J. A., and T. J. Divers. 1998. *Manual of equine emergencies: Treatment and procedures*. Philadelphia, PA: Saunders.

31
Black-Tailed and White-Tailed Deer

Sophia Papageorgiou, Darlene DeGhetto, and Jennifer Convy

NATURAL HISTORY: BLACK-TAILED DEER

The black-tailed deer (*Odocoileus hemionus*) is of the order Artiodactyla and family Cervidae. It is native to North America.

Description/ID

Black-tailed deer have a dorsal coat that is reddish or yellowish-brown (grayish in winter) and they have a cream to tan coat ventrally. The throat patch, rump patch, inside of the ears and inside of the legs are generally white. The ears are large, 4.75–6 inches in length. The tail is blackish or brown above, white below. Fawns have a tawny or reddish-brown colored coat with numerous white spots. Check the tail to differentiate black and white-tailed deer fawns. They stand 3–3.5 feet tall at shoulder and are 3.75–6.5 feet long with a 4.5–9-inch tail (Macdonald 1995; Nowak 1991).

Reproduction

One to two fawns born are born in the spring. Females have one fawn at their first breeding, with twins or triplets in subsequent years. Young are born after 6 1/2 months gestation. Rarely a dam may have triplets, one of which is much smaller than the other two and may not survive. This is important to note in a rehabilitation situation. The tiny fawn, in a group of triplets, may thrive with a nutritious diet and proper management, but that may not always be the case (Macdonald 1995).

Habitat and Foraging Technique

They live along forest edges, mountains, and foothills (Macdonald 1995).

Natural Diet

They eat herbaceous plants, huckleberry, salal, thimbleberry, twigs of Douglas fir, cedar, yew, aspen, dogwood, service berry, juniper, sage, and acorns (Nowak 1991).

Additional Information

Their activity level tends to be crepuscular. They have extremely sharp hooves. They have the ability to jump high fences (6 feet or more) and generally bed down in thick vegetation (Macdonald 1995; Nowak 1991; PAWS 2001).

Behavioral Considerations

Fawns exhibit "freeze behavior" when they are very young (one to three weeks old) and "flight behavior" when they are older than three weeks (Nowak 1991).

NATURAL HISTORY: WHITE-TAILED DEER

The white-tailed deer (*Odocoileus virginianus*) is of the order Artiodactyla and family Cervidae. It is native to North America.

Description/ID

White-tailed deer have a tan or reddish-brown dorsal coat color (grayer in winter), with a white band on the snout just above the nose. The abdomen, throat, and inside of the ears are white. They have a white ring around the eyes. Their tail is brown with a white edge above, white below. The top of the tail may have a dark stripe down the center. Fawns are tawny with numerous light spots. Check the tail to differentiate White- from Black-tailed Deer fawn. They stand 3–3.5 feet tall at shoulder and are 3.75–6.5 feet with a 6–13-inch tail (Macdonald 1995; Nowak 1991).

Reproduction

Females have one fawn at their first breeding, with twins or triplets in subsequent years. Fawns are born in the spring. Young are born after 6 1/2 months gestation. Rarely a dam may have triplets, one of which is much smaller than the other two and may not survive. This is important to note in a rehabilitation situation. The tiny fawn, in a group of triplets, may thrive with a nutritious diet and proper management, but that may not always be the case (Macdonald 1995).

Habitat and Activity Period

They inhabit farmland, brushy areas, woodlands, typically in lowland areas (Macdonald 1995; Nowak 1991).

Natural Diet and Foraging Techniques

White-tailed deer forage on green plants, acorns, beechnuts, woody vegetation, twigs, and buds especially of birch and maple (Macdonald 1995; Nowak 1991).

Additional Information

They are a predominantly nocturnal species. Like black-tailed deer, they have extremely sharp hooves, which can lacerate easily, and they have the ability to jump high fences (Macdonald 1995; Nowak 1991; PAWS 2001).

Behavioral Considerations

Fawns exhibit "freeze behavior" when they are very young (one to three weeks old) and "flight behavior" when they are older than three weeks (Nowak 1991).

RECORD KEEPING

Detailed records must be maintained as in all captive animal situations. Accurate daily recording of attitude, weight, temperature, heart and respiratory rate (if possible), food fed (measured), and amount eaten (measured). Monitoring stool production and consistency is important in young ruminants. All procedures, physical examinations, medications provided, or other information must be written in the animal's individual record file. Case number and tag numbers should be placed on all sheets of the animal's permanent record for identification purposes.

ASSESSMENT OF THE NEONATE

Age Determination

Age can be determined using the following guide:

Birth: Calves are spotted, umbilicus is fresh and wet within the first 12 hours. Hooves are very soft.
7–14 days: Umbilicus sloughs off. Hooves are firm.
1 month: Eyes are brown.
3–5 months: Spotted pelage fades.
4–6 months: Weaning and eating solid foods.

There are a number of successful methods used by different people to raise fawns. This text describes successful methods used over a number of years at the PAWS Wildlife Center (PAWS 2001). Readers may find other methods that work for their particular rehabilitation center.

Weight Estimation

If an accurate scale is not available, a simple tool to get an accurate weight for fawns is obtained by using a goat weight tape. These can be purchased at most feed stores. The goat measuring tape should be placed around the girth of the fawn just behind the point of the elbow at the axilla. The weight should be taken the first day the fawn presents to your facility. If the fawn is stressed or in shock, guesstimating the weight is okay to do until you have an opportunity to get a more accurate reading with the goat measuring tape (PAWS 2001).

Restraint and Handling

Care should be taken to properly restrain these animals in order to avoid fractured limbs, or hyperthermia, which may result in capture/stress myopathy.

Fawn Restraint

Cover the eyes of the animal with a towel or blindfold before handling (Spraker 1993; PAWS 2001).

Restrain fawns for routine procedures in lateral recumbency ensuring the fawn is lying with its left side down to decrease chances of bloat. The ideal position is sternal recumbency especially when the animal is recovering from sedation or anesthesia. Do not roll the animal onto its back to change positions; it may cause regurgitation and possibly inhalation pneumonia. The best way to roll an animal is to tuck the feet and legs under the animal and roll it over its sternum to place it on the opposite side, while supporting the head and neck in an upright position. Be sure to have proper control or restraint of all four feet and legs when handling the animal. Two people should always be involved in restraining the fawn for safety reasons and both should remain on the same side of the animal during its restraint.

Carrying a Fawn

Hold the fawn under one arm close to your side. With your free hand control the neck region to keep the fawn from rearing its head up and hitting the handler's face. Cover the fawn's eyes with a blindfold (soft towel) and pick it up under its belly with both arms. Have the second person stretch the rear legs straight out, taut and away from the handler's body to restrict kicking of the rear feet (PAWS 2001).

Generally, fawns will settle down with proper restraint and allow physical examination and any appropriate therapy. We have had great success performing all the above with appropriate restraint. Young/small fawns may also be restrained with inhalant gas anesthesia using Isoflurane with oxygen via a face mask, but only if the animal is stable enough to undergo anesthesia (see Fig. 31.1). This procedure should be done in the presence of a veterinarian after he or she has assessed the animal. Always remember to lubricate an animal's eyes with artificial tears when anesthetizing it. Light anesthesia may facilitate performing a complete physical examination, obtaining a blood sample, fecal, skin scrapings/samples, and placing an intravenous catheter in a cephalic vein to provide intravenous fluid therapy and medications, if necessary (PAWS 2001).

INITIAL CARE AND STABILIZATION

Perform a complete physical examination starting with the head and proceeding to the rump. Be sure to check the umbilical cord and treat with 7% tincture of iodine if moist or infected. Check all four sets of scent glands for maggot infestation. They include the tarsal, metatarsal, pedal, and preorbital glands. Rehydrate the fawn if necessary and obtain a fecal sample for analysis. Take the temperature and if possible draw a small amount of blood to check packed cell volume (PCV), total solids (TS), and blood glucose (BG) on arrival. Check the condition of the hooves. Observe the fawn while standing and walking for any musculoskeletal abnormalities (i.e., splayed legs, lameness, fractures) (PAWS 2001; Smith 1990).

FAWN FEEDING GUIDELINES

Always provide fresh cool water to the fawn(s) and be sure to have plenty of water sources available when you have multiple fawns in a pen.

NURSING TECHNIQUES

The most successful technique to have fawns accept the bottle is to sit with the individual fawn for 10–15 minutes at the beginning of each feeding and present it with the bottle and nipple. Encourage it to take the nipple and suckle by placing the nipple into the fawn's mouth. Gently squirt some of the milk

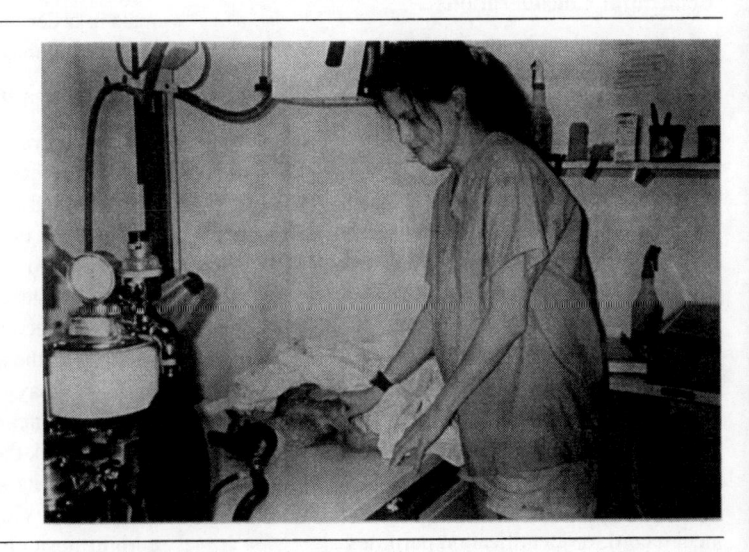

Figure 31.1 Fawn under anesthesia for physical examination.

into the fawn's mouth or onto the palm of your hand and encourage the fawn to take the milk, all the time trying to place the nipple into the mouth. You can also try to have a fawn suckle on your finger in order to stimulate the suckling response, then introduce the nipple into the mouth so that the fawn will subsequently suckle from the bottle. It may take a day or two to have the fawn on the bottle, but a fairly healthy fawn will accept the nipple and nurse after a few sessions of nipple training. Once the fawn is taking the bottle consistently it should be placed in a pen with conspecifics for appropriated socialization. Monitor the fawn for formula intake, weight gain, and thriftiness in the first few days of introduction with the other fawns. Be sure the fawn is taking formula, gaining weight, and thriving (PAWS 2001).

Newborn fawns less than 24 hours old need to receive a source of colostrum for absorbable immunoglobulins, which provide them with initial immune function and aid in the treatment of failure of passive transfer in newborn calves. The colostrum serves as an aid in the prevention of scours by supplying antibodies that block the K-99 *E. coli* disease process. PAWS Wildlife Center uses COLOSTRX (*Escherichia coli* antibody) bovine origin for 24–48 hours after a one- to two-day-old fawn presents. This can be purchased at local veterinary drug distributors and possibly livestock feed stores. PAWS Wildlife Center orders its supply from Provet in Mukilteo, WA (contact your local veterinary distributor to obtain this product). Follow directions on the label and use one bag (454 g powder, reconstituted per package instructions) per animal and give it orally via bottle or stomach tube (PAWS 2001; Smith 1990).

When fawns present to the center they are started on formula based on Table 31.1 (Deer Feeding Guide) and formulated as follows (LMR is Lamb Milk Replacer from Land O'Lakes) (PAWS 2001).

Day 1: straight oral lactated Ringer's solution (LRS)
Day 2: 3/4 LRS to 1/4 LMR
Day 3: 1/2 LRS to 1/2 LMR
Day 4: 1/4 LRS to 3/4 LMR
Day 5: 100% LMR and continue based on the age/feeding guide in Table 31.1.

TUBE FEEDING

Although not an ideal or safe situation, tube feeding may be the only solution to providing nutrition to an orphan and having it strong enough to begin suckling. This can be performed with a stomach tube, a light source, and the appropriate formula (see above). It will require two people, one to restrain the fawn and one to pass the stomach tube and gently pour the formula into the tube. The tube should pass easily into the stomach. In order to double check that it is in the stomach and not the trachea, palpate

Table 31.1 Deer Feeding Guide

Age in days/weeks	Body weight (kg)	Cc/ml	Frequency of feedings
1 day	2.5–3.2	94–122	5 × day
2 days	2.7–3.5	101–131	QID
3 days	2.9–3.7	109–141	QID
4 days	3.1–4.0	117–150	QID
5 days	3.3–4.2	124–159	QID
6 days	3.5–4.5	165–211	QID
7 days	3.7–4.	174–222	QID
8–14 days	3.9–6.5	184–304	TID
15–21 (2–3 weeks)	5.3–8.2	251–386	TID
22–28 (3–4 weeks)	6.8–10.0	317–467	TID
29–42 (4–6 weeks)	8.2–13.5	480	BID–introduce solid food
43–49 (6–7 weeks)	11.0–15.2	480	SID
50–99 (7–weeks)	12.5–27.7	480	SID–Start weaning seriously
8–10 weeks			Weaned
4–6 months			Released about late October or Early November

the neck. You should feel two firm, tubular structures. One is the trachea and the other is the tube within the esophagus. If you do not palpate two tubes, then recheck and visualize the trachea and tube or remove the tube and begin all over again. Once the formula has been delivered, kink the tube and gently remove it. Be very careful to check that the tube has been passed into the stomach and not the trachea (leading to the lungs). If tubed improperly (into the trachea), the animal will die very quickly as a result of having its lungs flooded with fluid, which will cause it to drown. This procedure should be performed by trained personnel in a quiet place, free from external stimuli (PAWS 2001; Smith 1990).

Special Note: The Deer Feeding Guide (Table 31.1) is a loose guideline as we raise deer in a herd of typically 10 to 15 fawns. This makes feeding and weaning difficult to standardize per individual. Therefore, the herd sets the feeding guideline and the older deer may need to remain on bottle-feeding longer than is ideal (i.e., beyond optimum weaning time) in order to allow the younger deer to remain in the herd and still achieve their adequate nutritional needs from the fawn formula. We do not manually separate individual deer from the herd for bottle-feeding unless medical reasons prevail. The younger deer will wean earlier and remain more afraid of humans if allowed to remain as part of the herd. This is an important philosophy to follow especially if you plan to release the fawns back into the wild. To appease the larger deer that need to be off formula but still come to the bottle rack, offer a bottle of water instead of milk while the smaller deer are still suckling milk. This will keep the larger deer from throwing a "tantrum" and they eventually decide browse and grain are better than water. They will stop suckling and begin consuming the solid food. This is also a weaning technique that can be used on the entire herd to truly wean them from the bottle if it is difficult to provide feed at two different growth levels (i.e., if the facility does not have two pens suitable for different-aged fawns) (PAWS 2001).

HOUSING BY AGE AND DEVELOPMENTAL STAGE

During the neonatal stage, or on initial presentation, place the fawns in airline kennels within a quiet pen or enclosed room, and move them into larger housing as they develop and mature. A concrete run enclosed on all six sides (preferably a combination of concrete with chain link), with a concrete floor and lined with plenty of towels and blankets to provide warmth, is necessary initially. It should be easily cleaned and maintained while fawns are being assessed, treated, and conditioned to bottle-feeding. This space should be at least 4 ft square and free from direct drafts and inclement weather conditions.

Provide an external heat source if the animal is young, weak, or not thermoregulating well. Once it is stable, thermoregulating well, and drinking from a bottle, you may place it with conspecifics (same species) in protected outdoor stalls. Move them into small outdoor paddocks as they mature. Eventually they should be housed in a fairly large pen or large cervid paddocks. Be sure to have padlocks on pen doors or gates. Enclosures should also have a double door system and lean-to type shelters to accommodate animals in inclement weather, and be designed for minimal human contact.

The larger cervid paddocks should have walls that are predator proof and provide adequate visual and sound barriers from humans. Once the animal is stable and assessed as healthy, it may be moved out with other fawns into a paddock/enclosure with natural substrate (dirt/ground cover/plants/foliage) on the ground and vegetation that is appropriate for deer browsing and native to the area. Bottle racks should be mounted at appropriate heights for all the animals to reach in one or two areas of the enclosure. The bottle racks should be accessible from the outside and be easy to clean and maintain (see Fig. 31.2). Minimal exposure to humans should be protocol once the animals are drinking consistently from bottles on their own. Be sure to discourage any taming of the animals, especially if they are to be released back into the wild. A full-grown buck that is at all tame or lacks fear of humans is a very dangerous animal and can easily injure someone.

IMMUNE STATUS AND SPECIAL NEEDS

Fawns must have their age assessed and be given certain inoculations on presentation. Clostridia toxoid injections, vitamin E with selenium, and vitamin A and B injections must be given after the initial exam provided the animal is healthy and stable (see Vaccinations below). If the fawn is ill or traumatized, these injections may be postponed for a day or two. The assessment may be performed by a veterinarian (Smith 1990).

If the animal appears to be too small or very weak, it may not have nursed at birth, and plasma transfusions may be necessary. Plasma may be given via oral gavage (tube fed) if it is a few days old or IV catheter if it is older to provide immunoglobulins that are necessary to protect the fawn until its own immune system begins to function and mature. This treatment may need to be repeated (Smith 1990).

Vaccinations

The following vaccinations may be given:

1. Quatracon 2X (Actinomyces pyogenes, *Pasteurella multicoda, Escherichia coli, Salmonella*)
   Dose: 3 ml/4.54 kg SQ
   Frequency: Give one injection upon arrival and repeat in five days if the fawn develops diarrhea, or repeat in ten days if no diarrhea occurs for a total of two injections.
   This product is ordered from Provet in Mukilteo, WA.
2. Clostridium Perfingens Types C&D Antitoxin
   Dose: 10 ml SQ (in several different sites)
   Frequency: Give 48 hours after arrival or at one week of age and repeat in five days if the fawn develops diarrhea, or repeat in ten days if there is no diarrhea; for a total of two injections.
3. Clostridium Types C&D Bacterin Toxoid
   Dose: 2 ml SQ
   Frequency: Give at four weeks old (over 8 kg) and repeat in 21 days for a total of two injections.

Vitamin and Mineral Supplements

Myosel-E (selenium) may be given in a dose of 0.02 ml/kg IM. Give on arrival or at one week of age (the animal should be over 3.5 kg). Note: Giving additional vitamin E and selenium depends on the quality of soil, the nutrient levels in the feed, and geographical variation in soil content or from your hay distributor. Contact your local large-animal veterinarian to determine the needs for this type of supplementation in your area.

Cervids require a large amount of space once grazing. Heat lamps may be needed outdoors initially, especially if raising a single animal. Indoor bedding should be provided and towels or large blankets may be used. Fresh straw is good outdoor bedding (Fig. 31.2).

TIPS FOR WEANING FROM FORMULA TO SOLID FOOD

Once the fawns are two to three months old, they should be eating primarily solid food with supplemental bottles. Goat chow (Purina), calf manna (Manna Pro), and alfalfa hay should be introduced once they present to the center. Begin weaning the bottle-feedings if the fawns appear healthy and have had solid food available along with their bottle-feeding. Once fawns are taking the bottle consistently, they should begin nibbling on the solid food diet. Natural browsing foods and foliage indigenous to your region should always be present, along with a plentiful supply of fresh, clean water (PAWS 2001).

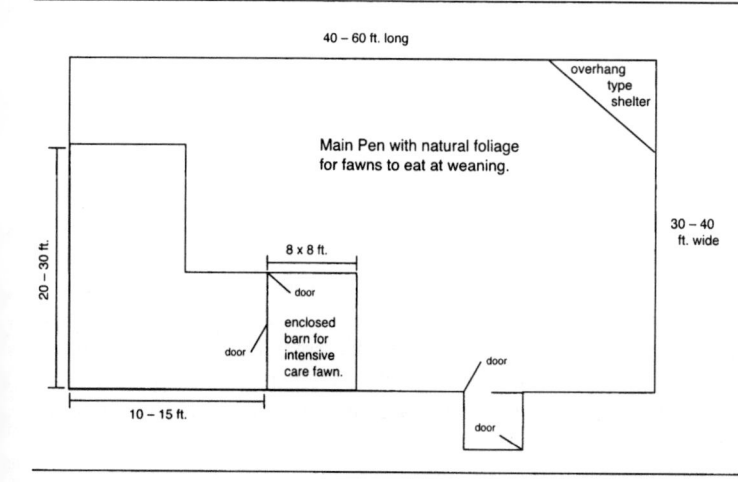

Figure 31.2 Outdoor fawn pen with separate pens and barn area.

COMMON MEDICAL PROBLEMS

The medical problems of deer are presented here in order of the most common presentation. Special Note: During oral antimicrobial therapy, give Probios (CHR Hansen Biosystems) microbial products or some type of bovine oral gel (e.g., Probiocin, available from Pro-Vet, Mukilteo, WA, or your local feed store) for ruminants at the recommended label dose to maintain healthy rumen and gut flora.

Navel Ill (Omphalitis/Omphalophlebitis)

Newborn and very young animals may have infections that begin from the umbilical area. This structure is rich with blood vessels and can be open to the environment (as a result of trauma or an overzealous dam chewing the umbilicus too close to the baby's abdomen). Infectious organisms may enter the animal's bloodstream and quickly spread systemically. The umbilicus will generally be red, inflamed, and hot to the touch. There may be a purulent or bloody discharge from the area. An animal may feel febrile and be lethargic or depressed.

Treatment includes swabbing/dipping the umbilicus in 7% tincture of iodine solution two to three times a day for four to five days or until clinical signs resolve. If the animal has signs of systemic disease (fever, inappetence, lethargy), place it on oral or injectable broad-spectrum antibiotics (trimethoprim sulfadiazine, 55 mg/kg initially, then 27 mg/kg PO SID for 7–14 days). If giving antibiotics orally, administer Probiocin (or any appropriate gut protectant product) to aid the gastrointestinal tract in maintaining appropriate gut flora. If the fawn is not improving in 36–48 hours, it should be worked up for secondary problems such as pneumonia, peritonitis, or septicemia (Plumb 1998; Smith 1990).

Fluid therapy (lactated Ringer's or Normosol-R with or without 2.5% dextrose) may be administered subcutaneously if the animal has systemic signs of illness. A complete blood count (CBC) and chemistry panel may need to be submitted to a laboratory for analysis (Cotter 1993). If possible, a packed cell volume (PCV), blood glucose (BG), and total serum protein should be done if enough blood can be obtained without stressing the animal.

Be sure to check the umbilicus daily for resolution of signs and monitor the animal for appetite, water consumption, attitude, and weight gain. If the umbilicus is oozing purulent material, be sure to do a culture and submit to the lab for a culture and sensitivity, along with the additional tests listed above, and consult with a veterinarian (Plumb 1998; Smith 1990).

Trauma

Fractures

Fractures in the young fawns occur from automobile accidents, animal attacks (primarily dogs), fence entanglements, and other trauma. Fractures of the ribs, long bones, pelvic girdle, and skull are seen most frequently. Radiographs should be performed on all fawns with fractures once they are stable. This may require waiting a day or two for the animal to stabilize. Keep fawns with suspected fractures confined in large airline kennels or very small enclosures. Seek veterinary assistance for treatment and stabilization of fractures.

Radiographs should be taken with the animal under light sedation to decrease the stress level of the patient. Small fawns can be anesthetized with isoflurane/O_2 using a facemask and the radiograph taken. Larger fawns may require injectable immobilization with ketamine (2.0 mg/kg IV to effect)/valium (0.4 mg/kg IV) or xylazine (Rompun, 0.044–0.11 mg/kg IV slowly or 0.01–0.33 mg/kg IM), which can be reversed with yohimbine (0.125 mg/kg IV) (Plumb 1998).

Female fawns with pelvic fractures should not be released, and may need to be euthanized because of the likelihood of dystocia or suffering during breeding season later in life. Females with pelvic fractures should be evaluated by a wildlife veterinarian who can determine a final plan for the animal. For males with pelvic girdle fractures, the type and extent of the fracture(s) need to be evaluated by a veterinarian in order to establish a plan for repair or euthanasia (Morgan 1992; PAWS 2001; Smith 1990).

Capture Myopathy

This is a physiologic phenomenon that occurs through a cascade of metabolic reactions. The outcome may be an irreversible condition leading to the animal's death. Capture myopathy generally occurs after a stressful event in well-muscled animals species (hoofstock, waterfowl, etc.). If a fawn has been attacked or chased by dogs, or hit by a car, it may be suffering from capture myopathy. Aggressive fluid therapy, broad-spectrum antibiotics, and regulating temperature are the mainstays in treating this condition. Most treatment is unrewarding once the capture myopathy progresses (Spraker 1993).

Metabolic Abnormalities

Shock

Shock is usually a result of being hit by cars or attacked by dogs. The animals present with severe hypovolemia and hypoglycemia (see Hypoglycemia below). Animals have pale mucous membranes and glazed/glassy appearing eyes, are recumbent, may have an elevated temperature and a prolonged capillary refill time. If head trauma has occurred, the animal may have seizures, slip into a coma, have problems thermoregulating, or be hypoglycemic.

Administer warm fluids and medication under the direction of a veterinarian. Treatment consists of shock dose fluids via IV catheter. The shock dose of fluids we use is 90 ml/kg IV of Normosol-R or lactated Ringer's solution (Morgan 1992; Murtaugh 1994). Fluids with 5–10% dextrose, once shock dose fluids have been given, should be started IV if the BG level is less than 60 g/dl. Intravenous antibiotics and IV short acting steroids (Solu-Delta Cortef, 0.2–1 mg/kg IV or 1–4 mg/kg IV) can be given as well. If the animal is having seizures, oral Karo syrup and/or IV dextrose may need to be given in lieu of shock dose fluids until the animal stops seizing, then shock dose fluids may be administered (see Hypoglycemia below). Monitor the temperature and treat accordingly (see Hyperthermia and Hypothermia below). It is best to have traumatized/shocky fawns evaluated by a veterinarian at the time of presentation. When the animal is stable, blood samples and radiographs should be taken to check for fractures or any organ abnormalities (Morgan 1992; Plumb 1998; Smith 1990).

Hypoglycemia

Young animals have higher blood glucose (BG) requirements than most adults of their species. If an animal has low blood glucose levels on presentation, less than 60 g/dl, quickly apply Karo syrup to the gums and then give dextrose via gavage (stomach tube) (10–20 ml/kg of 20% dextrose) or subcutaneously (SQ). If giving dextrose SQ, give only a concentration of 2.5% dextrose. Immediately consult a veterinarian to assist in organizing a treatment plan for ongoing therapy and placing an IV catheter. Once the BG has been corrected and the animal is stable, proper management with environmental control, nutrition and additional oral, SQ, or IV fluid therapy can maintain the patient until its metabolism takes over (Morgan 1992).

Animals that are hypoglycemic may begin to have seizures. If a fawn is presented to you and begins to seize, administer 1–2 ml diazepam rectally and provide glucose immediately by rubbing Karo syrup on the gum line of the fawn's mouth. Do not continue to use valium if an animal has low blood glucose levels. You must correct the blood glucose level to stop the seizures. If the blood glucose level is normal and the seizures continue, the animal should be given diazepam IV dosed to effect and assessed for central nervous system damage. At this point a veterinarian should be evaluating the animal and formulating a treatment plan.

Hyperthermia

Hyperthermia occurs when heat production exceeds heat loss (Ettinger and Feldman 1995). Normal body temperature for fawns is 99–101°F (37–38.3°C). The following is a list of causes of hyperthermia: fever, infection/sepsis/abscess, environment (heat/humidity), dehydration, medications, anxiety, seizures, malignant hyperthermia (associated with capture myopathy as seen in traumatized exotic hoofstock), dyspnea, or fever of unknown origin (Ettinger and Feldman 1995).

There are four general stages of hyperthermia: hyperthermia (overheating), heat exhaustion, heat prostration, and heat stroke. A hyperthermic and heat exhausted patient will pant and have open-mouth breathing, tachycardia/arrhythmias, elevated rectal temperature, hot appendages, and headache. As the temperature continues to elevate and heat prostration sets in, nausea, muscle weakness, cramps, tachycardia, and tachypnea are seen. If the temperature is elevated to the point of causing heat stroke, cellular damage sets in and disseminated intravascular coagulation occurs. At this point the animal may not be saved (Ettinger and Feldman 1995; Morgan 1992).

Therapy for hyperthermic patients depends on determining the cause and level of hyperthermia. The following treatment regimen is a guideline for the four categories of hyperthermia outlined above.

Mild temperature elevations: Begin with passive cooling using environmental temperature regulation and temperature monitoring, plain caging (no newspaper or towels) (Ettinger and Feldman 1995; Morgan 1992; PAWS 2001).
Heat exhaustion: Cool distal area of limbs, set up a fan, and give subcutaneous fluids at room temperature. Cool the animal slowly to avoid hypothermia.

Heat prostration: Intravenous fluid therapy (crystalloids) based on 8% dehydration calculations or if shocky use shock dose (90 ml/kg large animals, 60 ml/kg smaller animals) and run fluid line in cool water, place cool-water-soaked towels on cage floor, fan outside cage, wet down the body surface with tap water, monitor the temperature. Once you are two degrees above normal temperature, stop all external cooling therapy and maintain fluids (without cooling mechanism). Continue temperature monitoring until the temperature is normal and the animal is stable. Be sure the animal does not become hypothermic (Ettinger and Feldman 1995; Morgan 1992; PAWS 2001).

Heat stroke: A veterinarian should be consulted immediately to assess and treat a fawn at this stage of overheating. Treatment with aggressive intravenous fluid therapy (crystalloids—LRS or Normosol-R, and possibly colloids—using plasma, hetastarch, dextrans, or Oxyglobin) will be necessary. Begin with crystalloids. Run the fluid line in cool water, cool the body with a normal temperature water bath, apply alcohol to peripheral limbs, and monitor for seizures. Perform a blood glucose level check and treat according to hypoglycemia section above. The animal may not respond and may have irreversible cellular and metabolic damage even in the face of aggressive therapy with plasma transfusions and medications. Monitor temperature regularly and treat as outlined above in heat prostration. Humane euthanasia may be necessary if the temperature is uncontrollable (Ettinger and Feldman 1995; Morgan 1992; PAWS 2001; Plumb 1998).

Hypothermia

Hypothermia occurs when heat loss exceeds heat production. The following are causes of hypothermia: exposure to inclement elements (ice, snow, etc.), anesthesia/sedation, overaggressive treatment of hyperthermia, sepsis, hypoglycemia, medications, head trauma, debilitation, and shock/trauma (Ettinger and Feldman 1995).

A hypothermic patient has pale mucous membranes, cold appendages, low rectal temperature, and tachycardia/cardiac arrhythmias (Ettinger and Feldman 1995).

Therapy for rewarming the patient depends on determining the cause and level of hypothermia. There are four categories of hypothermia: minimal, moderate, substantial, severe. The following treatment regimen is a guideline for the four categories of hypothermia (Ettinger and Feldman 1995; Morgan 1992).

Minimal: Passive rewarming using blankets, towels, and environmental control.

Moderate: Active surface rewarming using, if available, circulating hot water blankets, hot water bottles, heated water-filled latex gloves ("bed buddies"), radiant heat warmer (heat lamp), hair dryer.

Substantial: Contact a veterinarian to initiate therapy and formulate a plan.

Severe: Contact a veterinarian to initiate therapy and formulate a plan; may be irreversible (Ettinger and Feldman 1995).

Sepsis/Septicemia

Neonates suffer from various infectious agents (primarily bacterial) that cause sepsis. Environmental conditions such as overcrowding, unsanitary enclosures, contamination of the environment or feed can cause bacterial infections. Stress can lead to sepsis through ulcers allowing bacteria to gain access to the blood stream. Bacteria that commonly cause problems are *E. coli, Clostridia* spp., *Pasteurella* spp., and *Salmonella* spp., coronavirus, cryptosporidia, and others (Smith 1990).

Clinical signs may include fever (or in the case of extreme sepsis, low temperature), swollen joints, umbilical infections/omphalophlebitis, diarrhea, or seizures. A complete blood panel (CBC and chemistry panel) should be submitted for evaluation prior to beginning antibiotic therapy. In-house PCV/TS/BG should be done immediately (Cotter 1993; Ettinger and Feldman 1995; Smith 1990).

Treatment is similar to that for domestic species. Place cephalic IV catheter and provide aggressive IV fluid therapy with IV broad-spectrum antibiotics (see Navel Ill and Hypoglycemia above for fluid/drug doses). A veterinarian should be directly involved in assessing the animal and formulating a treatment plan. Antibiotic therapy should be continued for two weeks or longer depending on the resolution of signs or type of infection. Be sure to maintain the animal's nutritional support and continue to monitor blood values until it normalizes. Attempt to determine the cause of the infection and correct the underlying problems causing the sepsis. Septic fawns may not respond to even the most aggressive therapy. The fawn's individual immune system, age, nutritional state, and nature of sepsis along with treatment and supportive care will determine if it responds and does well (Smith 1990).

Gastrointestinal System Problems

Indigestion: (Ruminitis/bloat/vagal indigestion/obstruction)

The following conditions may cause indigestion: improper formula, moldy feed, inappropriate amounts of concentrated feed, stress causing ulcers leading to gastrointestinal upset, diaphragmatic hernia, or foreign bodies (Smith 1990).

Clinical signs of these conditions include abdominal distention, inappetence, fever, pain and discomfort, abnormal or scant feces, or inability to eructate. If a fawn has these signs it should be evaluated immediately by a veterinarian. Keep the animal sternal to avoid complications of regurgitation (PAWS 2001; Smith 1990).

Treatment may require placing an IV catheter followed by fluid therapy, IV antibiotics (broad-spectrum, cefazolin or ampicillin at 10 mg/kg), or passing a stomach tube and relieving the bloat (gas or ingesta). Prudent use of pain medication (flunixin megulamine at an initial dose of 2.2 mg/kg IV or IM, then decrease to a dose of 1.1 mg/kg every 8–12 hours for a few doses, not for prolonged use), abdominal radiographs, and performing an abdominocentesis are also required.

A simple case of bloat may be relieved by passing a stomach tube, and following up with supportive care and reintroducing the proper diet. But complications may necessitate additional therapy (see below).

With simple bloat, the diet should be appropriate for the age level of the fawn, and feedings should begin with small amounts frequently. The animal should be monitored until it is eating normally for its age and weight. If the fawn continues to have difficulty and rebloats, it may require microbial cultures orally such as Probiocin (see Sources below), or transfaunation of microflora from another fawn. Additional treatment would require placing an IV catheter followed by fluid therapy and IV antibiotics (broad-spectrum—cefazolin or ampicillin at 10 mg/kg). Contact a veterinarian to prepare a treatment plan (PAWS 2001; Plumb 1998; Smith 1990).

If a bloated animal is in distress and showing signs of difficulty breathing, it should be seen by a veterinarian immediately. In the meantime, if the bloat is not relieved by placing a stomach tube, then the rumen should be trocarized by a trained technician or veterinarian. This is done by puncturing the left side rumen areas (generally the distended area) with a sterile needle and releasing air. With small fawns I have used a sterile 18-gauge needle. Placing two or three needles in close proximity assists in allowing the air to escape quickly. If time permits, a quick sterile scrub should be done prior to trocarization. Regular trocars are often too large for these small fawns. The 18-gauge needles should work well (PAWS 2001; Smith 1990).

In cases that do not appear to resolve with initial treatment outlined above, the fawn may need to be surgically explored to look for gastrointestinal perforations, torsions, or other abnormalities. If you suspect a complicated bloat situation, inform a veterinarian as soon as possible (PAWS 2001; Smith 1990).

Diarrhea/Scours

Diarrhea can be characterized as acute or chronic and must be differentiated as originating in the small or the large bowel. Most of our patients present as acute cases of diarrhea and have either small or large bowel abnormalities. Initial treatment of diarrhea, until it can be further characterized is fluid therapy, diet change, and possibly broad-spectrum antibiotics (Ettinger and Feldman 1995; PAWS 2001).

Acute diarrheas in fawns are generally caused by a number of factors including "stress, bacteria, viruses, parasites, improper diet/nutrition, drugs/medications and toxins" (Ettinger and Feldman 1995). Chronic diarrheas may be caused by uncorrected acute diarrhea problems and rectal anatomical abnormalities (strictures, masses) and can be seen in younger patients, infections (bacterial or viral), ulcers, toxins, or metabolic diseases (hepatic, renal) (Ettinger and Feldman 1995; Smith 1990).

Clinical signs include dehydration, inappetence, lethargy, bloat, loose/runny stool, fever, +/– painful abdomen on palpation, +/– gaseous bowel loops, weight loss, tenesmus, and dyschezia (constipation) (Ettinger and Feldman 1995; Smith 1990).

Diagnostics include fecal analysis (direct and flotation), evaluation for giardia (direct microscopic check or ELISA tests), and hemaoccult tests. CBC, radiographs, fecal cytology, fecal cultures, and serologic tests for infectious diseases may be necessary to determine the cause and characterize the type of diarrhea, especially if the diarrhea does not resolve with diet modification and simple fluid therapy. In fawns, diarrhea is generally caused by parasites (coccidiosis), inappropriate diet, or stress (Ettinger and Feldman 1995; Smith 1990).

Treatment should be targeted at the underlying cause of the diarrhea. Young/baby animals should have diets reviewed and corrected and should be given SQ fluids—crystalloids at appropriate dehydration/shock/maintenance doses—until they can be placed on the appropriate diet and clinical signs resolve. They may require systemic antibiotics if they are significantly compromised and appear debilitated. (Trimethoprim sulfas are good for fawns at a dose of 55 mg/kg initially, then 27 mg/kg PO SID for 7–14 days.) Fecal examinations should be done on all patients with diarrhea and appropriate anthelminth therapy instituted (see Parasites below). Fluid therapy and dietary correction are the primary mechanisms to correct most of the acute diarrheas we see at the wildlife center. Coccidia can be treated with Albon (sulfadimethoxine) at an initial dose of 55 mg/kg, then 27.5 mg/kg once a day for ten days. Recheck fecal examinations must be done after treatment is completed and as new animals are added to the group. A low burden of endoparasites may be tolerated as long as the animals are healthy, gaining weight, and having normal stools (Morgan 1992; Smith 1990).

Use Corrective Scour Base paste (Schuyler) mixed with Probios (Hansen) microbial products feed granules. Mix 300 ml paste: 1 tsp granules. Administer 6–10 ml orally twice a day for five to seven days. This product may be stopped once the animal has normal, firm stool (PAWS 2001).

Chronic diarrheas are more difficult to treat. A veterinarian should evaluate the animal if it has this problem.

Parasites

Endoparasites

The most common parasite problem in young deer is coccidia species. They are treated with Albon at an initial dose of 55 mg/kg, then a dose of 27.5 mg/kg once a day for ten days. Recheck fecals should be done to ensure that the herd is maintained coccidia free or at a low enough burden to maintain good health and appropriate weight gains (Bowman 1999; Plumb 1998).

Other types of parasites such as cryptosporidia or nematodes may occur, but these are less likely in these young patients. If cryptosporidia is suspected a veterinarian should assess the animal and the others in the herd and begin appropriate therapy (PAWS 2001; Smith 1990).

Ectoparasites

Sarcoptic mange is caused by sarcoptes mites; small arthropods visible by microscope. Clinical signs are diffuse alopecia +/– patchiness of the fur. Diagnosis is obtained by skin scraping. The mites are visible under 4x or 10x power on the microscope. Treatment is with ivermectin injections. Discuss treatment plan and doses with the veterinarian. Generally one subcutaneous injection of ivermectin at 0.300 mg/kg can be given with a follow-up dose three weeks later (Bowman 1999; Plumb 1998).

Ticks can be found in debilitated animals and should be removed using a hemostat clamp while the animal is sedated. Generally, a very small number of ticks may live on the animal but they should not be present in overwhelming numbers. If that is the case, they are a result of the animal's being debilitated. The animal may need to be treated with an appropriate dip to eliminate all ticks.

Occasionally, fleas or lice may be present. If they are in large enough numbers a light flea bath may be used to treat them. Special flea and lice topical sprays are available in most feed stores. Check with a veterinarian before using these products on the fawn.

Ringworm is contagious to humans, but is generally not a severe problem in fawns. It is a fungal disease and the lesions are characterized by a reddish ringed worm appearance on the skin in an area of alopecia. Consult a veterinarian if ringworm is suspected. For further information, see Ectoparasites in Chapter 23.

Ocular Lesions

Corneal ulcers, foreign bodies, lens luxations, and blindness can be a result of trauma due to car accidents or dog attacks. Lens luxations and other complicated ocular lesions should be evaluated by a veterinary ophthalmologist because the animal must be able to see well with both eyes in order to be released back into the wild (Plumb 1998; Slatter 1990).

RELEASE CRITERIA AND RELEASE SITE

The deer must be weaned and able to forage solely on natural food types before releasing them. Fawns should have developed a natural/healthy fear of humans, flee at the sight and sound of humans, and not vocalize (as in begging for food or attention) toward humans. The fawns must possess the physical ability for strong flight to maneuver around and over trees and logs. The fawns' athletic abilities should be assessed by trained individuals prior to capture, transport, and release. The release should be arranged in conjunction with local wildlife officials in your area. At PAWS Wildlife Center a staff naturalist coordinates the particulars of the release with local Washington State Fish & Wildlife officials.

Female fawns/does that have sustained pelvic fractures should be fully assessed by a veterinarian trained in wildlife rehabilitation medicine. Generally, these animals should be humanely euthanized because they would not be able to go through normal parturition if released back into the wild and would likely die as a result of dystocia while attempting to give birth. This is a sensitive situation and should be discussed with the animal's long-term well-being in mind. If the animal is to remain in captivity, she should probably have an ovariohysterectomy.

ACKNOWLEDGMENTS

We would like to thank Dr. John Huckabee for his contribution and for training us to care for orphan fawns. We are especially thankful for his expertise with the medical problems. We would also like to thank the staff, volunteers, and veterinary externs at PAWS Wildlife Center who assisted in all the medical, nursing, and orphan care responsibilities, which made it possible to treat and raise numerous fawns and to write this chapter during 1999–2000.

SOURCES OF PRODUCTS MENTIONED

Hansen Biosystems, 9015 W. Maple St., Milwaukee, WI 53214-4298; 1-800-247-6782; www.chbiosystems.com

Land O'Lakes, Fort Dodge, IA

Manna Pro: St. Louis, MO; 1-800-690-9908; www.mannapro.com

Probiocin: Pro-Vet, Mukilteo, WA

Purina Mills: 1-800-778-7462; www.Purinamills.com

Schuyler Labs, 1000 MaComb Road, Rushville, IL 62681; 1-217-322-4324

REFERENCES

Bowman, D. D. 1999. *Georgis' parasitology for veterinarians*. Philadelphia, PA: Saunders.

Cotter, S. M. 1993. Pathophysiology of the hemiclymphatic system, course syllabus. Fall. North Grafton, MA: Tufts University School of Veterinary Medicine.

Ettinger, S. J., and E. C. Feldman. 1995. *Textbook of veterinary internal medicine*. 4th ed. Philadelphia, PA: Saunders.

Macdonald, D., ed. 1995. *The encyclopedia of mammals*. New York: Facts on File.

Morgan, R. V., ed. 1992. *Handbook of small animal medicine*. 2d ed. Philadelphia, PA: Saunders.

Murtaugh, R. 1994. Principles of medicine, course syllabus. Spring. North Grafton, MA: Tufts University School of Veterinary Medicine; Section on Small Animal Fluid Therapy.

Nowak, R. M. 1991. *Walker's mammals of the world*, vol. 2. 5th ed. Baltimore: The Johns Hopkins University Press.

PAWS wildlife rehabilitation manual. 2001. Lynnwood, WA: PAWS Wildlife Center.

Plumb, Donald C. 1998. *Veterinary drug handbook*. 3d ed. Ames: Iowa State University Press.

Slatter, D. 1990. *Fundamentals of veterinary ophthalmology*. 2d ed. Philadelphia, PA: Saunders.

Smith, B. P., ed. 1990. *Large animal internal medicine*. St. Louis: C.V. Mosby.

Spraker, Terry. 1993. *Zoo and wild animal medicine, current therapy 3*, edited by Murray E. Fowler. Philadelphia, PA: Saunders.

32
Exotic Ungulates

Kelley Greene and Cynthia Stringfield

NATURAL HISTORY

The bovids and cervids we will discuss in this chapter include gerenuks (*Litocranius walleri*), black duikers (*Cephalophus niger*), red-flanked duikers (*Cephalophus rufilatus*), zebra duikers (*Cephalophus zebra*), southern pudus (*Pudu pudu*), Chinese water deer (*Hydropotes inermis*), axis deer (*Axis axis*), giraffes (*Giraffa camelopardalis*), pronghorns (*Antilocapra americana*), and Speke's gazelles (*Gazella spekei*). The average birth weights for these animals are as follows: gerenuk, 3.48 kg; black duiker, 1.75 kg; red-flanked duiker, 1.00 kg; zebra duiker, 1.44 kg; southern pudu, 0.65 kg; Chinese water deer, 0.82 kg; axis deer, 3.00 kg; giraffe, 63 kg; pronghorn, 2.85 kg; and Speke's gazelle, 1.50 kg. Of these species, only a few give birth seasonally. Pronghorn give birth in late May through June, usually to twins. Chinese water deer have multiple births, usually in June. Litters average one to three fawns.

RECORD KEEPING

Infant arrival data charts are kept listing parentage, parent's history with infants, birth weight, condition, reason for hand rearing, and birth weight. Daily charts are maintained recording diet, feeding times and amount consumed, daily weights, medications and supplements, stool quality, and behavior toward cagemates. Developmental milestones are also noted such as first consumption of solid foods, rumination, and the appearance of horns or antlers.

EQUIPMENT

Plastic 8-oz Evenflo human baby bottles (Pyramid) and human "preemie" nipples with the hole slightly enlarged with a hot needle work well for most of the smaller antelope and deer. Some infants are fussier to start with and a joey teat (Coreen Eaton) works very well. We switch them over to a preemie nipple as soon as they are nursing well, as the joey teat does not hold up to the rigors of an older nursing infant. Giraffe calves do well using a lamb's nipple to begin with, and finish up with a calf nipple on a 2-liter plastic bottle (Nasco). All feeding equipment is washed in hot soapy water and then left to soak in a chlorine bath (1 cup bleach to 3 gallons water) between feedings. Rinse very thoroughly.

CRITERIA FOR INTERVENTION

Hoofstock calves may be pulled for hand rearing for many reasons, such as maternal neglect or aggression, illness or weakness of the calf or dam, or failure to nurse. It is very important that the newborn receive maternal colostrum within the first 12 to 24 hours after birth, and infants are watched very closely during this period. Skittish species are routinely hand reared at some institutions to temper an explosive flight response.

ASSESSMENT OF THE NEONATE

Upon arrival at the nursery, the calf is weighed, the umbilicus is dipped in Betadine solution, and a quick physical examination is given by the veterinarian. Generally the vet will confirm the sex, examine the palate, listen to the heart and lungs, and draw a blood sample to check IgG, blood glucose, and total protein levels. It is important to determine whether or not passive transfer of maternal antibodies has occurred through absorption of colostrum. If not, the veterinarian may choose to give the dam's (or a closely related species) plasma intravenously. Ungulates are almost totally dependent on colostral intake for immunity at birth. Ideally, neonates should get 6–10% of their body weight in colostrum per day for the first 48 hours, and if possible should get 4–5% of body weight in colostrum within the first two hours of life. For example, give 40–50 ml colostrum per kilogram body weight orally within the first two hours. We prefer to have the neonates nurse this amount, and give them up to 12 hours to nurse before tube feeding them the colostrum.

INITIAL CARE AND STABILIZATION

The infant is placed in a small, quiet stall, bedded with wood shavings covered with towels. The towels make it easier to monitor stool and urine output, and also help to prevent accidental shavings ingestion. In the case of duikers and deer, we prefer to bed them on towel-covered alfalfa, as shavings stick to wet noses. The same applies to weak or injured infants of all small species. Giraffe calves are bedded on shavings covered with straw.

Ambient building temperature is kept at about 70°F (21°C) and spot heat is provided. We use 250-watt heat lamps hung well out of the animal's reach. A hypothermic animal may be warmed using heat lamps or heating pads (under supervision) or bath towels warmed in a microwave. Normal body temperature is 100–101°F (37.8–38.3°C). Dehydrated animals may be given warmed subcutaneous fluids. The veterinarian should evaluate the degree of dehydration and give fluid amounts determined by the percent of dehydration multiplied times the body weight.

FORMULAS AND SUPPLEMENTS

All hoofstock neonates are started on cow's colostrum. Raw colostrum is purchased from a local dairy. It is then pasteurized and cultured, and antibody levels are measured using a colostrometer. We use the highest mg/ml colostrum for the youngest infants. After pasteurization, colostrum can be frozen, labeled, and dated for later use for up to one year. Packaging it in small, sterile, whirl-pack bags allows us to thaw only what we will use in a 24-hour period.

Neonates are fed 100% cow's colostrum for the first 72 hours. Then they are offered 50% cow's colostrum and 50% formula for the next 72 hours. At that time the ratio changes to 10% cow's colostrum and 90% formula until the animal is 21 days old. Straight formula is fed from three weeks of age until weaning.

Table 32.1 Ungulate Formula Guidelines

Species	Formula
Gerenuk	Evaporated goat's milk 1:1 distilled water
Speke's gazelle	
Pudu	
Chinese water deer	
Axis deer	
Redflanked duiker	Fresh, whole cow's milk
Black duiker	
Zebra duiker	
Giraffe	
Pronghorn	Evaporated (not condensed) cow's milk undiluted

Formulas for various hoofstock species are simple and easily obtained from most grocery stores (see Table 32.1).

Supplementation begins at seven days of age. Neonates are given 500 IU vitamin E acetate. We use a powdered formulation of vitamin E acetate, 1/4 tsp (1 g) 500 IU/g powder once daily in the first morning bottle (Western Medical Supply).

We also give a pinch of Probios granules (CHR Hansen Biosystems) in each bottle to seed the gut with beneficial bacteria. Infants fed a canned formula are also offered Hi-Vite drops (CHR Hansen Biosystems) at the rate of one drop per 50 ml of formula in each bottle.

Giraffe calves, due to their size, get 1 tsp (5 ml) vitamin E once daily. In addition, due to their rapid growth rates, we supplement giraffe calves with Lixotinic (Pfizer) as an iron supplement starting with 15 ml and increasing to 30 ml once daily and calcium lactate tablets (648 mg), 2.4 g to start, increasing proportionally with body weight as the calf grows (Rugby).

Formula is heated to body temperature using a warm-water bath. Microwaving is less desirable for heating as formula may heat unevenly and burns may occur. Formula should feel warm on your wrist. Some infants are more particular than others are when it comes to formula temperature. Formula may be rewarmed during a feeding session if the animal is fussy, but any formula that was heated and not consumed that feeding must be discarded.

WHAT TO FEED INITIALLY

The first feeding offered to the newborn is boiled distilled water. We offer half the amount we would offer of formula. Infants often resist attempts to bottle-feed and can put up quite a fight. Aspiration of formula can be a problem. This first feeding allows the keeper to evaluate the infant's feeding response without the risk of aspiration of actual formula. We then offer colostrum at the second feeding attempt.

NURSING TECHNIQUES

While the desire to suckle is natural, receiving formula through a rubber nipple from a human "mother" is not (Fig. 32.1). We start our infants in a very small stall (4 ft by 4 ft or 1.2 m by 1.2 m) that is quiet and free of distractions. Often, reduced lighting can be helpful.

With smaller species of deer and antelope, stimulation of the perianal area while hovering over the animal will elicit a "feeding response," usually slight lip smacking and swallowing, and sometimes nuzzling the keeper's chin or neck. In some species, duikers in particular, punching the keeper's chin or body with their muzzle is a good response. Some animals will suckle on the keeper's hair, forehead, and nose searching for a teat. Sometimes at this point, just slipping the nipple into the infant's mouth will result in an empty bottle and a full stomach. Those are the easy ones. Generally, infants that have not nursed at all from their dams are this simple to start. The longer the calves stay with the mother, the more difficult the keeper's job will be to get them to accept a bottle.

Sometimes infants are unresponsive to stimulation. These babies need to be gently restrained and have the nipple placed into the mouth until they suckle. Often the first suckle happens quite by mistake as the animal resists, but it usually catches on quickly. Generally speaking, most of the smaller species are nursing well in 24 to 48 hours. Pronghorn as a rule are extremely flighty and it often takes them several days to really master the idea of a keeper as "mom."

Hand-reared deer and antelope must be stimulated manually to urinate and defecate at first, but will usually eliminate on their own in a week or two. Meconium is passed for the first 24 to 48 hours, followed by yellow to orange pasty milk stool and normal pellets once solids are being consumed. The umbilicus is dipped in Betadine solution (povidone-iodine) twice daily until the stump drops off, or for about one week. Giraffe calves keep their umbilical stump for up to six weeks, but we discontinue Betadine treatments after one week.

Giraffe calves pose different problems when they are learning to nurse from a bottle. Because the animal at birth is sometimes taller and heavier than the keeper, convincing the animal that you are the food source may be challenging. The usual methods don't apply here. This baby instinctually searches for a teat in a location that is taller than it is. We have had hungry calves licking the stall walls in search of milk, refusing to have anything to do with the five-foot-tall keeper. We have had the best results using a stepladder and extending our arms above our head under a towel. The babies seem to like to get up under something to search for a nipple. We used an umbrella to stimulate one calf. Another liked to suckle on a curly wig. Whatever works! You cannot be shy about looking ridiculous. Be creative about finding whatever item it takes to get the individual excited about nursing. We have also had some luck in starting the nursing process in infant giraffes while they are recumbent. If you can catch the individual lying down, sometimes it will start to suckle if you cover its face with your arm and body and place the nipple in its mouth.

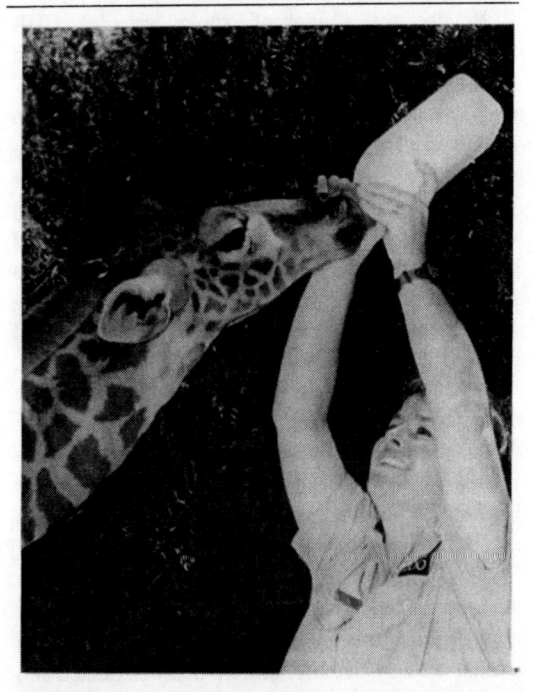

Figure 32.1 Feeding giraffe calves may be a challenge.

TUBE FEEDING

We generally avoid tube feeding ruminants whenever possible. The act of suckling and swallowing allows the milk to bypass the rumen and go directly to the abomasum where it can be digested. The risk of tube feeding is that the milk goes into the rumen where it cannot be processed and it sours. Bacterial infections may result. Occasionally, and as a last resort, we have tube fed giraffe calves that were difficult to start. The tube is placed midway down the esophagus to avoid aspiration but to allow swallowing. Sodium bicarbonate (20 ml of 8.4% injectable product) is poured down the tube first to stimulate closure of the rumen and allow milk into the abomasum. About one liter of formula per feeding is gravity fed into the tube via a funnel. The animal is manually restrained in a sternally recumbent position with the neck vertically supported. It takes several strong people to restrain the calf, and it helps to cover its eyes with a towel. The process is stressful and is avoided if possible. Attempts are continued between tubings to convince the calf to nurse from a bottle. It may take a few days to one week for the animal to consistently nurse from the bottle.

FREQUENCY OF FEEDING

The smaller species of antelope and deer are initially fed six times in 24 hours at three-hour intervals. We feed at 9 A.M., noon, 3 P.M., 6 P.M., 9 P.M., and midnight. This schedule continues until weaning begins at 60 days of age, at which point one feeding per day is eliminated each week. We usually start by eliminating the last night feeding. Weaning is usually completed by day 95. Solid foods such as alfalfa hay and acacia browse are offered free choice from the start. At one month of age, we begin to offer ADF-16 herbivore pellets (5/32-in size) (O.H. Kruse) and Mazuri browser maintenance pellets.

Animals housed with older cagemates tend to pick up on solid foods earlier. Rumination is usually seen by three to four weeks. Giraffe calves often feed best at four-hour intervals. They seem to take more formula overall when offered a larger amount, less often.

AMOUNTS TO FEED

Amounts fed to start with vary and are determined by the animal's birth weight. See Table 32.2. Increases are made at 72 hours, 144 hours (6 days), and then weekly until the maximum is reached at about 45 days. We increase no more than 20% at a time. For example, a 3-kg gerenuk would start out at 70 ml six times daily reaching a maximum formula intake of 160 ml six times daily at 45 days.

Giraffe calves follow generally the same routine, starting out at about one liter of formula per feeding five to six times per day and reaching the maximum of about 12 liters per day in about four to five feedings. Giraffe calves reach the maximum later than 45 days, and are weaned at about eight months. Each giraffe that we have worked with was different, and each worked out a feeding schedule that worked well for it. They can sometimes be gluttons and if given too much formula they can be slower to accept solid foods. They are always slower than parent-reared calves to try solids. Chopped apple and carrot over pellets can be helpful in encouraging consumption of solid foods.

EXPECTED WEIGHT GAIN

Calves are weighed daily, after the first morning bottle, for as long as they will tolerate it. It is not uncommon for infants to lose weight initially, but they should start an upward trend within a day or two if they are nursing well. Smaller antelope species, such as duikers, will gain 0.3–0.5 kg on average by seven days of age. Medium-sized species can expect to gain 0.5 to 1 kg by seven days of age. Giraffe calves can gain 10 kg during the first week.

HOUSING

Infants are housed indoors in a warm, quiet stall until they are nursing reliably from a bottle. It is advantageous to isolate newborns initially from each other so they are not distracted by cagemates during this period. They need time to bond with the keeper. Sometimes infants are more interested in "nursing" from each other than they are in nursing from the bottle. This is particularly true of the duiker species, and does occur even after infants are nursing well from the bottle. If it becomes excessive, we have had some success using Bitter Apple to discourage this behavior. Sometimes it becomes necessary to keep the offenders separated. Overstimulation of genitals or the perineal region by cagemates may cause diarrhea in the recipient.

Once infants are nursing well, we allow them access to an outdoor yard to encourage exercise. Often newborns have weak pasterns and fetlocks but they will straighten out in a day or two with exer-

Table 32.2 Exotic Ungulate Feed Chart

Body weight (kg)	Formula % of weight	Per feeding (cc)	Number of feedings	Daily total (cc)	Per feeding (cc)	Number of feedings	Daily total (cc)
.50 kg	18%	15 cc	× 6	= 90 cc	13 cc	× 7	= 91 cc
1.00	17	30		180	25		175
1.50	16	40		240	35		245
2.00	15	50		300	45		315
2.50	14	60		360	50		350
3.00	14	70		420	60		420
3.50	13½	80		480	70		490
4.00	13½	90		540	75		525
4.50	13	100		600	85		595
5.00	13	110		660	90		630
5.50	12½	120		720	100		700
6.00	12½	120		720	100		700
6.50	12	130		780	110		770
7.00	12	140		840	120		840
7.50	11½	150		900	130		910
8.00	11½	150		900	130		910
8.50	11	160		960	140		980
9.00	11	160		960	140		980
9.50	11	170		1020	150		1050
10.00	10	170		1020	150		1050
11.00	10	190		1140	160		1120
12.00	10	200		1200	170		1190
13.00	10	220		1320	190		1330
14.00	10	230		1380	200		1400
15.00	10	250		1500	210		1470
16.00	10	270		1620	230		1610
17.00	10	280		1680	240		1680
18.00	10	300		1800	260		1820
19.00	10	320		1920	270		1890
20.00	10	330		1980	290		2030
21.00	10	350		2100	300		2100
22.00	10	370		2220	310		2170
23.00	10	380		2280	330		2310
24.00	10	400		2400	340		2380
25.00	10	420		2520	360		2520
26.00	10	430		2580	370		2590
27.00	10	450		2700	390		2730
28.00	10	470		2820	400		2800
29.00	10	480		2880	410		2870
30.00	10	500		3000	430		3010
31.00	10	520		3120	440		3080
32.00	10	530		3180	460		3220
33.00	10	550		3300	470		3290
34.00	10	570		3420	490		3430
35.00	10	580		3480	500		3500

cise. Sunshine and fresh air are beneficial, and social interaction with other animals is also important.

COMMON MEDICAL PROBLEMS

The most serious hurdle a newborn ungulate must overcome occurs in the first 24 hours. They must receive passive transfer of immunoglobulins from colostrum, or receive a plasma transfusion. Septicemia and death may follow if they are untreated (Parish 1996). (See also Chapter 31, under Common Medical Problems, for additional information.)

The most commonly seen problem in hand-reared ungulates is diarrhea. Most infants face a bout with diarrhea at some point early in their lives. We always collect a fecal sample for analysis to determine whether or not the diarrhea is caused by internal parasites or other bacterial pathogens. Viral disease may also be a culprit and must be ruled out. Sometimes antibiotic treatment is necessary. We have been successful in treating nonspecific diarrhea by feeding psyllium such as Equi-Aid (Equi-Aid Products, Inc.), in their bottles. This helps to firm up the feces. It is offered in tiny amounts, usually just a pinch in their bottles a few times a day for the smaller species.

Occasionally, the effects of diarrhea must be supported with additional oral fluids, such as Pedialyte (Ross), or even just extra water. Subcutaneous fluids may be necessary if the diarrhea is severe or if the animal is inappetent (Naylor 1996). Often the problem will clear up when the animal is consuming solid foods regularly.

Giraffe calves sometimes have trouble with constipation. It has been our experience that manual stimulation to defecate is usually not successful. It is common for a giraffe calf to go several days between stools. Glycerin suppositories or milk of magnesia have been helpful in moving things along if needed. This has only been a problem while the animal is young and only consuming formula.

Animals receiving no maternal care may present hypothermic, hypoglycemic, and weak. These problems must be immediately corrected with heat and fluid therapy (Koterba and House 1996). (For further information see Chapter 31, under Common Medical Problems.)

Vaccination protocols should be tailored to the species, diseases problematic to them, and the institution. The ability to handle or dart the animal at varying ages must be considered.

SOURCES OF PRODUCTS MENTIONED

Coreen Eaton, 914 Risky Lane, Wentzville, MO; 1-314-828-5100

Equi-Aid Products, Inc., Phoenix, AZ 85027

Hansen Biosystems, 9015 W. Maple St., Milwaukee, WI 53214-4298; 1-800-247-6782; www.chbiosystems.com

Mazuri: 1-800-227-8941; mazuri@purina-mills.com

Nasco Farm and Ranch, 4825 Stoddard Rd., Modesto, CA 95356-9318; 1-209-545-1600; www.nascofa.com

O.H. Kruse Grain and Milling, 321 South Antonio Ave., Ontario, CA 91762; 1-800-729-5787

Pfizer Animal Health, Animal Health Group, Whiteland Business Park, 812 Springdale Drive, Exton, PA 19341; 1-800-877-6250; www.pfizer.com/ah

Pyramid International, Inc., Ravenna, OH 44266

Ross Products Division, Abbott Laboratories, Columbus, OH 43215-1724; 1-800-986-8510; www.abbott.com, www.ross.com

Rugby Laboratories, Inc., Duluth, GA 30097
Western Medical Supply, 1-800-242-4415

REFERENCES

Koterba, Ann M., and John K. House. 1996. Supportive care of the abnormal newborn. In *Large animal internal medicine*, edited by B. P. Smith. 2d ed. St. Louis: Mosby Year Book.

Naylor, Jonathan M. 1996. Neonatal ruminant diarrhea. In *Large animal internal medicine*, edited by B. P. Smith. 2d ed. St. Louis: Mosby Year Book.

Parish, Steven M. 1996. Ruminant immunodeficiency diseases. In *Large animal internal medicine*, edited by B. P. Smith. 2d ed. St. Louis: Mosby Year Book.

Appendix
Resources for Products Mentioned

BABY SCALES AND PLATFORM SCALES

Tanita Corporation, 5200 Church Street, Skokie IL 60077; 1-708-581-0250; 1-800-TANITAS

Technidyne Corp.; 1-800-654-8073

Weigh-Tronix, 19821 Cabot Blvd., Hayward, CA 94545; 1-800-350-8550

COLOSTRUM REPLACERS

Cow's colostrum replacer, Colostrum Plus, Jorgensen Laboratories, Inc., Loveland, CO 80538; 1-800-525-5614; www.jorvet.com

Seramune immunoglobulins for horses, Sera, Inc., Shawnee Mission, KS; 1-913-541-1307

Wombaroo Food Products, PO Box 151, Glen Osmond SA, Australia 5064

COMMERCIAL BLENDERS

Waring Commercial One Gallon Blender, Waring Products Division, Dynamics Corporation of America, New Hartford, CT 06057

DIETARY AND VITAMIN SUPPLEMENTS

Bo-Se: Vitamin E and Selenium injectable, Schering-Plough Animal Health Corp., Union, NJ 07083

Calcium Lactate (648 mg): Rugby Laboratories, Inc., Duluth, GA 30097

Calcium gluconate 10%: Calciquid, Econolab

Dyna-Taurine: Liquid lecithin base taurine supplement for veterinarian use; Harlmen Corporation, PO Box 371073, Omaha, NE 68114; Voice/FAX 1-800-393-0794; E-mail info@harlmen.com

Ferret Drops: Tomlyn Company, 711 S. Harding Hwy., Buena, NJ 08310; 1-800-866-5582; www.tomlyn.com

Hi Vite Drops: CHR Hansen Biosystems, 9015 W. Maple St., Milwaukee, WI 53214-4298; 1-800-247-6782; www.chbiosystems.com

Lixotinic: Pfizer Animal Health (North American Region), Animal Health Group, Whiteland Business Park, 812 Springdale Drive, Exton, PA 19341; 1-800-877-6250; www.pfizer.com/ah

Mazuri Vita-Zu Mammal Tablet 5M26 Vitamin Supplement; 1-800-227-8941; mazuri@purina-mills.com

Nutri-Cal: Tomlyn Company, 711 S. Harding Hwy., Buena, NJ 08310; 1-800- 866-5582; www.tomlyn.com

Poly Vi Sol (baby multivitamin): Mead Johnson & Company, Evansville, IN 47721

ViSorbin (liquid iron supplement); Animal Health, Exton, PA 19341, Division of Pfizer Inc., New York, NY 10017

DIETS FOR OMNIVORES

Primate Chow Purina Lab Diet, www.Purina.com

DIETS FOR YOUNG CARNIVORES

Hill's AD: Hills Diets; 1-800-445-5777; www.sciencediet.com

Science Diet Feline Growth: Hills Diets; 1-800-445-5777; www.sciencediet.com

ZuPreem Feline Diet: Premium Nutritional Products, Inc., PO Box 2094, Shawnee Mission, KS 66202; 1-913-438-8900; FAX 1-913-438-1881; www.zupreem.com

DIETS FOR YOUNG HERBIVORES

Calf Manna, Manna Pro St. Louis;1-800-690-9908; www.mannapro.com

High-fiber 25% ADF herbivore pellet: O. H. Kruse Grain and Milling, 321 South Antonio Ave., Ontario, CA 91762; 1-800-729-5787

High milk content pellet: Perfection Brand Milk Pellet; O.H. Kruse Grain and Milling, 321 South Antonio Ave., Ontario, CA 91762; 1-800-729-5787

Low-fiber 16% ADF herbivore pellet: O. H. Kruse Grain and Milling, 321 South Antonio Ave., Ontario, CA 91762; 1-800-729-5787

DIGESTIVE AIDS

Lactase: Lactaid, McNeil Consumers Health Care, Ft. Washington, PA; 1-800-522-8243; Lac-Dose, Rugby Laboratories, Inc., Norcross, GA 30071

Probios feed granules: CHR Hansen Biosystems, 9015 W. Maple St., Milwaukee, WI 53214-4298; 1-800-247-6782; www.chbiosystems.com (From Western Medical Supply; 1-800-242-4415)

Psyllium: Equi-Aid, Equi-Aid Products, Inc., Phoenix, AZ 85027

FEEDING TUBES

Kalajian Company, Long Beach, CA; 1-562-424-9749

Kendall Sovereign Feeding Tube and Urethral Catheter, the Kendall Company, Mansfield, MA 02048; 1-800-962-9888

Ryan Herco, 1819 Junction Ave., San Jose, CA 95131-2101; 1-800-848-1411

Sherwood Medical, St. Louis, MO 83103 through Kendall Corp.; 1-800-962-9888

FORMULAS

Biolac: Geoff and Christine Smith, PO Box 93, Bonnyrigg, NSW, Australia 2177

Buckeye Mare's Milk Plus, Buckeye Feeds, Dalton, OH; 1-800-321-0412

Enfamil: Mead Johnson & Company, Evansville, IN 47721

Enfamil with Iron: Mead Johnson & Company, Evansville, IN 47721

Ensure/Ensure Plus: Ross Products, Abbott Laboratories, Abbott Park, IL; 1-800-227-5767; www.ensure.com

Esbilac: Milk replacer for puppies by PetAg, Inc., 261 Keyes Ave., Hampshire, IL 60140; 1-800-323-6878; www.petag.com

Foal Lac: PetAg, 30 W. 432, Rt. 20, Elgen, IL 60120; 1-800-332-0877; www.petag.com

Formula 32/40 by Fox Valley Animal Nutrition, Inc., PO Box 146, Lake Zurich, IL 60047; 1-800-679-4666

Goat's Milk Esbilac: Milk replacer for puppies with sensitive digestive systems by PetAg, Inc., 261 Keyes Ave., Hampshire, IL 60140 1-800-323-6878; www.petag.com

Grober's Elephant Calf Milk Replacer: Grober Inc., 162 Savage Drive, Cambridge, Ontario, N1T 1S4, Canada; Ph:519-622-2500; 888-937-3392, or Toll Free 1-800-265-7863 (in Canada and USA); www.grober.com

Just Born: Milk replacer for puppies and kittens by Farnam Pet Products, A Division of Farnam Companies, Inc., Phoenix, AZ 85013; 1-800-234-2269; www.farnam.com

KMR: Milk replacer for kittens by PetAg, Inc., 261 Keyes Ave., Hampshire, IL 60140; 1-800-323-6878; www.petag.com

Lactol: Milk replacer for puppies and kittens manufactured by Sherley's Limited, Homefield Rd., Haverhill, Suffolk CB9 8QP U.K.; Voice: 01440 715700; FAX: 01440 713940; E-mail: sherleys@dial.pipex.com

LitterMilk, powdered pig milk product made by Land O' Lakes, St. Paul, MN; 1 800 328 4155

Mare's Match: Land O' Lakes, St. Paul, MN; 1-800-328-4155

Mother's Helper: Lambert Kay, Division of Carter-Wallace, Inc., Cranbury, NJ 09512-0187

Nuturall: Milk replacer for puppies and kittens by Veterinary Products Laboratories, PO Box 34820, Phoenix, AZ 85067-4820; 1-888-241-9545; www.vpl.com

Similac: Abbott Laboratories, www.similac.com

Staged kangaroo milk replacers: Wombaroo Food Products, PO Box 151, Glen Osmond SA, Australia 5064

Wombaroo diet: Perfect Pets Inc., 23180 Sherwood Road, Belleville, MI 48111-9306; 1-734-461-1362; FAX 1-734-461-2858; E-mail GSCHROCK1@aol.com

Wombaroo Food Products, PO Box 151, Glen Osmond SA, Australia 5064; 08-8379-1339; wombaroo@adelaide.on.net

Zoologic Milk Matrix: Nutritional Components, Powdered milk replacers for mammals. A division of PetAg, Inc., PO Box 396, Hampshire, IL 60140; 1-800-323-0877; FAX 1-847-683-3251; E-mail techservice@petag.com.

HARD TO FIND SPECIALTY FORMULAS AND HAND-REARING EQUIPMENT

Geoff Schrock Perfect Pets Inc., 23180 Sherwood, Belleville, MI 48111; 1-800-366-8794 or 1-734-461-1362; FAX 1-734-461-2858; E-mail GSchrock1@aol.com; www.frozenrodents.com

Grober Inc., 162 Savage Drive, Cambridge, Ontario, N1T 1S4 Canada Tel: 1-519-622-2500; Toll Free 1-800-265-7863 (in Canada and USA); FAX 1-519-623-8120; www.grober.com

PetAg, Inc., 261 Keyes Ave, Hampshire, IL 60140; 1-800-323-6878; www.petag.com

Wombaroo Food Products, PO Box 151, Glen Osmond SA, Australia 5064; 08-8379-1339; wombaroo@adelaide.on.net

HEATING PADS

Wombaroo Food Products, PO Box 151, Glen Osmond SA, Australia 5064

Wet/dry heating pad: Osborne Industries, 120 N. Industrial Avenue, Osborne, KS 67473; 1-800-255-0316

HUMIDIFIERS

Fine-mist humidifier: Durocraft, Durocraft Corporation, 490 Boston Post Road, Sudbury, MA 01776-9102

IMMUNOGLOBULIN TESTING

Immunoglobulin levels using an Equi-Z test: V.M.R.D., Inc., PO Box 502, Pullman, WA 99163

Immunoassays: SNAP Foal IgG Test, IDEXX Corp., Westbrook, ME 04092

INCUBATORS

Detailed information for making a homemade water-based incubator in the article "Simple Things That Make A Difference: Making Water-based Incubators" See Graboski, R. 1995. *Journal of wildlife re-habilitation* 18(2):16–17.

Animal Intensive Care Unit (AICU): 30 lb table top acrylic forced air incubator by Lyon Electric Company, Inc., 1690 Brandywine Ave., Chula Vista, CA 91911; 1-619-216-3400; FAX 1-619-216-3434; E-mail lyonelect@cts.com; www.lyonelectric.com

Intensive Care Systems: Portable water-lined warmers by Thermo Care, PO Box 6069, Incline Village, NV 89450; 1-800-262-4020; FAX 1-775-831-1230; E-mail: staff@thermocare.com

Isolette Infant Incubator: Used Air Shields Incubator, Rankin Biomedical Corporation, 9580 Dolores Dr., Clarkston, MI 48348; 1-248-625-4104; FAX 1-248-625-1070; E-mail: rankin@tir.com

Nursery Hospital Intensive Care Units and Incubators for pets: Petiatric Supply Company, www.petiatric.com

Thermocare, Inc., PO Box 6069, Incline Village, NV 89450; 1-800-262-4020

LACTOSE AND GLUCOSE ADDITIVES

Reagent grade powdered dextrose: Sigma Chemical Co., PO Box 14508, St. Louis, MO 63178

Powdered edible grade lactose: AMPC, Inc., 2325 North Loop Dr., Ames, IA 50010

NIPPLES AND BOTTLES

Syringes and feeding bottles: Catac, Bedford, England

Nasco Farm and Ranch, 4825 Stoddard Rd., Modesto, CA 95356-9318; 1-209-545-1600; www.nascofa.com

Fisher Scientific, Inquiry Department, 600 Business Center Dr., Pittsburgh, PA 15205-9913; 1-412-490-8300 (1 liter polyethylene laboratory bottle)

Lixit bottles, lixit.com, 1-800-358-8254

NUK nipples: Gerber Products Company, c/o Consumer Affairs, 445 State Street, Fremont, MI 49413-0001; 1-800-443-7237; www.gerber.com

Playtex Company; www.Playtex.com; 1-800-222-0453

Evenflo Company, Inc., 1801 Commerce Dr., Piqua, OH 45356; 1-800-233-5921; www.evenflo.com

Joey teats: Coreen Eaton, 914 Riske Lane, Wentzville, MO 63385; 1-314-828-5100; E-mail: wxicof@juno.com.

Four Paws Pet Nurser (conical shaped nipple): Four Paws Products Limited, 50 Wireless Blvd., Hauppauge, NY 11788; 1-516-434-1100; www.fourpaws.com

Pet-Ag nurser, variety of nipples and bottles: PetAg Inc., Hampshire, IL 60140; 1-800-323-0877; www.Petag.com

Mead Johnson Nutritionals: Nipples,1-812-429-6339; FAX 1-812-429- 7189; 24-hour toll-free fax-on demand 1-888-606-7737; www.meadjohnson.com

Wombaroo Food Products, PO Box 151, Glen Osmond SA, Australia 5064

Geoff and Christine Smith, PO Box 93, Bonnyrigg, NSW, Australia 2177

REHYDRATION SOLUTIONS

Pedialyte: Ross Products Division, Abbott Laboratories, Columbus, OH, 43215-1724; www.abbott.com

Biolyte: Pharmacia and UpJohn Co., Kalamazoo, MI 49001

SYRINGES AND CANNULAS

BD Company, 1 Becton Drive, Franklin Lakes, NJ 07417; 1-201-847-6800; www.BD.com

Jorgensen Laboratories, 1450 N. Van Buren Ave., Loveland, CO 80538; 1-800-525-5614; 400-cc syringes

Sherwood Medical Ballymoney, N. Ireland; 140-cc Monoject catheter tip syringes

Index

A

abscesses, seals, 140
Alpaca Registry, Inc., 40
alpacas, 39
American Association of Swine Veterinarians (AASV), 33
anemia, 148, 168, 175–176, 201
antibiotic therapy, elephants, 227
artificial pouches, 55, 64
Atlantic walrus, 150
Aviarios del Caribe Sloth Rescue and Rehabilitation Center, 81
axis deer, 256
aye-ayes, 106

B

baby bottles, foals, 24
bacteremia, foal risk, 25
bathing, kittens, 22
bats
    birth weights, 96
    blended mealworm diet, 101
    breeding cycle, 96
    captive versus wild release, 102–103
    container temperature requirements, 99
    defecation stimulation, 98
    equipment, 96
    feeding frequency, 97
    food amounts, 97
    housing, 98–100
    initial care/feeding, 97
    intervention criteria, 96–97
    medical problems, 101–102
    milk replacement formulas, 97
    nursing, 97
    rabies concern, 96
    record keeping, 96
    solid food introduction, 100–101
    species identification importance, 96
    weaning, 100–101
    weight gain targets, 97–98
bears. See black bears and polar bears
betadine solution, umbilicus dip, 256, 258
black bears
    activity period, 170
    age determinations, 171
    anemia, 175–176
    behaviors, 171
    birth weight, 170
    breeding cycle, 170
    demodectic mange, 174–175
    denning, 170
    diarrhea, 177
    distribution pattern, 168
    ectoparasites, 174–175
    endoparasites, 174
    epistaxis, 178–179
    food amounts, 172–173
    foraging techniques, 170
    foreign bodies, 176–177
    habitat, 170
    handling guidelines, 173–174
    housing, 173
    hypoglycemia, 177–178
    immune status, 174
    initial care, 171–172
    mange, 174–175
    medical problems, 174–179
    nursing, 172
    ocular lesions, 178
    parasites, 174–175

record keeping, 171
rehabilitation diet formula, 172
release guidelines, 179
restraints, 173–174
ringworm, 174
sarcoptic mange, 174
septicemia, 178
shock, 178
tagging, 179
trauma, 175
vomiting, 178
weaning diet formula, 172
black duikers, 256
black-tailed deer, 244 See also deer
blended mealworm diet, bats, 101
bloat, 101, 197
bonbo, 125
brooders, pig housing, 31–32
burrows, rabbit housing, 6, 9

C

cages
    bats, 98–100
    lemurs, 110–111
    macaques, 121
    opossum housing, 53, 54
    rabbits, 6
    seals, 138–139
    sloths, 85
    squirrels, 93
    sugar gliders, 59
canine distemper virus (CDV), 164, 199–200
capture myopathy, deer, 250
cataracts, macropod health problem, 72
cats
    birth weight, 19
    breeding cycle, 19
    cleaning/bathing, 22
    crates, 21–22
    defecation stimulation, 19–20, 22
    feline imunodeficiency virus (FIV), 22
    feline leukemia virus (Felv), 22
    food amount guidelines, 20–21
    housing, 21–22
    litter box introduction, 22
    medical problems, 23
    milk replacement formula, 21
    nursing techniques, 19–20
    record keeping, 19
    solid food introduction, 22
    syringes, 19
    tube feeding, 19–20
    weaning, 19, 22
    weight gain targets, 21
cecotrophs, rabbits, 11
chimpanzee, 125
Chinese water deer, 256
chlorine bath, feeding equipment, 256
combs, piglet parasite removal, 31
constipation. See species section
cotton top tamarin, 114
cottontail rabbit, 5
crates, cats, 21–22
cynomolgus macaque, 118

D

deer
    carrying fawns, 246
    E.coli disease, 247
    feeding guide, 247
    goat weight tape, 245
    housing, 248–249
    immune status, 248–249
    initial care/stabilization, 246
    medical problems, 250–254
    neonate assessment, 245–246
    nursing, 246–247
    record keeping, 245
    release criteria, 254–255
    release site, 254–255
    restraining, 245
    tube feeding, 247–248
    weaning, 248, 249
dehydration
    bat medical problem, 101
    exotic felids, 217
    ferrets, 205
    foal risk, 25
    foxes, 167
    lactated Ringer's solution (LRS), 7
    macaques, 123
    pigs, 30
    raccoons, 199
    seals, 140
demodectic mange, 174–175, 196
diarrhea. See species section
disbudding (horn removal), goat kids, 37
domestic rabbit, 5
Duchess Fund, 33

E

E. coli infections, 38, 247
East African black rhinoceros, 236
eastern cottontail, 5
eastern grey kangaroo, 63
ectoparasites, 164, 174, 174–175, 195–196
elephants
    antibiotic therapy, 227
    behaviors, 227
    birth weight, 221
    body temperature, 221
    breeding cycles, 221
    caretaker selection criteria, 224
    constipation, 225
    diarrhea, 225
    equipment, 221
    feeding frequency, 224
    fluid therapy, 226–227
    food amounts, 223–224
    herpesvirus infection, 225–226
    immune status, 224
    immunoglobulin transfer, 224–225
    initial care, 221–222
    intervention criteria, 221
    medical problems, 225–226
    metabolic bone disease, 115
    milk replacement formula, 222
    milking the dam, 223
    neonate assessment, 221–222
    nursery location, 224
    nursing, 222–223
    physical development, 227
    record keeping, 221
    rickets, 225
    skin dryness, 226
    solid food introduction, 227–228
    sunburn, 226
    supplements, 222
    trauma, 226
    umbilical infection, 226
    vaccinations, 227
    weaning, 228
emaciation, foxes, 167–168
enclosures. See housing and cages
endoparasites, 163, 174, 185, 254
epistaxis, black bears, 178–179
European rabbit, 5
exotic felids
    bottle-feeding, 213
    calcium deficiency, 217
    dehydration, 217
    diarrhea, 217
    feeding strategies, 214–215
    housing, 213–214
    hypoglycemia, 217
    hypothermia, 216–217
    immunoglobulin transfer, 215–216
    intervention criteria, 207
    medical problems, 216–217
    milk replacement formulas, 207–213
    respiratory infections, 216
    socialization, 217–218
    umbilical stump treatment, 216
    weaning/enrichment diet, 208–213
    weight gain targets, 215
exotic ungulates
    ambient temperatures, 257
    amounts to feed, 259
    equipment, 256
    feeding schedule, 258–259
    formulas/supplements, 257
    initial care/stabilization, 257
    medical problems, 261
    neonate assessment, 256
    normal body temperature, 257
    nursing, 258
    reasons for hand rearing, 256
    record keeping, 256
    tube feeding, 259
    umbilicus dip, 256, 258
    weight gain, 259

F

failure of passive immune transfer (FPT), South American camelids, 40
fawns. See deer
feeding
    bats, 97–98
    black bears, 172–173
    cats, 19–21
    elephants, 222–224, 227–228
    exotic felids, 207–213, 214–215
    fawns, 246–248
    ferrets, 204–205
    foals, 25–28
    foxes, 160, 162
    goat kids, 35–36
    great apes, 127–128
    hedgehogs, 78
    lemurs, 107–109

macaques, 119–120
macropods, 65–67, 68
nondomestic equids, 230–232, 233
opossums, 46–51, 52
pigs, 31–32
polar bears, 184–187
puppies, 14–16
rabbits, 7–9
raccoons, 193, 194
rhinoceros, 239–240
sea lions, 145–146, 147–148
seals, 135–138, 139–140
sloths, 82–84
squirrels, 91–93, 94
South American camelids, 40–42
sugar gliders, 56–59
tamarins, 115
ungulates, 258–259
walrus, 150–155, 156
felids. See exotic felids
fenbendazole toxicity, raccoons, 196
ferrets
    birth weight, 204
    dehydration, 205
    diarrhea, 205
    feeding, 204–205
    feeding/housing jills, 203–204
    hypothermia, 205
    medical problems, 205
    nursing, 204–205
    nutrition importance, 203
    parenting methods, 203–204
    weaning, 204, 205
fleas, raccoons, 196
fluid therapy, elephants, 226–227
foals
    bedding materials, 27
    birth weights, 24
    birthing cycle, 24
    body temperatures, 25
    constipation relief, 25
    equipment, 24
    feeding frequency, 27
    food amount guidelines, 27
    grafting onto nurse mares, 24–25
    heart rates, 25
    housing, 27–28
    immune status, 28
    initial care, 25
    intervention criteria, 24–25
    mean time to first urination, 25
    medical problems, 28–29
    milk replacement formulas, 25–26
    neonate assessment, 25
    nursing, 26–27
    record keeping, 24
    selenium deficiency avoidance, 25
    socialization, 27–28
    solid food introduction, 28
    tube feeding, 27
    umbilicus sizing/evaluation, 25
    weaning, 28
    weight gain targets, 27
foreign bodies, black bears, 176–177
formulas
    bat, 97
    black bear, 172
    cat's, 21
    elephant, 222
    exotic felid, 207–213
    fox, 160
    goat, 35
    great ape, 127
    heating guidelines, 257
    lemur, 106–107
    macaque, 119
    macropod, 65–66
    mare, 25–26
    nondomestic equid, 230–231
    opossum, 48–49
    pig, 31
    polar bear, 185–186
    puppies, 14
    rabbit, 7–8
    raccoon, 193
    rhinoceros, 238–239
    sea lion, 143–144
    seal, 133–134
    sloth, 81–83
    South American camelids, 40–41
    squirrel, 91
    storage guidelines, 14
    sugar glider, 56–57
    tamarin, 114
    ungulates, 257
    walrus, 150–152
foxes
    activity periods, 158, 159
    age determination, 159
    anemia, 168
    behavior characteristics, 158, 159
    breeding cycle, 158, 159
    canine distemper virus (CDV), 164
    dehydration, 167
    diarrhea, 165–166
    ectoparasites, 164

emaciation, 167–168
endoparasites, 163
foraging techniques, 158, 159
fractures, 167
habitat, 158, 159
handling concerns, 160
housing, 161–162
hypoglycemia, 166–167
immune status, 163
infectious diseases, 164–165
initial care, 159–160
medical problems, 163–168
nursing, 161
ocular lesions, 168
parasites, 163–164
parvovirus (canine viral enteritis), 164–165
rabies, 165
record keeping, 159
rehabilitation diet formula, 160
release guidelines, 168
restraints, 160, 163
septicemia, 167
shock, 167
trauma, 167
tube feeding, 161
vaccination protocols, 163
weaning diet formula, 160
fractures, 167, 198, 250

G

gastrointestinal parasites, raccoons, 195
gastrointestinal problems, deer, 253
gastrointestinal (GI) tract infections, hedgehogs, 79
gerenuks, 256
giraffes. See exotic ungulates
goat kids
    body temperature, 35
    bottle-feeding, 35–36
    castration, 37
    colostral antibodies, 37
    daily milk intake, 35
    described, 34
    disbudding (horn removal), 37
    herd reintroduction, 38
    housing, 36–37
    medical problems, 38
    milk replacement formulas, 35
    nursing, 35–36
    record keeping, 34–35
    solid food introduction, 37
    tattooing, 37
    tetanus antitoxin, 37
    tube feeding, 36
    umbilical cord care, 37
    weaning, 37
    weight gain targets, 36
golden lion tamarin, 114
grafting, nursing foals, 24–25
gram scale (postal scale), rabbits, 5
gray fox, 158–159
great apes
    24-hour watch, 126
    air temperature requirements, 129
    bonding timeframe, 126
    described, 125
    equipment, 125–126
    feeding frequency, 127–128
    group reintroduction, 130
    growth curve, 129
    housing, 129
    initial care, 127
    intervention criteria, 126
    medical problems, 129–130
    milk replacement formula, 127
    neonate assessment, 127
    nursing, 126, 127
    protocols, 125
    record keeping, 125
    suck knobs, 126
    toy introduction, 129
    tuberculosis concerns, 125
    vaccination guidelines, 125
    ventral vertical nursing, 126
    weaning, 127–128
Greby's zebra, 229
guanaco, 39
gut worms, hedgehogs, 79

H

hair loss, bats, 102
harbor seals, 132
hares, 5
Hartmann's mountain zebra, 229
heart rates, foals, 25
heat prostration, deer, 252
heat sources, rabbits, 6
heat stroke, deer, 252
hedgehogs
    adult appearance, 76–77
    adult feeding guide, 79
    biological data, 77

colostrum needs, 78
equipment, 77
feeding, 78
housing, 78–79
initial care, 78
medical problems, 79–80
record keeping, 77
scientific and common names, 76
weaning, 79
helminthosis, macropod diarrhea cause, 72
herpesvirus infection, elephants, 225–226
hoofstock neonates, cow's colostrum, 257
horn removal (disbudding), goat kids, 37
housing. See also cages
    bats, 98–100
    black bears, 173
    cats, 21–22
    deer, 248–249
    elephants, 224
    exotic felids, 213–214
    foals, 27–28
    foxes, 161–162
    goat kids, 36–37
    great apes, 129
    hedgehogs, 78–79
    lemurs, 109, 111
    macaques, 120–122
    macropods, 67–68
    nondomestic equids, 232–233
    opossums, 51, 53
    pigs, 32
    polar bears, 187
    puppies, 16–17
    rabbits, 5–6, 9
    raccoons, 193–194
    rhinoceros, 240–241
    sea lions, 146–147
    seals, 138–139
    sloths, 85
    South American camelids, 42
    squirrels, 93
    sugar gliders, 59
    tamarins, 116
    ungulates, 259–261
    walrus, 155–156
hyperthermia, deer, 251
hypoglycemia
    black bears, 177–178
    deer, 251
    exotic felids, 217
    foal risk, 25
    foxes, 166–167
    goat kid risk, 38
    raccoons, 198–199
    seals, 140
hypothermia
    deer, 252
    exotic felids, 216–217
    ferrets, 205
    foal risk, 25
    goat kid risk, 38
    macaques, 123–124
    rabbit nest area temperature, 9
    rabbit warming methods, 7
    seals, 140

I

inappetence, sea lions, 148
indigestion, 197, 253
International Llama Registry, 40
International Species Information System (ISIS), 63
irritable bowel syndrome, macropods, 71

J

joeys
    growth cycle, 63
    intervention criteria, 64–65

K

kangaroos, 63
kindling, defined, 5

L

lactose intolerance, great apes, 130
lemurs
    body temperature, 109
    breeding cycle, 104
    defecation stimulation, 111
    equipment, 105
    feeding frequency, 108–109
    food amounts, 108–109
    housing, 109, 111
    initial feeding, 107
    intervention criteria, 105
    medical problems, 112
    milk replacement formulas, 106–107

neonate assessment, 105–106
nursing, 108
pathogen exposure avoidance, 111
record keeping, 105
reintroducing to their mother, 112
socialization, 111
solid food introduction, 111
supplementation versus hand rearing, 104–105
weaning, 111
weight gain targets, 109–110
litter box, kitten introduction, 22
litter trays, opossums, 50
llamas, 39
lowland gorilla, 125
lung worms, hedgehogs, 79

M

macaques
    air temperature requirements, 121
    birth weight, 118
    breeding cycles, 118
    cercopithicine herpes 1, 118
    equipment, 118
    feeding frequency, 120
    group reintroduction, 124
    housing, 120–122
    incubators, 120–121
    intervention criteria, 118
    maternal abuse concerns, 118
    measles virus (rubeola), 118
    medical problems, 123–124
    milk replacement formulas, 119
    neonate assessment, 119
    nursing, 119
    record keeping, 118
    self-feeders, 121–122
    tube feeding, 119–120
    weaning, 123
    weight gain target, 120
macropods
    active immunity, 68–69
    artificial pouches, 64
    body temperatures, 65
    breeding cycle, 63
    captive versus wild, 72–73
    cataracts, 72
    developmental milestones, 67
    equipment, 63–64
    feeding, 66
    food amounts, 66–67
    housing, 67–68
    infectious diarrhea causes, 71–72
    initial care, 65
    intervention criteria, 64–65
    medical problems, 70–72
    milk replacement formula, 65–66
    noninfectious diarrhea causes, 70–71
    nursing, 66
    passive immunity, 68–69
    pneumonia, 72
    pouch emergence, 69
    pouch liners, 64
    pouch young assessment, 65
    record keeping, 63–64
    solid food introduction, 69–70
    tube feeding, 66
    weaning, 69–70
    weight gain targets, 67, 69
malnourishment, great apes, 130
mange, 174–175, 196
medical problems
    black bears, 174–179
    cats, 23
    deer, 250–254
    elephants, 22–225
    exotic felids, 216–217
    ferrets, 205
    foals, 28–29
    foxes, 163–168
    goat kids, 38
    great apes, 129–130
    hedgehogs, 79–80
    lemurs, 112
    macaques, 123–124
    macropods, 70–72
    nondomestic equids, 233–234
    pigs, 33
    puppies, 17
    rabbits, 11–12
    raccoons, 195–201
    rhinoceros, 241–242
    sea lions, 148
    seals, 140–141
    sloths, 88
    South American camelids, 42
    squirrels, 94
    sugar gliders, 60–61
    tamarins, 116–117
    ungulates, 261
    walrus, 156
membranes, bats, 102

metabolic abnormalities, deer, 251
metabolic bone disease (MBD), 115, 197
Modified-Jurgelski Diet, opossums, 51–52

N

nasogastric tubes, foals, 24, 25
National Committees on Potbellied Pigs, 33
natural history, rabbits, 5
naval ill (Omphalitis/Omphalophlebitis), deer, 250
nematode infestation, seals, 141
neonatal diarrhea goat kid risk, 38
nondomestic equids
    birth weights, 229
    equipment, 230
    feeding frequency, 232
    food amounts, 232
    group reintroduction, 234
    housing, 232–233
    initial care, 230
    initial feeding, 231
    intervention criteria, 230
    medical problems, 233–234
    milk replacement formulas, 230–231
    nursing, 231–232
    record keeping, 229–230
    solid food introduction, 233
    supplements, 230–231
    weaning, 233
nontoxic browse, sugar gliders, 59
northern elephant seals, 132
nursing
    bats, 97
    black bears, 172
    elephants, 222–223
    foals, 26–27
    foxes, 161
    goat kids, 35–36
    great apes, 126, 127
    kittens, 19–20
    lemurs, 108
    macaques, 119
    macropods, 66
    nondomestic equids, 231–232
    rabbits, 8
    sea lions, 145
    sloths, 83
    South American camelids, 41
    squirrels, 92
    sugar gliders, 57
    tamarins, 115

ungulates, 258
walrus, 152–153

O

occular lesions, 168, 178, 201, 254
Opossum Society of the United States (OSUS), 45
opossums
    breeding cycles, 45
    cage setup, 53
    defecation stimulation, 46
    disinfectant uses, 51
    feeding, 46–51, 52
    housing, 51, 53
    initial care, 46
    intervention criteria, 45
    litter training, 50
    milk replacement formula, 48–49
    Modified-Jurgelski Diet, 51–52
    orphan care guidelines, 45
    outdoor cages/runs, 53, 54
    rehydrating before syringe feeding, 47, 50
    release guidelines, 53–54
    solid food introduction, 51
    syringe feeding, 47, 50
    tube feeding, 46–47
    warming before rehydrating, 46
    weaning, 50–51
    weighing, 46
orangutan, 125

P

Pacific walrus, 150
parama wallaby, 63
parasites
    bat medical problem, 102
    black bears, 174–175
    deer, 254
    foxes, 163–164
    hedgehogs, 79–80
    pig inspection, 30–31
    raccoons, 195
    sea lions, 148
    seals, 140–141
parvovirus (canine viral enteritis), 164–165, 200
pelvic fractures, deer, 250
pesticides, bat poisoning concern, 102
pigs
    bedding materials, 32

bottle-feeding, 31–32
breeding cycle, 30
brooders, 31–32
castration issues, 33
deworming, 31
equipment, 30
feeding, 31–32
housing, 32
initial care, 31
intervention criteria, 30
loose stool treatment 31
medical problems, 33
milk replacement formula, 31
neonate assessment, 30–31
pan feeding, 31
parasite inspection, 30–31
rehydration methods, 30
solid food introduction, 32–33
weaning, 32–33
weight gain targets, 32
playpens, pig housing, 32
pneumonia, 72, 140–141, 148
poisons, bat medical problem, 102
polar bears
    birth weights, 181
    body temperature, 182, 184
    breeding cycle, 181
    described, 181–182
    development stages, 187
    environmental stimulation sensitivity, 187
    feeding frequency, 186
    housing, 187
    initial care, 182–186
    intervention criteria, 182
    milk replacement formulas, 185–186
    record keeping, 182–183
    serum dosages, 184–185
    solid food introduction, 187
    umbilicus care, 184
    weaning, 187
pouch liners, 59, 64
preputial sucking, raccoons, 196
products mentioned, sources, 262–265
pronghorn, 256
Przewalski's horse, 229
puppies
    age assessment, 13
    amounts to feed, 16
    bedding, 17
    elimination, 16
    equipment, 13

    feeding, 14–16
    formula selection, 14
    formulas/supplements, 14
    housing, 16–17
    humidity, 17
    immune status of hand raised, 17
    initial care/stabilization, 14
    medical problems, 17
    neonate assessment, 13
    nursing, 15
    reasons for hand rearing, 13
    record keeping, 13
    socialization, 18
    tube feeding, 15–16
    umbilicus used for age assessment, 13
    weaning, 17

R

rabbits
    birth weight, 5
    body temperature, 7
    cecotrophs, 11
    equipment, 5–6
    fear vocalizations, 9
    feeding frequency, 8–9
    food amount guidelines, 9–10
    handling guidelines, 9
    hindgut fermentation, 11
    housing, 9
    initial feeding, 8
    intervention criteria, 6
    medical problems, 11–12
    milk replacement formulas, 7–8
    neonate assessment, 6
    nursing, 8
    record keeping, 5
    size differences, 5
    solid food introduction, 9–11
    stimulating defecation, 8
    tube feeding, 8
    warming methods, 7
    water consumption, 10–11
    weaning, 5, 9–11
    weighing, 5
    weight gain targets, 9
rabies, 96, 165, 200–201
raccoons
    activity periods, 191
    age determinations, 192

anemia, 201
behaviors, 191
bloat, 197
breeding cycle, 191
canine distemper virus (CDV), 199–200
dehydration, 199
demodectic mange, 196
deworming, 194–195
diarrhea, 198
ectoparasites, 195–196
endoparasites, 195
fenbendazole toxicity, 196
fleas, 196
fractures, 198
gastrointestinal parasites, 195
habitat, 191
handling techniques, 191–192
housing, 193–194
hypoglycemia, 198–199
indigestion, 197
infectious diseases, 199–201
initial care, 192
juvenile diet formula, 193
mange, 196
medical problems, 195–201
metabolic bone disease (MBD), 197
milk replacement formulas, 193
occular lesions, 201
parasites, 195
parvovirus (canine viral enteritis), 200
physiological parameters, 191
preputial sucking, 196
rabies, 200–201
release guidelines, 201
restraints, 191–192
ringworm, 195–196
septicemia, 199
shock, 199
ticks, 196
trauma, 197–198
tube feeding, 193
vaccination protocol, 194–195
vomiting, 201
weaning diet formula, 193
radial immunodiffusion (RID) test plate, South American camelids, 40
rat-kangaroos, 63
ravel-free fabric, opossum handling, 45, 50
red fox, 158
red kangaroo, 63
red-flanked duikers, 256

red-necked wallaby, 63
rehydration fluids, piglets, 30
resources, products mentioned, 262–265
respiratory disorders, bat medical problem, 102
respiratory infections, exotic felids, 216
rhesus macaque, 118
rhinoceros
    bedding, 240
    biological data, 236
    body temperature, 237
    feeding, 240
    formulas, 238–239
    housing, 240–241
    initial care/assessment, 237
    medical problems, 241–242
    nursing, 239–240
    record keeping, 236–237
    reintroduction to adult groups, 242
    San Diego Wild Animal Park (SDWAP), 236
    supplements, 239
    trouble indicators, 237
    weaning, 241
    weight records, 2136–237
rickets, elephants, 225
ring-tailed lemurs, 104
ringworm, 174, 195–196
ruffed lemurs, 104
ruminants, tube feeding cautions, 259

S

salmonellosis, walrus calves, 156
San Diego Wild Animal Park (SDWAP), 229, 236
sarcoptic mange, 85, 94, 174
scrotal hernias, great apes, 130
sea lions
    birth weight, 143
    blood drawing, 148
    breeding cycles, 143
    captive versus wild release, 148
    feeding, 145–146
    food amounts, 146
    force-feeding fish, 147
    housing, 146–147
    immune status concerns, 147
    intervention criteria, 143
    medical problems, 148
    milk replacement formulas, 143–144
    nursing, 145
    record keeping, 143

solid food introduction, 147–148
tube feeding, 145–146
weaning, 147
weight gain targets, 146
seal pox virus, 141
seals
    24-hour watch, 133
    birth weight, 132
    breeding cycles, 132
    equipment, 132
    feeding frequency, 137–138
    housing, 138–139
    initial care, 131
    intervention criteria, 132–133
    medical problems, 140–141
    milk replacement formulas, 133–134
    record keeping, 132
    rehydration before formula introduction, 133
    solid food introduction, 139–140
    supplements, 134–135
    tube feeding, 135–137
    weaning, 139–140
    weight gain patterns, 135
self-feeders, macaques, 121–122
sepsis, 129, 252
septicemia, 167, 178, 199, 252
shock, 167, 178, 199, 251
siamang, 125
sifakas, 104
skin diseases, hedgehogs, 79
skin dryness, elephants, 226
skin rashes, macaques, 124
sloths
    birth weight, 81
    body temperatures, 85
    breeding cycles, 81
    feeding frequency, 83–84
    food amounts, 84
    handling techniques, 85–86
    housing, 85
    immune status, 85–86
    medical problems, 88
    milk replacement formulas, 81–83
    nursing, 83
    record keeping, 81
    reintroduction to an exhibit, 88
    release issues, 88
    sarcoptic mange, 85
    solid food introduction, 86–88
    stuffed animal as surrogate mother, 85–86
    toilet tree introduction, 85
    weaning, 86–88
    weight gain targets, 84–85
Somali wild ass, 229
South American camelids
    birth weights, 39
    birthing times, 39–40
    body temperature, 40
    breeding cycle, 39
    congenital defects, 42
    equipment, 39
    feeding frequency, 41–42
    FPT (failure of passive immune transfer), 40
    housing, 42
    initial care, 39–40
    initial feeding, 40–41
    intervention criteria, 39
    medical problems, 42
    milk replacement formulas, 40–41
    nursing, 41
    premature birth indicators/causes, 40
    radial immunodiffusion (RID) test plate, 40
    record keeping, 39
    solid food introduction, 42
    umbilical cord care, 40
    weaning, 42
    weight gain targets, 42
southern white rhinoceros, 236
spaying, female piglets, 33
Speke's gazelles, 256
spiny hedgehogs, 75
squirrel pox (Fibromatosis), 94
squirrels
    age determinations, 90–91
    birth weights, 90
    body temperature, 91
    caloric requirements, 91
    captive versus wild release, 94–95
    equipment, 90
    feeding frequency, 92
    food amounts, 92–93
    gastrointestinal (GI) problems, 94
    housing, 93
    initial care, 91
    initial feeding, 91–92
    injury types, 94
    intervention criteria, 90–91
    medical problems, 94
    milk replacement formulas, 91
    neonate assessment, 91
    nursing, 92
    record keeping, 90

solid food introduction, 93–94
weaning, 93–94
subcutaneous drips, piglet rehydration, 30
sugar gliders
    air temperature guidelines, 56
    artificial pouches, 55
    breeding cycle, 55
    captive versus wild, 61
    colony reintroduction techniques, 61–62
    dietary component definitions, 60
    equipment, 55–56
    feeding, 57–58
    food amounts, 58
    growth milestones, 57
    hand-raising records, 55–56
    housing, 59
    immune status, 59
    initial care, 56
    intervention criteria, 56
    life expectancy, 55
    medical problems, 60–61
    medications, 60–61
    milk replacement formulas, 56–57
    nontoxic browse, 59
    nursing, 57
    pouch liners, 59
    socialization, 61–62
    solid food introduction, 59–60
    stress-free environment importance, 56
    toys, 59
    weaning, 59–60
    weight gain targets, 58–59
sunburn, elephants, 226
syringe feedings, opossums, 47, 50

T

tagging, black bears, 179
tamarins
    air temperature requirements, 116
    body temperature, 114
    breeding cycles, 114
    equipment, 114
    food amounts, 115
    housing, 116
    initial care, 114
    initial feedings, 115
    intervention criteria, 114
    medical problems, 116–117
    milk replacement formulas, 114

    neonate assessment, 114
    nursing, 115
    record keeping, 114
    reintroduction to family group, 116
    stuffed toy as surrogate mother, 116
    umbilicus treatment, 114
    weaning, 116
    weight gain targets, 115
tammar wallaby, 63
tattoos, goat kids, 37
temperature stress, macropod diarrhea cause, 70
ticks, raccoons, 196
towels, ungulate bedding, 257
Triple J Farms, radial immunodiffusion (RID) test plate, 40
true lemurs, 104
tusk infections, walrus, 156

U

ungulates. See exotic ungulates

V

vicuna, 39
viral infections, seals, 140

W

wallabies, 63
walrus
    birth weight, 150
    breeding cycle, 150
    caloric value determinations, 154–155
    equipment, 150
    feeding frequency, 154
    food amounts, 154
    housing, 155–156
    immune status, 156
    initial feeding, 152
    intervention criteria, 150
    medical problems, 156
    milk replacement formulas, 150–152
    nursing, 152–153
    record keeping, 150
    salt water requirements, 156
    solid food introduction, 156
    supplements, 152
    tube feeding, 153–154

weaning, 156
weight gain targets, 155
western grey kangaroo, 63
white-tail deer, 244–245
wing injury, bats, 101

Y

yeast, macropod diarrhea cause, 71

Z

zebra duikers, 256
zoonotic disease, 5, 79